'Doctors for Export'

Clio Medica

STUDIES IN THE HISTORY OF MEDICINE AND HEALTH

VOLUME 99

The titles published in this series are listed at *brill.com/clio*

'Doctors for Export'

Medical Migration from Ireland c.1860 to 1960

By

Greta Jones

BRILL
RODOPI

LEIDEN | BOSTON

Cover illustration: A political cartoon from a supplement to the *Weekly Freeman* (July 2nd 1881). Flanked by an elderly woman and man, Erin, the female personification of Ireland, holds a chart showing the great loss of Irish population due to famine and emigration. Below the cartoon the text: "A terrible record. Erin - In forty years I have lost, through the operation of no natural law, more than Three Millions of my Sons and Daughters, and they, the Young and the Strong, leaving behind the Old and the Infirm to weep and to die. Where is this to end?"
Attributed to John Fergus O'Hea, (ca. 1838–1922). Shelfmark: Political Cartoons 3 (122). Courtesy of Bodleian Library, University of Oxford: John Johnson Collection.

Library of Congress Cataloging-in-Publication Data

Names: Jones, Greta, author.
Title: Doctors for export : medical migration from Ireland c.1860 to 1960 / Greta Jones.
Description: Leiden ; Boston : Brill, 2021. | Series: Clio medica, 0045-7183 ; vol. 99 | Includes bibliographical references and index.
Identifiers: LCCN 2021030084 (print) | LCCN 2021030085 (ebook) | ISBN 9789004324459 (hardback) | ISBN 9789004324466 (ebook)
Subjects: LCSH: Medical personnel, Foreign. | Emigration and immigration–Health and hygiene. | Physicians–Ireland.
Classification: LCC R697.F6 J66 2021 (print) | LCC R697.F6 (ebook) | DDC 610.6909415–dc23
LC record available at https://lccn.loc.gov/2021030084
LC ebook record available at https://lccn.loc.gov/2021030085

Typeface for the Latin, Greek, and Cyrillic scripts: "Brill". See and download: brill.com/brill-typeface.

ISSN 0045-7183
ISBN 978-90-04-32445-9 (hardback)
ISBN 978-90-04-32446-6 (e-book)

This book is printed on acid-free paper and produced in a sustainable manner.

Contents

Acknowledgements

First thanks to the Wellcome Trust whose generosity allowed this study to be undertaken. Thanks also to the readers of this manuscript whose comments were wise and helpful.

I owe a particular debt of gratitude to the librarians and archivists of the Royal College of Surgeons in Ireland and to the Council of the College who gave me permission to examine their manuscript collection relating to the history of the College. Most of all a special thanks to Mary O'Doherty of the College whose assistance and guidance was invaluable.

I also benefited from the help and advice of Harriet Wheelock, archivist of the Royal College of Physicians of Ireland. Other librarians and archivists greatly assisted. They include the staff of the Queen's University Medical Library, Queen's University's McClay Library, and the University Archivist. The Registrar's Office at Queen's were also very helpful as was the Belfast Central Library. I also very much appreciate the hospitality of the Central Catholic Library, Dublin who went out of their way to help.

The staff of Public Record Office of Northern Ireland greatly facilitated the research as did the staff and archivists in the National Archives in Dublin and the National Library, Dublin.

Further afield, I would like to thank Dr Caroline Morrison of Chicago who helped smoothed access to the American Medical Association's archives and to the staff at the AMA archive and the archivists at Rockefeller Archive at Tarrytown, New York State.

Fellow historians were also of great help, in particular Laura Kelly who, in the course of her own research on medical students in Ireland, was generous in her advice and who gave me many useful references. Professor David Wright has played an important part in the development of research on medical migration and brought me to Canada in 2012 for a conference at McGill University where I met other researchers in the field.

I benefited from the special knowledge of Professor Frank Geary of the Ulster University and Professor Leslie Clarkson of Queen's University Belfast to whom I offer thanks. Dr Patrick Maume also passed on references and suggestions from which I benefited. Anne Crowther, Marguerite Dupree, Anne Digby and Megan Vaughan are academics from whose ground work in the area I benefited greatly. Ailbhe Enright of the Medical Registration Council of Ireland kindly answered several of my questions.

Thanks also to Frank Huisman and Rosanna Woensdregt at Brill and to Jonathan Reinarz my editor. I am grateful to Oxford and Cambridge University Presses who allowed me to reproduce material from articles I published in their journals.

Many thanks to my mother-in-law, Dr Mary Bew, whose family produced a generation of Irish migrant doctors to Britain and the United States and who, herself, enrolled in the Indian Medical Service towards the end of the Second World War reaching the rank of Captain. Also her brother, Dr Anthony Leahy, who practised in Gateshead, England for over forty years. They both supplied many stories of their experience as Irish medical graduates on the move.

Figures and Tables

Figures

Tables

Abbreviations

AMA	American Medical Association
AMD	Army Medical Department
BAO	Bachelor of Obstetrics
BCh	Bachelor of Surgery
BMA	British Medical Association
BMJ	*British Medical Journal*
DEA	Department of External Affairs
DFA	Department of Foreign Affairs
DPM	Diploma in Psychological Medicine
DSM	Distinguished Service Medals
ECFMG	Educational Commission for Foreign Medical Graduates
EEC	European Economic Community
EFMG	Examination for Foreign Medical Graduates
EU	European Union
GDP	Gross Domestic Product
GMC	General Medical Council
HMSO	His/Her Majesty's Stationery Office
ILP	Independent Labour Party
IMA	Irish Medical Association
IMS	Indian Medical Service
JAMA	*Journal of the American Medical Association*
JIMA	*Journal of the Irish Medical Association*
LAH	Licentiate of the Apothecaries Hall
LGB	Local Government Board (Ireland)
LRCPI	Licentiate of the Royal College of Physicians of Ireland
LRCSI	Licentiate of the Royal College of Surgeons in Ireland
MB	Bachelor of Medicine
MD	Doctor of Medicine
MRC	Medical Research Council
NBME	National Board of Medical Examiners
NHS	National Health Service
NSPCC	National Society for the Prevention of Cruelty to Children
NUI	National University of Ireland
OBE	Order of the British Empire
OECD	Organisation for Economic Co-operation and Development
P & O	Peninsular and Orient Company
PRONI	Public Record Office Northern Ireland
QCB	Queen's College Belfast

QUB	Queen's University Belfast
RAMC	Royal Army Medical Corps
RBS	Royal Bank of Scotland
RCP	Royal College of Physicians
RCPI	Royal College of Physicians of Ireland
RCSI	Royal College of Surgeons in Ireland
RF	Rockefeller Foundation
RIC	Royal Irish Constabulary
RUI	Royal University of Ireland
TB	Tuberculosis
TCD	Trinity College Dublin
UCC	University College Cork
UCD	University College Dublin
UCG	University College Galway
UK	United Kingdom
UNESCO	United Nations Educational, Scientific and Cultural Organization
US	United States
USA	United States of America
VC	Victoria Cross
VHI	Voluntary Health Insurance
WHO	World Health Organization

Introduction

The serious academic study of migration is relatively recent. From a European perspective it is largely the outcome of the recent increase in the flow of people to Europe from areas previously only minimally involved in migration. But an important outcome of the research has been to correct this rather Eurocentric view of migratory patterns. Migration is ubiquitous throughout human history and much of it has occurred outside the immediate gaze of scholars in the developed world. The range of studies relating to migration is very wide indeed. It encompasses the examination of migration in populations in prehistory by the analysis of genes and cultural artefacts.[1] Cultural sociology has adopted the sociobiological concept of the 'meme'- a unit of culture but which migrates through societies by imitation rather than sexual reproduction.[2] In the latter half of the twentieth century, economics focussed upon migration as an aid or barrier to economic development giving rise to a debate on its costs or benefits to countries who sent migrants and to those who received them.[3]

This study is an historical examination of migration from one particular society – Ireland – set within defined time limits and relating to one professional group: doctors. Even here there are many possible organising principles which need to be taken into account. Migration can be voluntary or forced, though in many cases it involves elements of both. It can involve crossing continents, oceans, political borders or be local and regional. In his discussion of migration, Leo Lucassen points out that one of the greatest population flows of the last two centuries was the movement from town to city often within the borders of a state.[4] Migration can involve large groups of people or

1 See Elisabeth S. Vbra et al., eds., *Paleoclimate and Evolution with Emphasis on Human Origins* (New Haven: Yale University Press, 1995).

2 The origins of this debate are to be found in Edward O. Wilson, *Sociobiology: The New Synthesis* (Cambridge Mass.: Harvard University Press, 1975). Its continued influence is illustrated in a recent book, Alan C. Love and William Wimsatt, *Beyond the Meme: Development and Structure in Cultural Evolution* (Minneapolis: University of Minnesota Press, 2019).

3 From the 1960s a large amount of literature was produced on this theme. Recent overviews of the literature can be found in George J. Borjas and Barry R. Chiswick *Foundations of Migration Economics*, ed. Benjamin Elsner (Oxford: Oxford University Press, 2019) and Francesco Ortega and Giovanni Peri, *The Effect of Income and Immigration Policies on International Migration* (Cambridge, Mass.: National Bureau of Economic Research, 2012).

4 Leo Lucassen, 'Beyond the Apocalypse: Reframing Migration History', in *History, Historians and the Immigration Debate: Going Back to Where We Came From,* edited by Eureka Henrich and Julian M. Simpson (London: Palgrave Macmillan, 2019), pp. 33–51.

 | DOI:10.1163/9789004324466_002

relatively small cohorts and its consequences vary. New nations have emerged when millions left Europe from the sixteenth to the twentieth century to found settlements in North America, Australia and other parts of the world. Or its effects are individual or among small groups.

Medical historians are already aware of the importance of migration. The growth of public health systems and the study of epidemic disease was largely a response to the rapid gathering together of the poor in overcrowded cities.[5] Regional and seasonal migration has also attracted the historian of epidemic disease.[6] In addition there is a growing body of work which examines the psychological impact of migration including, for example, the high concentration in the asylum system of Irish immigrants to Britain in the nineteenth century and mental breakdown among migrants to the British West Indies in the nineteenth century.[7]

Historians of medicine are beginning to ask questions about another migration pattern. This is the movement of doctors, nurses and other medical personnel. In 1976 it was claimed that six per cent of all physicians in the world were living and working outside the country of their birth.[8] By 2007 an OECD Report calculated that in 2000 16 per cent of all doctors working in OECD countries were foreign-born and trained.[9] The first treatment of this phenomenon, largely in the 1960s and 1970s, was generally undertaken by students of contemporary economics and politics. They commented on the growing phenomenon but did so largely from the point of view of the market

5 Ibid.

6 Migration of workers, often within a state or region, and its effect of the spread of tuberculosis have been examined in Randall M. Packard, *White Plague, Black Labor: Tuberculosis and the Political Economy of Health and Disease in South Africa* (Berkeley: University of California Press, 1989), William Johnson, *The Modern Epidemic: A History of Tuberculosis in Japan* (Cambridge, Mass.: Harvard University Press, 1995), and Greta Jones, *"Captain of all these Men of Death": Tuberculosis in Nineteenth and Twentieth Century Ireland* (Amsterdam–New York: Brill/Rodopi, 2001).

7 See Catherine Cox, Hilary Marland and Sarah York, 'Itineraries and Experiences of Insanity: Irish Migration and the Management of Mental Illness in Nineteenth Century Lancashire', and Letizia Gramaglia, 'Migration and Mental Illness in the British West Indies 1838–1900: The Cases of Trinidad and British Guiana', in *Migration, Health and Ethnicity in the Modern World*, eds., Catherine Cox and Hilary Marland (London: Palgrave Macmillan, 2013).

8 "International Comments", *Journal of the American Medical Association*, 15 March 1976, vol. 235 no. 7, p. 1167.

9 Organisation for Economic Co-operation and Development (OECD), *'Immigrant Health Workers in OECD countries in the broader context of highly skilled migration,'* Report (OECD, 2007). There are 36 OECD countries across the world, predominantly developed or developing nations.

for health care, health planning and the impact on the economics of developing countries.[10]

The recent work of Simpson, and Bornat and others on Asian doctors in the United Kingdom have moved forward the study of migration.[11] They concentrate upon the experience of migrant South East Asian doctors coming to Britain in the 1960s and 1970s. They have charted their settlement patterns, the problems they experienced in creating a space for themselves in medicine and the disadvantages they suffered. However, they suggest that, in spite of the particular difficulties they experienced, forced to seek work in the less desirable locations and in areas of relative medical deprivation, they helped transform the culture of certain medical specialties and raise their effectiveness and prestige. Because the migration from South East Asia is relatively recent, many of these studies are underpinned by oral histories. These narratives help dig out the emotional and cultural aspects of the migrant doctor experience, an aspect which was central to many doctors' experience. The issues raised in constructing the history of the recent south Asian medical migrant also informs the subject of the present study of migration: Irish medical graduates.

This book is about the migrating Irish doctor roughly between 1860 and 1960. There are further chapters that extend the study into the decades of the 1970s and 1980s when doctor migration began to alter significantly in line with the patterns described by the World Health Organization, a movement of physicians from outside Europe to the developed world. This is not to suggest that medical migration only began in 1860. Ireland exported a considerable number of doctors in the centuries before then. Accepting the dictum that migration is ubiquitous and has many forms, medicine can be seen as a particularly peripatetic occupation. Students in past centuries moved between medical schools or took a variety of medical apprenticeships with prominent doctors

---

10 Brian Abel-Smith and Kathleen Gates, *British Doctors at Home and Abroad* (Welwyn: Codicote Press, 1964) and Oscar Gish, *Doctor Migration and World Health: the impact of the international demand for doctors in health services in developing countries* (London: Bell, 1971).

11 Julian M. Simpson, *Migrant Architects of the NHS: South Asian doctors and the reinvention of British general practice (1940s–1980s)* (Manchester: Manchester University Press, 2018) and Joanna Bornat, Parvati Raghuram and Leroi Henry, '"Without racism there would have been no geriatrics": South Asian Overseas-Trained Doctors and the Development of Geriatric Medicine in the United Kingdom, 1950–2000' in *Doctors Beyond Borders: The Transnational Migration of Physicians in the Twentieth Century*, eds., Laurence Monnais and David Wright (Toronto: University of Toronto Press, 2016), pp. 185–207; see also Sasha Mullally and David Wright, 'Connecting to Canada: Experiences of the South Asian Medical Diaspora during the 1960s and 1970s', in *Doctors Beyond Borders*, eds., Monnais and Wright, footnote 1.

sometimes in other countries. They improved their postgraduate education in the medical schools of cities in the world considered to excel in certain specialities and the most ambitious learned languages to acquire medical knowledge. Many Irish doctors before 1860 were on the move. They went to areas which had become European settlements to serve its growing European population; to cities and regions in the British Isles in need of doctors. They became missionaries and took with them a particular culture and ethos of medicine. They worked overseas for foreign firms and often put down roots in the country to which their profession called them. They went as members of the army or navy to parts of the world where the topography and disease patterns were often very different from Europe.

There is an existing body of work in this area of great value in the present investigation. One is the pioneering work of Laurence Geary who looked at the role of Irish doctors in moulding the European settlements in Australia in the early nineteenth century.[12] His study includes not just the part emigration to Australia played in the fortunes of the doctors themselves but their general contribution to moulding the colonies in which they worked. Geary regards the new colony as space in which not just the ambitions of many doctors could be realised but in which they played a broad role in consolidating the new settler communities. Along with Geary, Dupree's and Crowther's book examining a cohort of medical students in Glasgow and Edinburgh in the late 1860s and 1870s has also been important for this current research.[13] The students they selected were taught by the pre-eminent Scots doctor Joseph Lister, famous for his work on anti-sepsis. The book traced their undergraduate experience, subsequent careers and assessed the influence of Lister's anti-sepsis in their practice.

Crowther and Dupree's tracing of the careers of these graduates, including their migration patterns, was a template for this book. They dealt with a smaller number (1,938) and followed them from entry to medical school to graduation and beyond. This book deals only with graduates and a larger number (4,246) are examined. The time period it covers is longer from 1860 to around 1960 though it follows the story of Ireland's medical migration patterns into the following decades. But many of the methods and sources Crowther and Dupree used are the foundation for this book. Their work also had an Irish dimension. Their student Laura Kelly helped lay the foundations for the present work by

---

12 Laurence M. Geary, 'Australia Felix: Irish Doctors in Nineteenth-Century Victoria', in *The Irish in the New Communities* (*The Irish World Wide: History, Heritage, Identity*, vol. 2), ed. Patrick O'Sullivan (Leicester: Leicester University Press, 1992), pp. 162–79.

13 See M. Anne Crowther and Marguerite W. Dupree, *Medical Lives in the Age of Surgical Revolution* (Cambridge: Cambridge University Press, 2007).

a study of the eventual destination of the Irish medical students educated in Glasgow in the period.[14] The combined influence of these scholars created both a broad picture of the careers of these doctors taken from certain standard research tools – including the *Medical Register* and *Medical Directories* – and combines it with illustrative biographical detail, methods which have influenced this book.[15]

This research is also an attempt to answer the kind of question which would have been familiar to the development economists of the late twentieth century; namely what was the cost or benefit of migration to the Irish doctor and to Ireland itself? As well as the economic balance sheet what was the impact of migration upon class, culture and learning in Ireland? And this leads to a further reflection. Ireland was only one among a number of nations which exported doctors. To what extent was its experience of medical migration unique or are there similarities or patterns to which it conforms when considering medical migration as a whole?

Indispensable in constructing the answer to these questions is the work done by social and economic historians on the medical market place and also upon the social history of the professions in the nineteenth and twentieth century. In particular Anne Digby, Jeanne Peterson and Hilary Marland have already addressed the question of doctor's incomes in the nineteenth and twentieth century.[16] Megan Vaughan's work was of particular interest since the doctors she described were also migrants.[17] The subject of migrant doctors has also engaged the attention of Anne Digby.[18] Hopefully this puts the book in the venerable tradition of historical work on class, income and the professions in the nineteenth century.[19]

---

14 Laura Kelly, 'Irish Medical Students at the University of Glasgow 1859–1900' (M.Litt thesis, University of Glasgow, 2007). Laura Kelly has also contributed two works on Irish medical history of great usefulness to this work; see bibliography.

15 This method has also been used in R.S.J. Clarke, *A Directory of Ulster Doctors (who qualified before 1901)*, 2 vols. (Belfast: Ulster Historical Foundation, 2013).

16 Anne Digby, *Making a Medical Living: Doctors and Patients in the English Market for Medicine 1720–1911* (Cambridge: Cambridge University Press, 1994); M Jeanne Peterson, *The Medical Profession in Mid-Victorian London* (Berkeley: University of California Press, 1978); Hilary Marland, *Medicine and Society in Wakefield and Huddersfield* (Cambridge: Cambridge University Press, 1987; republished 2008).

17 Megan Vaughan, *Curing their Ills: Colonial Power and African Illness* (London: Polity Press, 1991).

18 Anne Digby, 'Shaping New Identities: General Practitioners in Britain and South Africa', in, *Medical Identities; Healing Well Being and Personhood'*, ed. Kent Maynard (New York–Oxford: Berghahn Books, 2007).

19 W.D. Rubenstein, *Men of Property: The Very Wealthy in Britain since the Industrial Revolution* (London: Croom Helm, 1981).

The book aims to produce a work conscious of the impact of globalisation. Here the development literature on development characteristic of the late twentieth century has helped. But other expositions of the exercise of global power in medicine have been important. In particular, whilst Empires often facilitated medical migration, the rise of American influence in medicine particularly characterised the twentieth century. For this the classic work of Ludmerer on the transformation of American medical education and other work on the philanthropy of the Rockefeller Foundation (RF) in helping spread the gospel of the medical reforms have been a vital underpinning.[20] Nonetheless this book begins and ends with Ireland and relies upon the work of Irish historians on emigration and other political and medical issues.

1 Irish Emigration

In 1913 an editorial in the nationalist newspaper *The Leader* commented rather disparagingly on the number of doctors produced by Irish medical schools. They asked the question, "To where do all the medical practitioners that are raised in Ireland go?"[21] Over fifty years later the extent and nature of Irish doctor emigration was still unclear. The 'Report of the Commission on Higher Education' in the Republic of Ireland in 1967 commented that:

> Medical school authorities informed us that it was particularly difficult to place a figure on the rate of emigration of Irish doctors. A survey of the pattern of emigration over a long period involving the tracing of many individuals would be required to obtain accurate information and, in particular, to isolate the numbers of doctors who emigrate permanently. This we have not had the opportunity of doing.[22]

The genesis of this book was, in part, an attempt to answer the question raised by the Commission on Higher Education. How many medical graduates left Ireland to pursue a career outside Ireland, why and to what destinations did

---

20 Kenneth M. Ludmerer, *A Time to Heal: American Medical Education at the Turn of the Century to the Age of Managed Care* (New York: Oxford University Press, 1999). See Marcos Cueto, ed., *Missionaries of Science: The Rockefeller Foundation and Latin America* (Bloomington: Indiana University Press, 1994).

21 *The Leader*, 18 January 1913, p. 1.

22 'Report of the Commission on Higher Education 1960–7', vol. I (Dublin: Stationery Office, 1968), p. 246. They suggested that, in the preceding decade, emigration was around 25 per cent of all medical graduates from the Republic.

they go? But it has a wider remit. Doctor migration from Ireland cannot simply be subsumed under the general narrative of Irish emigration. This narrative is generally that of the cataclysm of the Famine during and after which emigration from Ireland, which had been a feature of earlier Irish decades, became a flood. Kerby Miller calculates that around 2.1 million Irish left their native country between 1845 and 1855 and that Ireland's population fell from 8.5 to 6 million in that decade.[23] A significant proportion who survived the Famine went on emigrating thereafter. By 1926 Ireland's population was around half of what it had been before the Famine, slightly more than 4 million.[24] The coming of political independence to the twenty-six counties of Ireland did not reverse the process. Emigration continued, a situation which accelerated in the 1950s. Kerby Miller argues that emigration in the nineteenth century was the product of de-industrialisation, rural decline and bourgeois stagnation. Thus it was a particular feature of the poor rural west of Ireland. Also, compared with other countries with a high rate of emigration, females comprised a majority of Irish emigrants. Ulster was an exception. There emigration, to a much greater extent than elsewhere in Ireland, was skilled, male and petty bourgeois.[25]

So pervasive has been the image of the poor, rural Catholic west in the history of Irish emigration that historians like Akenson have been at pains to remind us that, until the Famine, emigration was dominated by the Protestant north-east. He also points out that subsequent studies tend to underestimate the continuing importance of emigration from this part of Ireland.[26] But overall emigration studies since the Famine have confirmed a pattern of emigration in line with Kerby Miller's thesis. The Famine was the catastrophe that caused a sharp fall in Ireland's population, which subsequently never recovered to its pre-Famine levels. There were still emigrants from Ireland who had some capital, social position and skills after the Famine, but these were far fewer than the poor, rural, unskilled and landless.

Where did the emigrants go? Kerby Miller estimates that between 1856 and 1921 total emigration from Ireland reached 3.6 million, of which 3,054,000 went to the United States, while "about 209,000 sailed to Canada. An additional 289,000 emigrated to Australia and New Zealand and 60,000 went to South Africa."[27] There was also a stream of emigrants to Britain. Some of this

---

23 Kerby A. Miller, *Emigrants and Exiles: Ireland and the Irish Exodus to North America* (Oxford: Oxford University Press, 1985), p. 291.

24 Ibid., p. 346.

25 Miller, *Emigrants and Exiles*.

26 Donald Harman Akenson, 'The Historiography of the Irish in the United States of America', in *The Irish in the New Communities*, ed. O'Sullivan.

27 Miller, *Emigrants and Exiles*, Table 1, p. 569.

was preparatory to taking a longer journey overseas, often to the United States. But in the nineteenth and twentieth centuries there was significant long-term Irish settlement in Britain. Akenson quotes official figures that suggest that between 1876 and 1920 a total of 236,508 persons of Irish origin emigrated to Britain; but, as he points out, the official statistics undercount the real number. He quotes Cormac Ó Gráda's view that from 1852 to 1910 one fifth to one quarter of total Irish emigration, that is over a million, settled in Britain.[28]

By the late nineteenth century, emigration was absorbed into the nationalist rhetoric of a poor Catholic and Gaelic Ireland destroyed, betrayed and starved of people and resources. Nationalist narratives claimed that an independent Ireland would right this wrong and put an end to population decline. Emigration was, therefore, an emotive and highly political question.

2 Doctor Migration

Irish medical emigration was radically different. Because of this it has been less visible in the history of Irish emigration in the nineteenth and twentieth centuries. It was middle-class and composed of individuals who carried with them portable skills relatively scarce even in the countries to which they emigrated. Overall it was unimportant compared with Irish emigration in general. The available statistics demonstrate only a very small percentage of professionally qualified emigrants from Ireland. Statistics collected by the Free State's Government of those embarking from Irish ports in 1940–51 calculated that, of 213,420 emigrating in that decade, only 29,325 or 13.7 per cent were skilled, a category which includes a number of semi-manual or clerical occupations as well as the professionally qualified.[29]

Enda Delaney has also produced figures on the occupational structure of male emigrants for 1948–9 that gives the ratio of skilled workers as 3.3 per cent.[30] The proportion of Irish immigrants in Britain from a professional background was to rise by 1961 to around 5.6 per cent for males and 9.7 per cent for females. However, the professional occupations described are not exclusively

28 Donald Harman Akenson, *The Irish Diaspora: A Primer* (Toronto: P.D. Meany, 1996), pp. 195–6.

29 'Commission on Emigration and Other Population Problems 1948–54' (Dublin: Stationery Office, 1955).

30 Enda Delaney, *Demography, State and Society: Irish Migration to Britain, 1921–1971* (Liverpool: Liverpool University Press, 2000), Table 4.7, p. 189.

doctors, though the higher percentage of women emigrants in the professional category is undoubtedly because of the inclusion of nurses.[31] In spite of the relative invisibility of doctor emigration in the period, nonetheless it was significant for the medical profession. This study shows that of all the doctors produced in Ireland during 1860–1960, around 40 per cent emigrated.

Although most Irish emigration was unskilled, other emigrants besides doctors, before and after the Famine, carried some capital with them, whether in terms of ready money to invest at their destination, skills, professional qualifications or contacts with networks of family and friends in the country to which they travelled. They might therefore begin their exile with some advantages; and, even for those who left without these advantages, social mobility could be an important outcome of emigration. Kerby Miller points out the upward mobility of many Irish Americans. He suggests that, of the 5 million Irish Americans in the early twentieth century, many had achieved parity with or passed long standing American communities in terms of occupational advancement. But he also says that they were "yet still remarkably estranged from the dominant culture of their adopted country".[32] Part of this was, of course, remembrance of the Famine, nationalist dialogue and the concept of emigration as driven by poverty.

From the point of view of the Famine narrative, doctor emigration from Ireland was an anomaly. It was professional emigration, small in proportion to total emigration, and whilst this book will ask the question whether it was comparative poverty that drove Irish doctors abroad, these emigrants carried with them educational capital – a medical degree – and therefore were competing in a global medical marketplace. How did they fare financially and were their subsequent careers outside Ireland prosperous or not? Finally, what effect did medical emigration have upon Ireland itself? It was noted at the time and there are occasional references to the loss to Ireland of exporting its doctors. But there are even more robust defences of doctor emigration from medical schools, who often recommended emigration to their students. Sometimes medical emigration was criticised from the point of view of why Ireland needed so many doctors in the first place. *The Leader* in 1913 complained about "this island suffering from a plethora of persons rushing to be medical gentlemen whilst the industries of this country are partly allowed to lie fallow for the want of skilled labour".[33]

31 See Akenson, *The Irish Diaspora*, Tables 34 and 35, pp. 202–3.

32 Miller, *Emigrants and Exiles*, p. 493.

33 *The Leader*, 18 January 1913, footnote 1, p. 1.

3 The Internationalisation of Medicine

Irish medical emigration differs from the pattern of Irish emigration as a whole, but has a great deal in common with medical migration in other parts of the world. This study, as well as being a discussion on the particularities of medical emigration from Ireland, is also a discussion of the general issues that arise when doctors leave one country to practise in another. This immediately directs attention to the word 'globalisation', a term which has become well used since the end of the twentieth century. It carries more importance than it perhaps merits. There had always been movement of doctors across borders – both to practise their craft and for education. It may be that the nineteenth and twentieth centuries saw a rapid increase in the opportunities for doctor migration. It certainly saw developments which facilitated it and also some which threw obstacles in its path. However, Ireland was only one of many countries that was affected by these developments. Several countries produced and exported doctors during this period. Understanding Irish medical emigration, however, can contribute to understanding the nature of the phenomenon as a whole.

One of the most important issues for migrating doctors was accreditation. Was a nation prepared to accept doctors from other countries operating within its borders? The most important legislation affecting the ability of Irish doctors to emigrate was the Medical Registration Act of 1858 which applied to the whole of the United Kingdom and included on its lists Irish medical graduates. The General Medical Council (GMC) of the United Kingdom supervised the register. It inspected medical schools to ensure its graduates reached a standard of education which was good enough to allow admittance to the register. This allowed both practice in Britain and also in the British Empire and occasionally further afield. The GMC's *Medical Registry* remained the bible for Irish doctors contemplating emigration until in 1973 the accession of both the Republic of Ireland and the United Kingdom to the European Economic Community (EEC) made its provision redundant for Irish doctors.[34] Until then it was the most important point of reference. When twenty-six counties of Ireland became independent after 1922, the newly independent Irish government would, from time to time, receive a query from a foreign country about the right to practice in its jurisdiction but the answer was to refer to the list in the GMC's *Medical Register*.

The GMC published an intermittent series of reports, the first in 1910, advising the medical practitioner registered with them on the opportunities and

34 See Chapter 8. The Medical Practitioners Act of 1978 in the Republic of Ireland signalled the formal end of the GMC's position in Irish accreditation replacing it with that of Europe.

barriers to practice abroad.[35] Douglas M. Haynes has described the history of the GMC's negotiations to extend the opportunities for registration beyond Britain and the British Empire. Much of it was driven by the exigencies of health tourism or international relations but most negotiation was with newly independent ex-colonies like Canada and Australia.[36] However the list of countries permitting practice without any verified legal qualifications was small, and in successive editions the GMC advised doctors that the numbers in the category were diminishing. European countries, as they developed national regulatory bodies for medicine, placed restrictions upon the right of foreigners to practise. By the twentieth century certain European countries – Poland, Montenegro, Romania and Spain – required the doctor to become a naturalised citizen before he or she could practise. This condition also applied in various states of America.[37]

However, the growth of Empire in the nineteenth and twentieth centuries increased opportunities for the migratory doctor, notably in the Americas, Africa and Asia. Sometimes this was in places where a European power was the ruler and this simplified things for doctors contemplating working there. But in many places the advance of Empire was qualified, patchy, shared with others and based on predominant influence rather than outright annexation. In the 1933 edition of the GMC's guide, there is a peculiar patchwork of individual regulatory practices influenced by the global advance of Europe and America. In many of the countries under the suzerainty of European powers, doctors from Europe and then from the United States enjoyed access. As far as Empire was concerned, doctors – like traders – followed the flag.

Even where there was no formal colony as such, spheres of influence expressed through consulate authorities, as well as indigenous institutions, set the boundaries. Syria in 1933 allowed practitioners with a degree from any state that belonged to the League of Nations.[38] Iraq recognised the principal medical qualifications of the UK and USA and the major European medical

35 'Report as to the Conditions under which Medical and Dental Practitioners registered or legally qualified in their own country may practise abroad' (London: GMC, 1910). Subsequent guides were published in 1912, 1927 and 1933.

36 Douglas M. Haynes, *Fit to Practice: Empire, Race, Gender and the Making of British Medicine, 1850–1980* (Rochester, N.Y.: Rochester University Press, 2017). Italy and Japan were two countries which negotiated mutual recognition.

37 'Report as to the Conditions under which Medical and Dental Practitioners registered or legally qualified in their own country may practise abroad', 10th edition, (London: GMC, 1933), Table A, p. 7. For the difficulties encountered in the United States, see ibid., Table B, p. 8 and Chapter 7.

38 Ibid., p. 130. Syria was under French influence exercised through a League of Nations' mandate.

schools.[39] Japan allowed practice by British and Mexican subjects possessed of the qualifications of their respective counties and certified by the French consul.[40] In Persia those with "recognised authority but subject to agreement by the Persian medical authorities" were permitted to practise.[41] It was sometimes an issue in which government became involved, since organisations of indigenous doctors might pressurise their governments to legislate on the matter, or aspirant medical migrants ask the government of the country in which they wanted to practise what status and qualifications they would need.

Empire accelerated medical migration in another way. This was through the medical missions and the medical schools founded by them. They trained both missionaries and people indigenous to the country. Even in China, which was threatened by the colonising impulse from Europe and America but which still managed to protect a measure of its independence, medical schools on the Western model took root in the nineteenth century. This made Western medicine and Western doctors a familiar sight, at least to the educated middle class in these countries. A number subsequently made their way to European and American medical schools in the nineteenth and twentieth centuries. Missionary medicine was one of the factors which nourished the flow of medical students and doctors between Europe and its colonies, or from spheres of European and American influence in Asia and Africa to America and Europe.

However, medical migration, initially at least, was most easily facilitated to the colonies settled by substantial European populations. For Irish and British medical immigrants, this was predominantly Australasia and Canada. Registration with the General Medical Council of the United Kingdom was generally sufficient to allow practice. However, even here things were in flux. As these countries moved into the twentieth century, they developed their own medical schools and the shortage of doctors abated. Processes were underway in both Australasia and Canada to create federal medical bodies to oversee registration and medical standards, including advice on who should be admitted from abroad to practise. In 1912 a Canadian Medical Council was set up, though most Canadian states retained autonomy over the permission to practise, as did the Australian states where a similar process of creating federal medical bodies was underway.

The Lancet reported in 1920 on the recent legislation regulating the profession in the state of South Australia, which maintained that "no diplomas other

39 Ibid., pp. 69–70. Iraq was under British and French control.

40 Ibid., p. 72. Japan was independent of European control but certainly influenced by European thought and culture from the late nineteenth century.

41 Ibid., p. 110. Persia (Iran) had traditionally been under British and Russian influence.

than those of the United Kingdom will be accepted unless issued by a country giving reciprocal recognition to South Australian diplomas".[42] Well into the twentieth century, registration by the GMC was a powerful portable qualification across the world; but, as *The Lancet* commented, this could not altogether withstand the winds of economic depression and the problem of oversupply of doctors in the receiving country. They warned in 1920 "that it would be well for British graduates to have some definite prospect before looking to Australia as a possible field of work".[43]

If the Empire pulled the world together and created opportunities for emigration of doctors, so too did the prestige of Western medicine. By the middle of the twentieth century it was doctors trained in Western medical culture who carried with them the qualification which allowed them to move to a new country. It was by that measure that they would be evaluated by and received into the medical system of the host country. This had not always been the case. Irish doctors in India, for example, along with their peers, regarded the indigenous medical culture with a great deal more sympathy; and the flow of medical information went in both directions.[44] However, just as Leiden in the eighteenth century had represented a medical tradition of exceptional importance which attracted the ambitious medical student, so by the middle of the twentieth century European and American medicine formed a model which shaped medical education worldwide.[45]

This was particularly true for the United States after the First World War. American medicine had been lifted out of its previous chaotic state by the Flexner reforms of 1910, and its gospel was spread around the world by funding bodies such as Rockefeller and Carnegie, including in Ireland. A global culture was created defining what a leading medical education was considered to be. Just as migration for education in the early nineteenth century to France and Germany was considered to enhance the practitioner's skills, so American medical schools and the European schools which adopted their ideas shaped the pattern of medical migration. Failure to fully absorb the precepts of this reformed medical education could prove a problem for the aspirant medical migrant particularly to the United States itself.

---

42 *The Lancet*, 1920, vol. 1, p. 835.

43 Ibid., vol. 2, p. 1331.

44 See David Arnold, *Science, Technology and Medicine in Colonial India* (Cambridge: Cambridge University Press, 2000).

45 See Henri Krop, 'Medicine and Philosophy in Leiden around 1700: Continuity or Rupture?' and Wiep van Bunge's contributions in *The Early Enlightenment in the Dutch Republic 1650–1750*, ed. Wiep van Bunge (Leiden and Boston: Brill, 2003).

In other words, there was an increasing fusion of medical practice. The first World Directory of Medical Schools sponsored by the World Health Organization appeared in 1953. The authors claimed that no endorsement or criticism of anyone of the medical schools listed was intended. Nonetheless, the guide displayed certain assumptions about what constituted a medical school. Though often in different continents they all offered similar medical practices and cultures. This was a world in which familiarity with medical practice abroad and a set of assumptions by which it could be measured was part of preparation for medical life, and especially for a migratory one.

With the growth of international organisations in health and increasing state investment in health and medical education, a period after 1945 follows in which economists and specialists in developmental aid begin to examine the export of both healthcare and also doctors. The world market for medical practitioners begins to be discussed largely in terms of its economic impact. Sometimes the broad conclusions arrived at in the debates around migration in this period disguised the actual mechanisms of doctor migration. The debate on medical migration and development in the 1960s and 1970s overgeneralised the processes which sustained it. What an examination of Ireland contributes, therefore, is twofold. It is a story of an important and pervasive experience of the Irish medical system for well over a hundred years, which illuminates a significant part of Ireland's medical and social history. It also shows how the broader ideas about migration actually work out in practice; in other words, Ireland illustrates the more general variegated and complex nature of medical migration.

4 The Structure of the Book

This book is based on a sample of 4,264 migrant doctors between 1860 and 1960 taken from the graduate lists of Irish medical schools every five years between 1860 and 1960. A discussion of the methods used is provided in the Appendix. Of the sample, around 40 per cent emigrated over the hundred years of the study.

The majority went to general practice in Britain or into the medical services in the army, navy or the colonies. Only a relatively small proportion of the sample went to destinations outside. They include the traditional British colonies or ex-colonies, such as Australia, New Zealand and Canada. In Africa there were Irish doctors following European settlements in South Africa and East Africa. A smaller number still went to even more remote places, outside or only marginally under British influence, such as China, South America or Africa.

The book follows the flow of medical migrants and therefore most attention is given to the two main destinations: Britain and the Empire. Between 1860 and 1915 only twelve of the 703 migrants in our sample went to either Australasia or North America, that is less than 2 per cent. Between 1920 and 1940 out of the 540 who left, none went to Australasia and nineteen went to North America, about 3.5 per cent. However, in the period 1945–60 sixteen went to Australasia and ninety-four to North America out of just over 489 migrants for those years, that is over 22 per cent.

The concentration of this book on the two main emigrant flows does not diminish the interest of other migration patterns. For example, the history of Irish doctors in China, South America, the Middle East, Asia and Europe would be instructive. Though small relative to the other patterns of migration, they reveal the complexity of doctor experience in missions, trade, foreign policy, health tourism and expatriate communities, as well as the cultural and economic ripples occasioned by the rise of the European Empires in the nineteenth and twentieth centuries. But to paraphrase the Commission on Higher Education, to follow all these migration routes would be a major undertaking and it is beyond the scope of this book.

However, the rise in the proportion of doctors going to North America in the 1950s is of particular interest and is dealt with for that reason. First it reflects a trend observable in many countries after the Second World War, of the emergence of the United States as a central destination for medical migrants from all over the world. Second it illustrates two of the issues which affect migrating doctors and Irish medical migrants in particular. These are accreditation and medical education. Without accreditation a doctor cannot move to a new country. Medical education is the means to secure accreditation. In both respects doctors from the Republic of Ireland faced difficulties in the 1950s; but these were solved, as far as admission to the United States was concerned, by the end of the decade.

The final chapter of the book deals with a change in the experience of medical migration in the 1960s: the arrival in Ireland itself of a substantial number of medical migrants from outside Ireland. First they were seeking a medical education, but in later decades they were leaving their own country to make a medical living in Ireland. They changed Ireland from being primarily an exporter to also being an importer of, first, migrant students and then doctors. This chapter reflects upon the increasing volume of medical migration in the world at large and its impact on Ireland.

The book covers a crucial hundred years, in which time the migration patterns changed. The number of medical migrants between 1860 to the First World War was higher than the rate after the First World War. Making a medical living in Britain was even more important in the interwar period than before. After the Second World War the rise in emigration to North America increased. Medical migration changed over time, and alongside these changes are the major political and economic events in the history of Ireland itself: the evolution of different medical systems, north and south; the emergence of two jurisdictions in Ireland, one with a largely Catholic population and the other largely Protestant; the growing influence of the United States in medical education; and the increasing global extent of migration post 1945. However, throughout all the historical changes taking place in these hundred years, Irish medical graduates went on emigrating.

CHAPTER 1

The Medical Institutions of Ireland

In 1878 Charles Keetley observed that, "If the number of students be considered, the Medical School of Dublin is larger than that of London or indeed any other town of the United Kingdom."[1] In the year in which Keetley observed this, there were six medical schools in Ireland. They included the medical school of Trinity College Dublin (TCD), or the University of Dublin as it was also called, founded in 1654. Trinity was linked to the Royal College of Physicians of Ireland (RCPI), which was its examining and licensing board. Trinity and the Royal College of Physicians (RCP) were old and venerable institutions but Trinity had been founded to educate members of the Church of Ireland, which effectively excluded the majority of the Irish population which was Catholic. In the north-east of Ireland, there was also a high concentration of Presbyterians also excluded by their religion from graduating from Trinity. Nor, in the first part of the nineteenth century, could non-Anglicans hold fellowships in Trinity.[2] Consequently aspirant Irish doctors from other denominations either enrolled in private medical schools or went abroad for their education to Scottish medical schools or to the Continent. If they studied at Trinity's medical school, which was possible in the late eighteenth century, they had to graduate from other schools that recognised Trinity's courses, usually from Scottish schools. This was popular among the Presbyterians of the north, many of whom had historical and cultural links with Scotland. But it was also a route available to Catholics. One of the most famous Catholic physicians of the nineteenth century in Ireland, Sir Dominic Corrigan (1802–1880), took courses at Trinity and private medical schools in Ireland but graduated from a Scottish medical school.[3] However, some Catholics went abroad to Europe for their medical education.[4]

---

1 Charles Robert Bell Keetley, *The Student's Guide to the Medical Profession* (London: Bailliere Tindall and Cox, 1878), p. 81.

2 McDowell and Webb's history of TCD points out that religious tests on students were not enforced in the late eighteenth century and some Catholics and Dissenters did attend. However, posts in the University were open only to Anglicans and a tradition existed of expecting some outward show of conformity among students to the Established Church. This meant that the number of non-Anglican students at TCD was proportionately reduced; see R.B. McDowell and D.A. Webb, *Trinity College Dublin 1592–1952: An Academic History* (Dublin: Trinity College Press, 2004), pp. 247–8 (First published 1982 by Cambridge University Press).

3 Eoin O'Brien, *Conscience and Conflict: A Biography of Sir Dominic Corrigan 1802–1880* (Dublin: Glendale Press, 1983).

4 Fiona Clark and James Kelly, eds., *Ireland and Medicine in the Seventeenth and Eighteenth Centuries* (London: Routledge, 2010).

 | DOI:10.1163/9789004324466_003

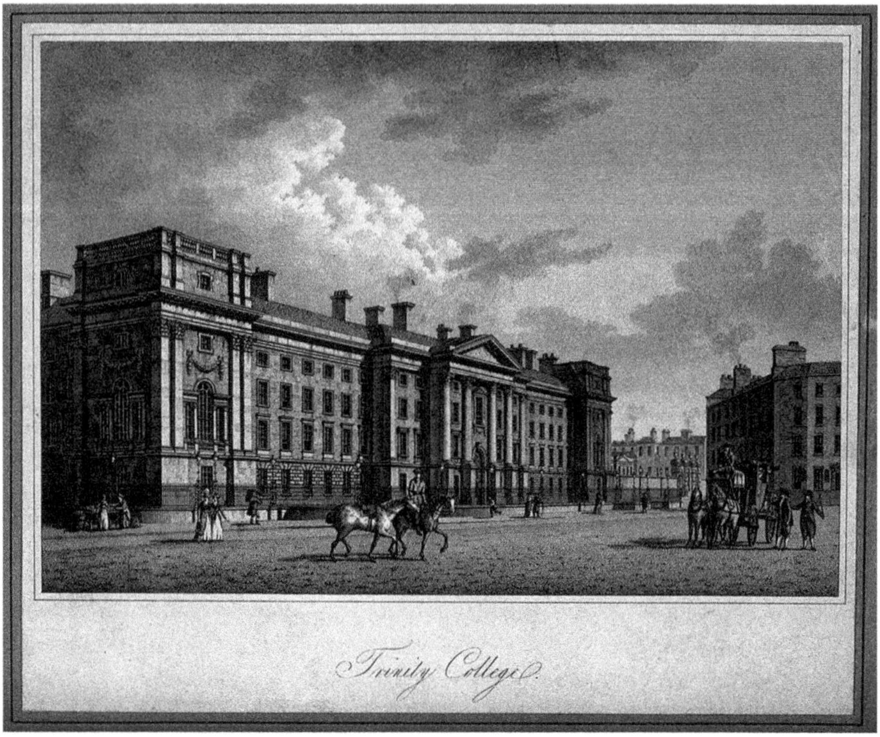

FIGURE 1 Trinity College, Dublin, Ireland. Line engraving after T. Jacobsen
SOURCE: WELLCOME COLLECTION. ATTRIBUTION 4.0 INTERNATIONAL (CC BY 4.0)

The religious question in education was a perpetual political issue throughout the nineteenth century, and it frequently affected medical education. However, in 1784 the College of Surgeons in Dublin was founded, and accepted medical students from all denominations. It also, like its counterpart in England, had a reputation for a more radical reforming attitude to medicine, and the Royal College of Surgeons in Ireland as it eventually became (RCSI) campaigned for the removal of the privileges enjoyed by Trinity and the RCPI. The battle in Ireland for medical reform echoed that of England, so much so that *The Lancet*, under Thomas Wakley, took up the Irish cause in the 1830s and 1840s. Out of this turbulent period in Irish medicine emerged two periodicals, the *Medical Press and Circular*, intended to become an Irish version of the radical and crusading *Lancet* and the *Dublin Journal of Medical Science*.[5] The Irish Medical Association (IMA) was also a product of this time: formed in 1839, it

5 The journal was founded in 1832 by Robert Kane as the *Dublin Journal of Medical and Chemical Science*. It changed its name between 1846–71 to the *Dublin Quarterly Journal of Medical Science* and between 1871–1925 to the *Dublin Journal of Medical Science*.

lapsed in 1846 but was revived in 1853. It published its own periodical, the *Journal of the Irish Medical Association* (*JIMA*).

In 1845 the British government recognised the justice of allowing non-Anglicans access to university education. Three Queen's colleges, at Belfast, Galway and Cork, were created with financial support from the state. They were to be strictly non-denominational. All three had medical schools. The Queen's Colleges proved controversial for the Catholic Church in Ireland, who wanted government support for an exclusively Catholic-run university and they warned Catholics against attending the three Queen's Colleges. Nonetheless the colleges began to attract Catholics, and many Catholic priests accepted in practice their parishioners' attendance at them as a necessary evil.

The Queen's Colleges were to prove an enduring feature of medical education in Ireland, though they metamorphosed from time to time. In 1879–80 the government brought the Queen's Colleges, the Catholic University and Trinity into a federal scheme, the Royal University of Ireland (RUI). In 1908 two of them, Cork and Galway, after another major reorganisation of tertiary level education, became, along with the Catholic University, constituent colleges of the National University of Ireland (NUI). At this point Trinity went its own way. As for Queen's College Belfast, its medical school survived in an independent university in Belfast, the medical school of the Queen's University. These changes in the university system all took place in an atmosphere of heightened political and religious dissension.

The reforms were intended to accommodate the sectarian divisions in Ireland. Because the Catholic Church was unhappy at mixed denominational education, in 1854 the Catholic University of Ireland was founded in Dublin, primarily through donations from the Catholic faithful. Though it tried during the next decades to persuade the government to fund it, it was unsuccessful and had to depend for its survival on charitable bequests and student fees. The Catholic University struggled in the initial years of its existence, surviving largely because of its medical school which was successful in attracting students. Crucial to this was the fact that that the RCPI and RCSI recognised the Catholic University's medical courses and graduated its students.

The Catholic University's medical school grew over the next fifty years, becoming first part of the Royal University of Ireland and finally the National University in 1908. At that point the Catholic University became University College Dublin (UCD) and a constituent of the National University of Ireland. The medical school of the Catholic University, now the medical school of UCD, was by 1908 the largest in Ireland.

The final medical school in Ireland was the Apothecaries Hall. This was a licensing body which, like the RCSI, taught and awarded medical licences. Its right to issue medical licences survived until 1971. In the 1950s and 1960s the nomenclature of Licentiate of the Apothecaries Hall (LAH) can still be found beside the names of medical practitioners in the *Medical Register* of the United Kingdom.

1 The Medical Registration Act 1858

In 1858 the Medical Registration Act was passed by the Westminster Parliament. This provided for the creation of a *Medical Register*. On this was recorded the names of those whom the medical profession regarded as properly trained and fit to practise. The Act set up the General Medical Council, drawn from senior members of the profession. Their remit was to run the register and to validate the education provided in medical schools. This was done by periodic visitations of medical schools by the GMC. Those graduating from schools approved by the GMC were eligible to have their names entered on the register. A third responsibility was to act as the disciplinary body within the profession. The GMC could suspend from the register or, in serious cases, strike off a doctor found guilty of breaching its disciplinary code. Medical graduates from all parts of the British Isles, including Ireland, were entered on the *Medical Register*.

Irish born and educated doctors may be found in the general UK list, the section reserved for practitioners in Ireland and the lists recording doctors serving in the army or colonial service or abroad. The 1858 Medical Registration Act was, therefore, a milestone on the road to the emergence of medicine as a profession in the British Isles. It set educational standards for those practising medicine which, over time, shaped the public's view of what it meant to be a doctor. Though enacted by statute, doctors now became a largely self-regulating profession. The GMC oversaw educational levels and disciplinary matters, and could represent and negotiate with the government on behalf of the profession.

The Act did not exclude those not on the register from practising medicine, but it did exclude them from certain posts in medicine and for misrepresenting themselves as qualified. Therefore the 1858 Act was initially a disappointment to many Irish doctors who had looked for legislation which banned the unqualified from practising at all. It meant that the battle which the medical professional had conducted before the Act of 1858 against the unqualified, or the 'quack' or 'coffinite', as they were often described in medical circles, went on. On the other hand, the Act heralded a significant improvement in the status and social position of the qualified doctor.

It also changed Irish medical education. By the middle of the nineteenth century the two colleges, the RCSI and RCPI, already had informal arrangements for combining their examinations and licensing procedures. This produced the famous medical designation in Ireland of Licentiate of the RCPI and the RCSI (LRCPI, LRCSI). A further Medical Act of 1886, however, laid down that a recognised medical degree must include medicine, surgery and obstetrics – the familiar three-sided qualification of MB (bachelor of medicine), BCh (bachelor of surgery) and BAO (bachelor of obstetrics). This gradually replaced the old MD (Doctor of Medicine) qualification familiar to an earlier generation. The Act also provided for the combination of licensing boards, and out of this change arose an examining structure set up by the two colleges RCPI and RCSI: the Conjoint Board.

Irish medical education remained different in certain respects from that in the rest of the British Isles. The GMC did not enforce absolute uniformity in education, but the Irish medical profession was always aware that too great a gap should not emerge between medical education in Britain and Ireland lest it endanger entry onto the United Kingdom *Medical Register*. Ireland's medical interests were looked after on the GMC by representatives drawn from the country's major medical institutions. Entry on the *Medical Register* meant access for Irish doctors to posts in England, Wales, Scotland and the British Empire. It was also, until the twentieth century, a passport to practise in many areas settled by the British overseas or even in more far flung places.

2 The Evolution of Irish Medical Education

Among the changes taking place in Irish medical education in the late nineteenth century were the decline in apprenticeships and private medical schools. They were replaced by the more familiar medical school situated within the university. E.D. Mapother calculated that of the 797 students he identified in Dublin in 1868, excluding the RCSI, 45 per cent were in private medical schools which prepared their pupils for the exams of the licensing bodies.[6] By 1905, however, some 86 per cent of first-year places of study were in the five medical schools attached to universities, and apart from the 14 per cent of first-year students who were being taught in the RCSI, the private school system had disappeared.

6 E.D. Mapother, *The Medical Profession and its Educational and Licensing Bodies* (Dublin: Fannin & Co., 1868), p. 161 states that 188 were at TCD, 161 at the RCSI, 90 at the Catholic University. The remainder were at the Carmichael (100), Dr Steevens' (80) or the Ledwich (178). Mapother (1835–1908) was consulting surgeon at St Vincent's Hospital. He was interested in public health and was appointed to the chair in hygiene at the RCSI in 1864. He led the eventual amalgamation of the RCSI, Ledwich and Carmichael Schools; see *Dictionary of Irish Biography* (Cambridge: Cambridge University Press).

TABLE 1 Number and percentage (in brackets) of first-year students in Ireland registered in the GMC, 1875–1935

School	1875	1885	1905	1910	1915	1920	1930	1935
RCSI	40 (15.15)	28 (8.3)	39 (13.6)	53 (13.9)	75 (15.8)	102 (18.3)	57 (16.8)	86 (16.35)
TCD	3 (0.1)	30 (8.9)	66 (23.07)	83 (21.7)	88 (18.6)	131 (23.5)	64 (18.87)	96 (18.4)
QCB	68 (25.7)	46 (13.7)	55 (19.2)	48 (12.6)	68 (14.4)	141 (25.3)	114 (33.6)	130 (24.9)
QCC	38 (14.39)	49 (14.6)	45 (15.7)	87 (22.8)	78 (16.5)	66 (11.85)	29 (8.55)	60 (11.5)
QCG	46 (7.4)	10 (2.9)	13 (4.5)	10 (4.5)	42 (8.5)	13 (2.3)	9 (2.26)	21 (4.0)
Catholic University/ UCD	18 (6.8)	25 (7.48)	68 (23.77)	100 (26.4)	121 (25.6)	104 (18.67)	66 (19.46)	128 (24.56)
Private medical schools	47 (17.8)	77 (23)	–	–	–	–	–	–
Hospitals	–	38 (11.3)	–	–	–	–	–	–
Apprenticeships	–	31 (9.28)	–	–	–	–	–	–
Other*	4 (1%)		–	–	–	–	–	–
Total students**	264	334	286	381	472	557 (552)	339	521

* Unclear in register. Often just county of residence given.
** The figure from the Medical Students' register is in brackets. There is an occasional discrepancy between the figures returned from medical schools and those given by the GMC. In these cases percentages are worked out using the figures from the medical schools.

SOURCE: BASED ON THE MEDICAL STUDENTS' REGISTER IN THE DIFFERENT PLACES OF STUDY IN IRELAND[7]

7 "Summary of the Number of Medical Students Registered during each year in each of the three divisions of the United Kingdom from the commencement of student's registration in 1865 to the end of the year 1915", and "Summary of the Number of Medical Students Registered during each year in each of the three divisions of the United Kingdom, from 1905 to 1936 inclusive", *The Medical Directory Medical and Dental Students' Register* (General Medical Council, 1936).

Private medical schools flourished in the early part of the nineteenth century, partly because medical professionals sought a route to increasing their income through founding a school. Among them were leading and distinguished luminaries of Irish medicine in the early nineteenth century. The Carmichael School was named after its founder Richard Carmichael, an important doctor in the early nineteenth century and a luminary of the RCSI. The name of the Ledwich School also resonates in the history of Irish medical education.[8] But gradually, together with medical apprenticeships, these private institutions went into decline. In 1885 the figure for those taking up apprenticeships or registering with private medical schools outside the RCSI was still 22 per cent.[9] The Ledwich and Carmichael, two of the most famous, go on appearing in the *Medical Register* as a place of education and also on the lists of those qualifying for the degrees of Cork, Galway and elsewhere into the 1890s. However, the private school became rarer, and although a few survived into the 1890s, they had disappeared by 1905. Apprenticeships also declined, although informal arrangements between distinguished consultants and private pupils still existed. However, the largest and most enduring private medical school was that of the Royal College of Surgeons in Ireland, which has survived and flourished to this day, largely given its right to issue licenses.

Another characteristic of Irish medical students and of medical students elsewhere in the British Isles in the nineteenth century was acquiring an education by peregrination.[10] The practice of moving between medical schools was becoming rarer but was still practised. The school in which you studied might not be the one from which you eventually graduated. A student could turn up in the graduate lists of, for example, the medical school of Queen's College Cork, having been taught mainly at the Ledwich or elsewhere. Some appeared in the institution at which they formally qualified to take their examination, but had received much of their education elsewhere. The medical education of Dominic Corrigan (1802–1880) illustrates this pattern. He began his education at Trinity medical school in 1820, but as a Catholic he could not graduate from there. He also took courses at both the Apothecaries Hall and the private medical school in Peter's Street, Kirby's Medical School. Finally he attended sessions

8 For the Carmichael and Ledwich medical schools, see John F. Fleetwood, *The History of Medicine in Ireland* (Dublin: Skellig Press, 1983).

9 Calculated from 334 first-year entrants; see Table 1.

10 This was common among mid-nineteenth-century medical students; see James Bradley, Anne Crowther and Marguerite Dupree, 'Mobility and Selection in Scottish University Medical Education 1858–1886', *Medical History*, vol. 40. no. 1, 1996, p. 9. The authors refer to students' "nomadic habits".

at Edinburgh from which he graduated in 1825.[11] Laura Kelly also mentions in her study of Irish medical students that Galway students would regularly go to Dublin hospitals to acquire surgical skills, given the relative dearth of hospitals in Galway itself; she notes the freedom of Irish students to wander into hospitals of their choice.[12]

Peregrination could be even further afield. The traditional links between Ireland, particularly the North of Ireland, and Scottish universities, though diminished by the expansion of higher education in Ireland, did not altogether disappear, even in the late nineteenth century.[13] The persistence could be attributed to family tradition, the relative nearness of Scotland, the perception that a licence to practise could be more easily obtained there and historical and religious links between Scotland and the Scots settlers of the north-east of Ireland. Crowther and Dupree's work on the cohort of graduates from the medical schools of Edinburgh and Glasgow suggests that 6 per cent of those who began their study of medicine in Glasgow in 1871 and 4 per cent in Edinburgh were Irish-born.[14] However, only a small proportion of Irish graduates educated in Scotland returned to Ireland. Crowther and Dupree state that 56 of their cohort were born in Ireland but only 12 practised there.[15] Similarly Laura Kelly followed the Irish graduates who trained in the Glasgow medical school between 1859 and 1900 to establish their destinations five years after graduating. Her conclusion is that only one in three of Irish-born graduates of Glasgow University's medical school returned to practise in Ireland.[16]

There are a number of shifts in venue that are very small and particular. A few examinees for an Irish qualification list a London school as the place in which they were educated. This was attributed at the time to the fact that Irish exams were easier and improved the chances of success for weaker students. This assertion must be treated with care. Medical schools in the late nineteenth and early twentieth centuries were in competition for students, and therefore some of their comments on each other should be treated carefully. Those educated in England and taking the exams of Irish institutions were, however, rare. By the end of the first decade of the twentieth century most students tended

---

11 O'Brien, *Conscience and Conflict*, p. 28.

12 Laura Kelly, *Irish Medical Education and Student Culture c.1850–1950* (Liverpool: Liverpool University Press, 2017), pp. 121–3.

13 See Kelly, 'Irish Medical Students at the University of Glasgow 1859–1900'.

14 Crowther and Dupree, *Medical Lives in the Age of Surgical Revolution*, Table 1.4, p. 23

15 Ibid., p. 253.

16 Kelly, 'Irish Medical Students at the University of Glasgow', p. 61 and Table 3.2, p. 62. Over 100 students were examined. See also P. Froggatt, 'The Irish Connection', in *The Influence of Scottish Medical Education*, ed. Derek A. Dow (Carnforth: Parthenon, 1988), pp. 63–76.

to spend their five years of medical education continuously within the portals of medical schools in universities: the National University of Ireland at Dublin, Cork and Galway, in the University of Dublin (TCD) or in Queen's University Belfast (QUB).[17] This left two independent schools outside the university system: the Royal College of Surgeons and the Apothecaries Hall.[18]

The Act of 1879 setting up the Royal University of Ireland (RUI), which came into being in 1880, was an attempt to meet some of the grievances of the Catholic University. In particular, the Royal University allowed some monies to be given to the Catholic University from the government. Additionally the Royal University could grant degrees in their own right, although medical students at the Catholic University generally still went the way of the Licentiateships of the Royal College of Physicians and the College of Surgeons. The system was a federal one with a governing body drawn from all the constituent colleges.

Nonetheless, the relationship between the Catholic University and the Royal University remained uneasy. There were various disputes about the philosophy syllabus set out in the examinations of the RUI, with the Catholic University finding it too much based on Locke and Hume.[19] Overall the Catholic Church felt the situation did meet their desire for a fully Catholic university. The Irish Universities Act of 1908, which created the National University, did not altogether satisfy the demands of the Catholic University, but it went a good way in that direction. It signalled a more denominational type of medical education in Ireland. Though the two remaining Queen's Colleges, of Cork and Galway, were founded as non-denominational institutions and formally retained that status they became increasingly Catholic in their student body and ethos.

3 The Hospitals

Ireland was well supplied with voluntary hospitals, the highest number of which were in Dublin. Dublin had ten general hospitals and five specialist

17 Qualified physicians in Ireland who styled themselves LRCPI (Licentiate of the Royal College of Physicians of Ireland) and LRCSI (Licentiate of the Royal College of Surgeons in Ireland) could have been educated in Trinity or another school, or more frequently had been students of the Royal College of Surgeons.

18 Kelly notes that some students could qualify more quickly through obtaining licences. This was consequently cheaper than the five years plus offered by medical schools. See Kelly, *Irish Medical Education and Student Culture c.1850–1950*, p. 27.

19 Greta Jones, 'Thomas Henry Huxley, the Catholic Church and the founding of the University of London', unpublished paper.

ones.[20] Several of the hospitals had been added in the nineteenth century as a result of Catholic charitable activity: including St Vincent's (1857) run by the Sisters of Charity, and the Mater Misericordiae (1861) run by the Sisters of Mercy. Thus, the situation in nineteenth-century Dublin by which Catholic medical students and graduates sought training or posts in Catholic hospitals and Protestants in Protestant hospitals intensified. Voluntary hospitals of whatever denomination received government grants in the nineteenth century, including some from Dublin Corporation, and they would regularly petition for money from government, describing their activities and the financial burdens under which they were operating.[21] The pleas were strengthened by the view of many in the medical establishment of the value of the medical culture in Ireland to the British Empire. As one commentator put it, "An Imperial objective is moreover fulfilled by the hospitals of Dublin, for in them are educated more surgeons for the army and navy than in those of England or Scotland."[22] It was also the general opinion that generous hospital provision put the poor of Dublin in a very advantageous position compared with the rest of the British Isles. The multiplicity of hospitals in Dublin lasted well into the twentieth century. One medical student training after the Second World War wrote, "Student life in the 1940s was so free and permissive that if you were a medical student you could wander into any Dublin hospital and attend the clinic of your choice, and the choice was dazzling."[23]

Nonetheless, there were problems.[24] The numbers of hospitals put a strain on finances as their use increased over the nineteenth century and they become a more routine part of the experience of being ill. Rationalisation and amalgamation of the Dublin hospitals became a recurrent theme in the twentieth century. But this was easier to discuss than achieve. Many hospitals became fiefdoms jealously guarding their territory. For the medical profession, their number increased the chances of professorships or consultancies. Even if the patients were drawn from both religious communities, the medical profes-

---

20 From E.D. Mapother, 'The Dublin Hospitals – their Grants and Governing bodies', *Journal of the Statistical and Social Inquiry Society of Ireland*, vol. V, Part XXXVII, 1869/1870.

21 See 'Fifth Annual Report of the Board of Superintendence of Dublin Hospitals' (Dublin: Alex Thom for Her Majesty's Stationery Office, 1862), Appendix 11, p. 18, and subsequent Annual Reports.

22 Mapother, 'The Dublin Hospitals – their Grants and Governing bodies', p. 131.

23 Joyce Delaney, *No Starch in My Coat: An Irish Doctor's Progress* (London: Cox & Wyman, 1971), p. 18.

24 For a recent overview of hospital provision, see Donnacha Seán Lucey and Virginia Crossman (eds.), *Healthcare in Ireland and Britain from 1850: Voluntary, Regional and Comparative Perspective* (London: Institute of Historical Research, 2014).

sion generally trained in the hospitals of their own religion and took consultancies in them too. Certainly the Catholic Church regarded the Catholic-run hospitals as an essential supplement to the medical education provided in the Catholic University.

Disinterested observers were inclined to see the disadvantages of the number of hospitals. This they considered led to chronic under funding, particularly in adapting to new medical technologies. A common complaint in the twentieth century was the lack of a research-based hospital in Ireland with laboratory and other research facilities. It also led to a disorganised and fractured medical education with a high amount of peregrination between different hospitals for medical students, in other words a rather *ad hoc* system.

Other parts of Ireland were less well supplied with hospitals than Dublin. Belfast, a thriving industrial city in the nineteenth century, had a voluntary hospital, the Royal Victoria, from the late eighteenth century. In 1883 it was joined by a Catholic voluntary hospital, the Mater. Another major Belfast hospital, the City Hospital, had its origin as a workhouse infirmary. Other smaller towns also replicated these developments, though the poorer and predominantly rural parts of the west of Ireland were not within easy reach of either hospitals or dispensaries.[25] The development of hospitals in Ireland was not altogether dissimilar to that in other parts of the British Isles, and even though the denominational aspect was strong in Ireland, it was not unknown in Britain too. A distinguishing factor in Irish health care, however, was the dispensary system, which grew throughout the nineteenth century and provided most routine medical care to the Irish population.

4 The Poor Law

Many Irish men and women could not afford the doctor. Doctors in fact had a sliding scale of fees, usually calculated on the rental value of the property in which their patient lived. The richer you were, measured by this, the more you paid the doctor. Alongside the more speedy, personalised and deferential service that the wealthy patient enjoyed came the ceremonies attached to waiting on a great or important person. By contrast, for the poor, medical care was often administered by the unqualified practitioner, or they relied upon home remedies supplied by a member of the family, or else they were thrown upon the Poor Law.

---

25 See Catherine Cox, 'Access and Engagement: The Medical Dispensary Service in Post-Famine Ireland', in *Cultures of Care in Irish Medical History 1750–1970*, eds. Catherine Cox and Maria Luddy (Basingstoke: Palgrave Macmillan, 2010), pp. 57–78.

In recognition of the special problem of the sick poor, various charitable institutions grew up before and during the eighteenth century to provide them with free medical care.[26] Even though public provision expanded in the nineteenth century, charities of this sort were still important in the ecology of Irish medical care. With the introduction of the New Poor Law into Ireland in 1838, however, a process began of increasing public provision of medical care for the poor. The infirmary attached to the workhouse took in the sick poor and, at times of epidemic, the infirmary was transformed into isolation wards for the afflicted.[27] The role of the workhouse infirmary expanded in the nineteenth century and eventually, with the reform of local government, they developed into institutions run by county councils. As well as the workhouse infirmary, networks of county hospitals were set up throughout Ireland by local government, with the help of charitable bequests.

More significantly for Ireland, under the 1851 Medical Charities Act charitable dispensaries were brought under the aegis of the Poor Law. Maintaining them became a responsibility of the boards of guardians elected under the 1838 Act to build and run the workhouses. Dispensaries treated outpatients, and medical provision could include a doctor's visit to one's home. Access to this service depended upon the presentation of a ticket issued by the local dispensary committee. The dispensary system grew very substantially in the nineteenth century and became important not just for the very poorest, but for substantial numbers of the non-pauper population. Between 1853 and 1872 the number of tickets issued allowing the holders to obtain care at the dispensary or a home visit from the dispensary doctor rose from 690,411 to 784,424, an increase which must be seen in the light of a falling population during that period.[28] The rise in the popularity of dispensaries among the general population led doctors to complain that they were treating some who could afford to pay the doctor, and this depressed levels of remuneration in the medical profession.

Nevertheless, the Poor Law medical service was close to the hearts of all Irish doctors because, for reasons which will become clear in the next chapter, they depended more than their brethren in other parts of the British Isles upon Poor Law and state employment. In exegeses on the state of the Irish medical profession in the nineteenth century, it was always an important topic.

---

26 See Ronald D. Cassell, *Medical Charities, Medical Politics: The Irish Dispensary and the Poor Law* (London: Royal Historical Society, 1997); and Laurence Geary, *Medicine and Charity in Ireland 1718–1851* (Dublin: University College Dublin Press, 2004).

27 See Virginia Crossman, *Poverty and the Poor Law in Ireland 1850–1914* (Liverpool: Liverpool University Press, 2013).

28 Helen Burke, *The People and the Poor Law in 19th Century Ireland* (Dublin: Women's Educational Press Ireland, 1987), Table 24, p. 247.

According to Mapother in 1868, in Ireland there were 786 medical officers for 716 dispensary districts, 163 workhouse physicians and 39 apothecaries. In addition, since 1845 Ireland had a publicly funded network of lunatic asylums. In 1868 these 20 public asylums employed 42 medical officers and ancillary medical staff.[29] Doctors were also employed in prisons and in police and army barracks. By the end of the nineteenth century doctors in the Poor Law service also had the opportunity of taking on the (usually part-time) role of the medical officer of health or sanitary superintendent.

Medical officers were appointed under the Public Health Act (Ireland) 1878. This was modelled on the landmark legislation in Britain in 1872 and 1875 which created a mandatory public health system. Both Belfast and Dublin, the largest cities in Ireland, had appointed sanitary inspectors and superintendents before the Act of 1878, and it was possible to acquire training in public health in Irish medical schools well before 1878. The first chair of hygiene was created in 1841.[30] Under the 1878 Act most medical officers of health were part-time and the distribution was patchy. Ironically Irish doctors with the Diploma in State Medicine who went to India probably contributed as much to public health there as in Ireland, though in much more extreme circumstances.

Appointments to the post of medical officer to the dispensary or workhouse were carried out under the general supervision of the Local Government Board (LGB Ireland) which oversaw the Poor Law. The day-to-day functioning of the Poor Law, including appointments of medical officers, was carried out by a committee appointed by the elected boards of guardians who looked after the Poor Law in their area. Although good relations often existed between the medical officers appointed to tend the sick poor and the board of guardians, sometimes there was friction. Eligibility to elect the board of guardians depended on whether you paid the poor rate. Whilst some subvention was received from the Local Government Board, much of the cost of poor relief fell on the poor rate, so there were financial tensions. Moreover, doctors often felt that some committees failed to acknowledge their social position and professional status. Added to this there was a strong denominational element to the whole process. Consequently, as one commentator put it in his advice for the new graduate applying for poor laws medical posts:

> The first thing he will discover is that as well as a medical and surgical qualification, he must also have a religious one; that is to say he must

29 Mapother, *The Medical Profession and its Educational and Licensing Bodies*, pp. 60–61.

30 See Fleetwood, *The History of Medicine in Ireland*, p. 77. A Diploma in State Medicine was created in TCD in 1871.

> belong to the sect suited for that particular appointment. He will very soon find out that a Catholic Astley Cooper would be perfectly ineligible with one Board of Guardians as a Protestant Benjamin Brodie would be with another and he will, therefore, do well to examine the list of electors carefully from a religious point of view before he incurs further expense.[31]

5 Professional Organisations in Ireland and Britain

The British Medical Association (BMA) was founded in 1832 to represent the interests of doctors. There were individual members of the BMA living in Ireland, and in 1874 a south of Ireland branch of the BMA was founded in Cork by Henry MacNaughton-Jones, then professor of gynaecology at the Queen's College.[32] In 1877 a Dublin branch was formed at the RCPI. The Dublin branch claimed 20 new members to add to the existing 93 individual members already in Dublin. By 1887 the number of branch members had risen to 200. In the early days the Dublin branch began to accumulate members outside Dublin in other counties. Other branches quickly followed and eventually four regional branches existed in Ireland: the Dublin area, the south, north and west. The foundation of branches as opposed to individual members was important for the BMA in Ireland: it could then act in concert in pursuit of Irish interests, and as the branches grew, it would have the right to nominate members to the Council of the BMA.

Relationships with the Irish Medical Association founded in 1839 were, initially at least, somewhat strained. The honorary secretary of the Dublin branch of the BMA attended a meeting of the IMA in 1877, where he claimed he had heard "some very discourteous and disparaging observations with regard to the BMA". He "was caused by this to leave the room and had written to ask for a retraction from Mr Macnamara".[33] This animosity did not persist. Many Irish doctors were members of both organisations, and the IMA and BMA cooperated to send joint deputations to the Secretary of State for Ireland or to Britain to protect or enhance Irish medical interests. The IMA needed the support of the local and national BMA, a support which over the years it received. If the IMA had a distinctive identity, it was as a champion of the doctors employed

---

31 'Religion and Nepotism in Medicine', *Journal of the Irish Medical Association* (*JIMA*), no. 23, 27 May 1868, p. 89.

32 For Henry MacNaughton-Jones's illustrious career, see Obituary, *BMJ*, 4 May 1918.

33 Royal College of Physicians of Ireland (RCPI) Archives, British Medical Association Archives, BMA/1/2 1877–1881, Minutes of the Council of the Dublin Branch, 25 June 1877.

in and dependent upon the Poor Law, or those in the poorer rural provinces of Ireland.

The IMA was very aware of the divide between the Dublin medical elite and the ordinary provincial practitioner. The Dublin branch of the BMA certainly embraced the mighty in Ireland's medical establishment. It included names familiar to historians of Ireland's medical and scientific history: T.W. Grimshaw, Ireland's Registrar General; E.D. Mapother; and Sir John Moore, who succeeded James Little as editor of the *Dublin Quarterly Journal of Medical Science*.[34]

The objective of the Irish branches of the BMA was that "it may be the means of strengthening the voice of the profession in Ireland and of bringing the Irish members into closer connexion with their Scottish and English brethren".[35] Apart from the considerable amount of business taken up, at least in the Dublin branch, by collecting late dues and organising the annual dinner, it had several aims. They were to scrutinise proposed medical legislation at Westminster, and to lobby for the inclusion or exclusion of Ireland. Or they looked at legislative proposals and asked for changes and modifications in the light of Ireland's particular circumstances. In 1880 the Dublin branch looked over the suggested changes to medical education which eventually passed into law in the Medical Act of 1886 and advocated the abandonment of two provisions: the exam at the end of the first year, and two years' experience in a recognised hospital in clinical medicine and surgery and obstetrics before the final qualifying exam.[36] The Irish BMA strongly supported Dublin Corporation's request for a local bill on public health, but watched carefully to protect and enhance remuneration for the additional medical work it might involve.[37]

The Irish Medical Association was founded in 1839, lapsed in 1846 but revived in 1853. Its revival was coincidental with the implementation of the Medical Charities Act of 1851, which reformed the Poor Law medical system. A major concern was representing dispensary and workhouse medical officers in Ireland, although its leadership claimed a broader role for itself. IMA membership fluctuated, and estimates in 1901 ranged from around 600 to 900. Even the higher figure meant that it represented approximately only half of dispensary and Poor Law officers in Ireland, and only around a quarter to a third of qualified physicians practising in Ireland. The Association's journal, the *Journal of the Irish Medical Association* (*JIMA*), appeared until 1871, when

34 See *Dictionary of Irish Biography*.
35 RCPI Archives, 25 January 1878.
36 Ibid., 19 March 1880.
37 Ibid., 16 April 1881.

it was published as a supplement to the *Dublin Medical Press and Circular.* In 1901 *JIMA* reappeared as an independent publication, circulating primarily to its members, and becoming an important mouthpiece for dispensary medical officers in that period.

The IMA was a means to mobilise those doctors dependent upon Poor Law employment to sustain their incomes, and they were most active in this area. They also voiced many of the grievances of the provincial doctors. Although the Irish medical profession were generally united on matters of remuneration and other professional concerns, there was an underlying tension between the poorer provincial doctor and what were considered to be their better-off urban counterparts. The practitioner in Ireland's rural west, who felt the brunt of the difficulties in making a medical living, was particularly militant against the dominance of Dublin. In correspondence to the Irish Medical Association in 1936, the letter-writer complained about "the utter contempt in which you in Dublin held us who are compelled to earn our living trudging through bogs and mountains in hail, rain and snow unknown and uncared for while you enjoy the feel of plush carpets, luxurious motors leaving you at the doorstep to sit in centrally heated houses".[38]

6 The Number of Doctors in Ireland

How many doctors were there in Ireland? The census is not a totally reliable guide, because several censuses after the 1858 Medical Registration Act continued to include anyone who designated themselves as a medical practitioner or curer whether their qualifications entitled them to be entered onto the *Medical Register* or not. Only in later censuses did it become routine to include only registered medical practitioners. Thus the 1911 census seems to show a decline in the number of medical practitioners, which for the reasons stated above was misleading. The 1911 census does show, however, an increase in the size of the medical sector as a whole, mainly because of a rise in the number of ancillary medical workers: nurses, midwives, pharmacists etc.[39]

38 John P. Shanley, 'The History of the Irish Medical Association', The Doolin Memorial Lecture, *Journal of the Irish Medical Association*, vol. 62, no. 385, July 1969, p. 242.

39 Around 10 per cent of the professional classes (9.7%) in the 1911 census were described as 'medical' (Information from Professor Frank Geary, University of Ulster, from a classification adapted from A. L. Bowley, *Wages and Income in the United Kingdom since 1860* (Cambridge: Cambridge University Press, 1937, and data from the Census of Population, Ireland). The percentage had increased 1901–11 from 3.2% to 9.7%, but largely because of an overall increase in ancillary medical staff, e.g., nurses, pharmacists. See also Charles Feinstein, 'New Estimates of Average Earnings in the United Kingdom 1880–1913', *Economic History Review* (New Series), vol. 43, no. 4, 1990, pp. 595–632.

The number of qualified medical practitioners in the Irish population was discussed by Rivington in 1879. He put the figure from the 1861 census as 2,357, and 2,420 in 1871, though wisely he concluded that "It is difficult to arrive at any trustworthy determination of the proper proportion of medical men to the population." Nonetheless he produced the figures in Table 2, based on the 1871 census.[40]

TABLE 2 Number of medical practitioners per 10,000 of the population, 1871

England and Wales	6.4
Scotland	5.2
Ireland	4.5
UK	6.0

SOURCE: RIVINGTON (1879)

In Rivington's view, the divergence in number of medical practitioners between Ireland and the rest of the British Isles was caused by her relative poverty. It was also his opinion that the gap was diminishing, and likely to diminish further.

The author's estimates of doctor numbers in Ireland and the rest of the British Isles in the twentieth century lend support to Rivington. Following 1871, the number of doctors per 10,000 of the population increased in Ireland until by the 1950s it was roughly comparable with other parts of the British Isles.

The question of numbers is important. First, the availability of health care is one measure of comparative wealth and poverty. The poverty of the west of Ireland is sometimes illustrated in histories by the scarcity of doctors there. Cormac Ó Gráda estimates that in 1851 there were 2.7 physicians per 10,000 of the population in relatively prosperous Leinster, but only 0.8 per 10,000 in the poor rural province of Connaught in the west of Ireland.[41]

A variety of reasons may account for this, but one of the most important is that medicine in the nineteenth century was determined by market forces, as it is to some extent today. Thus a combination of inability to pay for medical care and the difficulties of getting a medical living for the doctor in a particular area could combine to mean that a particular social class or region was wanting in terms of health care, regardless of overall figures for Ireland.

---

40 Walter Rivington, *The Medical Profession: Being the Essay to which was Awarded the First Carmichael Prize of £200 by the Council of the Royal College of Surgeons, Ireland* (Dublin: Fannin & Co., 1879), pp. 2–3.

41 Cormac Ó Gráda, *Ireland: A New Economic History 1780–1939* (Oxford: Clarendon Press, 1995), Table 8.4, p. 187.

TABLE 3 Number of doctors per 10,000 of the population in Great Britain and Ireland, 1911–61

Year	Great Britain	Ireland	Éire (26 counties)	Northern Ireland (6 counties)
1911	6.54	5.14	-	-
1921	6.5	-	-	-
1926	-	6.8	6.9	6.7
1931	7.4	-	-	-
1936	-	-	6.5	-
1951	9.8	10.1	9.8	10.7
1961	11.5	11.1	12.0	12.4

SOURCES:
FOR GREAT BRITAIN, 'REPORT OF THE ROYAL COMMISSION ON MEDICAL EDUCATION, 1965–8,' COMMAND PAPERS (CMD 3569), VOL. XXV, 1967–8, TABLE 1, P. 21
FOR ÉIRE, TONY FARMAR, *PATIENTS, POTIONS AND PHYSICIANS*, DUBLIN, 2004, TABLE 9.1, P. 190
FOR NORTHERN IRELAND, THE CENSUS OF 1926, 1951, 1971 AND THE 'REPORT ON HIGHER EDUCATION IN NORTHERN IRELAND,' BELFAST, HMSO, 1965 (CMD 475)

After taking this into consideration, however, Ireland was not, after the mid-nineteenth century, undersupplied with doctors. An examination of the comparative supply of doctors, in the context of development studies in the 1970s, pointed out that Ireland fell into the middle band of three bands as regards Gross Domestic Product (GDP). Its GDP measured less than the UK or USA, but more than an under- developed country. By the criterion of GDP, the authors calculated that Ireland should have a sustainable figure of 11 doctors per 10,000 persons in 1970. In fact it had 11.8.[42] Thus, whilst under-supplied in the middle of the nineteenth century, by 1911 Ireland was roughly comparable with Britain in the number of qualified doctors practising there, but doctors were unequally distributed across the country with some serious social consequences.

7 The Over-Production of Doctors in Ireland

More significant to the study of migration is that Ireland consistently throughout this period produced more medical students and graduates per population than other parts of the British Isles. In 1865 the GMC calculated that 36 per cent

42 Alfonso Mejia, Helena Pizuki and Erica Royston, *Foreign Medical Graduate: The Case of the United States*, WHO Division of Manpower (Lexington: Lexington Books, 1980), pp. 106–14.

of first year medical students throughout the British Isles were registered in Irish medical schools, although the percentage of Ireland's population to the population of the United Kingdom as a whole was around 20 per cent. Even in 1935, when Ireland's population had declined to around 9.5 per cent of the total population of the British Isles, 20 per cent, or one in five, of first-year medical students in the British Isles were studying in Irish institutions.[43]

TABLE 4 Percentage of medical students registered in first year by the GMC as studying in Ireland, to total number of UK medical students[44]

Year	**% of first-year medical students in Irish medical schools**	**Census year**	**% of Ireland's population to total UK population**
1865	35.7	1861	20.0
1890	12.04	1891	12.4
1910	25.2	1911	9.6
1935	20.0	1931 and 1936–7	9.48

SOURCE: COMPUTED FROM CENSUS AND *MEDICAL AND DENTAL STUDENTS' REGISTER*, GENERAL MEDICAL COUNCIL, 1936.45

There is, in fact, a remarkable continuity in the medical student body in Ireland. In 1875 there were approximately 1,274 medical students in Ireland (probably an underestimate, because it is difficult to know the numbers in private medical schools or working as apprentices). Davis Coakley, in his history of Trinity College medical school, quotes the census of 1901 which gave 1,331 medical students.[46] In 1938–9 there were around 1,503; in 1948–9, 1,489; and in 1964–5, 1,376.

There was wastage of students along the way: some who failed to qualify the first time round and retook their exams, sometimes more than once. These were

43 See 'Summary of the Number of Medical Students Registered during each year', 1936, p. 15.

44 There was a sharp drop in entrants to medical school in the early 1890s. First-year entrants fell to below 200 in 1892, 1893 and 1894. This fall in numbers has also been noted by Kelly, *Irish Medical Education and Student Culture c.1850–1950*, p. 24. She suggests that the attempt to abolish night-time teaching may have been among the reasons, because the practice had allowed students to study and work at the same time.

45 'Summary of the Number of Medical Students Registered in 1865 to the end of the year 1915', GMC, 1936, p. 15; and 'Summary of the Number of Medical Students Registered from 1905 to 1936 inclusive', ibid., p. 18.

46 Davis Coakley, *Medicine in Trinity College Dublin* (Dublin: Trinity College Dublin, 2014), p. 184.

known colloquially as 'chronics'.[47] However, overall the dropout rate among final-year Irish students was roughly comparable with Britain: 34 per cent of Irish students failed to qualify; in England it was 27.35 per cent; and in Scotland 30.9 per cent.[48] However it was also the case that it was relatively common for Irish students who failed first time round to return to the challenge.

How many of these graduates emigrated to make a professional living? The following tables are based on a longitudinal study looking at the destination of graduates from Irish medical schools every five years, beginning in 1860 and ending 1960: a sample of over 4,000.[49] There were fluctuations according to period, for example in the number of medical graduates produced. During 1860–95 a sample of 754 graduates was produced by the five-yearly graduate cohorts examined, but in the period 1900–15 this dropped to 618.[50] But during 1920–40 the numbers from the cohorts in those decades had more than doubled to 1,400. There were also external factors bearing upon the opportunities for emigration in each period. However, a total of around 40 per cent of graduates from Irish medical schools settled outside Ireland over the period 1860–1960. In the early part of the period before the First World War the figure was higher, around 50 per cent.

TABLE 5 Destination of medical graduates from Ireland by percentage (raw numbers in brackets)[51]

Years	In Ireland	Unregistered	Percentage outside Ireland	Total number of students
1860–95	32% (244)	15% (112)	53% (398)	754
1900–95	37% (228)	14% (85)	49% (305)	618
1920–40	47% (660)	14% (200)	39% (540)	1400
1945–60	51% (750)	16% (235)	33% (489)	1474
Total 1860–1960	44% (1882)	15% (632)	41% (1732)	4246

SOURCE: *MEDICAL REGISTER* OF THE UNITED KINGDOM FOR THE RELEVANT YEARS. SEE APPENDIX

47 Kelly, *Irish Medical Education and Student Culture c.1850–1950*, pp. 146–7.
48 See 'Report by the Statistical Committee of the General Medical Council containing a Summary of Statistics regarding Medical Students in the year 1871', p. 10.
49 Details are laid out in the Appendix.
50 See Digby, *Making a Medical Living*.
51 See Appendix for a study of over 4,264 medical graduates from Irish schools 1860–1960.

TABLE 6 Proportion of medical graduates outside Ireland working in the army, navy, colonial civil service, British colonies or ex-colonies

Period	Number outside Ireland	Number in army, navy, colonial civil service, British colonies or ex-colonies	Percentage of total emigrants in army, navy, colonial civil service, British colonies or ex- colonies
1860–95	398	170	43%
1900–15	305	121 (exc.19 banks)	40%
1920–40	540	98	18%
1945–60	489	140	29%
Total	1732	529	31%

SOURCE: SEE APPENDIX

The two major destinations for Irish medical graduates seeking work outside Ireland were Britain and the British Empire.

Denominational politics played an important part in Irish medical history. By the first decade of the twentieth century, religious segregation of medical students had increased. In 1875 16 per cent of medical students were being educated in two institutions, the Catholic University and Trinity College Dublin both with historic connections to different religious denominations. By 1905 it was 47 per cent.[52] Although the Queen's Colleges of Cork and Galway were formally and constitutionally non-denominational by statute, their incorporation into the National University of Ireland in 1908 and the departure of Queen's College Belfast and Trinity College signalled a growing influence of Catholicism in their atmosphere.

Was religion a factor in determining migration? Certainly, professional disappointment was sometimes a reason for migration out of Ireland, an outcome to which the sectarian divisions of Ireland often contributed. However, the evidence is that all schools, whatever their denomination, experienced emigration. Both TCD and Queen's College Belfast, whose student bodies were largely, though not exclusively, Protestant experienced high levels of emigration.

52 'Summary of the Number of Medical Students Registered in 1865 to the end of the year 1915', GMC, 1936, p. 15.

TABLE 7 Destination of Irish medical graduates from the main Irish medical schools 1860–1960, based on ten-year registration check (see Appendix Table 22)

	UCD 1910–60	RCSI 1860 -1960	QUB 1860–1960	TCD 1860–1960	Cork 1860–1960	Galway 1860–1960
In Ireland	375	334	554	324	193	102
Unregistered	120	120	105	169	45	73
Outside Ireland	231	449	378	459	128	87
British Isles	167	259	257	274	95	55
Total	726	903	1037	952	366	262
Percentage outside Ireland	32	50	36	48	35	33

In all schools in Ireland the numbers of doctors produced were more than could be absorbed within Ireland itself. Even when the proportion of doctors per population was rising and beginning to approach levels in other parts of the British Isles, Ireland's medical graduates still exceeded what could be absorbed into Ireland itself. Over-production of doctors was built into Irish medical culture. The Irish medical profession was well aware that more doctors were produced each year than Ireland could absorb, and also that the sustainability of this over-production depended on emigration. Student accounts of their education often refer to the expectation that they would have to leave Ireland. Michael P. Flynn who graduated in 1940 from UCD recalled: "It was an established pattern for decades that the surplus Irish medical graduates went to England, with a portion going to more distant English-speaking countries."[53] In fact, though Flynn emigrated, he eventually returned to Ireland to make a distinguished career there in public health.

Aidan McCarthy, a graduate of University College Cork (UCC) in 1938, was more forthcoming about the reasons for the difficulty of getting a job in Ireland:

> [It was] because all specialised appointments were controlled by local medical professional nepotism and the jobs were very limited in number; the situation was not helped by the fact that these so-called dispensary jobs were occupied by doctors well into their eighties – settled, well liked and with no intention of retiring. The result was that nearly eighty percent

53 Michael P. Flynn, *Medical Doctor of Many Parts: Memoirs of a Public Health Practitioner and Health Manager, Spanning Sixty Years of Social Change* (Dublin: Colourbooks Ltd, 2002), p. 4.

of newly qualified doctors had to cross the water to England and Wales where medical work was plentiful, particularly in the armed services.[54]

8 Conclusion

Medical emigration from Ireland was necessitated by the over-production of doctors. More doctors were educated in Ireland than could be absorbed within Ireland. But Ireland's requirements, it must be emphasised, were determined for much of the period by the fact that the majority of medical practitioners operated in a private health care market. However, even during periods when investment in health in Ireland increased and more doctors were absorbed as opportunities within Ireland expanded, emigration continued to be a significant part of the experience of newly graduated doctors. This was also true of Northern Ireland after 1945 and the introduction of the National Health Service (NHS) there in 1949. The NHS provided free medical care for all citizens, and the demand for doctors increased. However, graduates from Queen's University medical school continued to emigrate.[55]

Was there no opposition to the flow of doctors out of Ireland? There were a few who questioned or disapproved of it. John Stephen McArdle, a consultant at St Vincent's, gave a paper on emigration in 1902 in which he is quoted as saying, "This awful Emigration will affect Medical men very materially, for if the present state of things continues, in a few years the only complaint left us to deal with will be senile decay."[56] But Surgeon McArdle was talking about general emigration rather than medical emigration itself. He was a nationalist, and high levels of emigration from Ireland would, in the view of Irish nationalism, be cured by independence from Britain. As a consequence of independence, the Irish economy would revive and lead to Ireland being able to sustain a much larger population than under the British, including presumably more doctors. Meanwhile, however, another nationalist doctor, Thomas Myles, advised medical students that emigration, far from being a burden to them, might be their making.[57] So long as overproduction was built into the medical

54 Aidan MacCarthy, *A Doctor's War* (Cork: Collins Press, 1979).

55 See Chapter 8 for a discussion of this.

56 Reported in *St Stephen's: A Record of University Life*, 18 November 1902, p. 172. John Stephen McArdle (1859–1928) was Professor of Surgery at the Catholic University and a fellow of the Royal Academy of Medicine in Ireland. He was President of the IMA 1906–8.

57 Thomas Myles (1857–1937) was President of the RCSI 1900–2. He was knighted in 1902. He founded the Protestant Home Rule Association in 1886. In 1901 he addressed the students of the RCSI on the benefits of emigration; see *Journal of the Irish Medical Association*, vol. 1, no. 12, December 1901, pp. 89–91.

school system, medical emigration was inevitable and most luminaries of Irish medicine accepted that this would be the case.

After independence for the twenty-six counties of the south of Ireland in 1922, the prediction that the population would stabilise and possibly increase proved wrong. The Irish population continued to fall, and a high level of general emigration was one of the reasons, though not the only one.[58] Doctor migration also continued. Once or twice there were intimations that the market for Irish doctors abroad might be drying up and that the yearly production of doctors was overtaking the opportunities for emigration. The *Irish Times* in 1936 complained that "During 1935 more than 400 new students were entered upon the books of the Medical Council. When in four years' time they emerge, the Free State will be able to absorb only fifty of them." Nonetheless the *Irish Times* felt that the intensifying fight to acquire professional qualifications was inevitably the outcome of hard times. At least the length of the medical degree gave students the opportunity to pause before the need to find a medical post.[59]

Deans, registrars and the leaders of Irish medical education were well aware of the over-supply of medical graduates. Medical schools knew that they were producing for export, and even the government of Ireland in 1960, in the first major attempt to reform university education, including medical education, conceded that the medical schools had always produced a number of students for whom emigration was inevitable.[60] The question, therefore, is why? What part in the political economy of medicine was played by emigration? Further, did emigration amount to a loss or gain for graduates unable to practise their profession in Ireland and forced or lured to seek a position elsewhere?

58 Another reason was the low rate of marriage and late marriage, especially among rural farmers.

59 'Free State Medicine', *Irish Times*, 17 February 1936.

60 See 'Report of the Commission on Higher Education, 1960–7', vol. 1, p. 246.

CHAPTER 2

Making a Medical Living

There were two contrasting views in Ireland about the economic state of the medical profession in the nineteenth century.[1] In 1904, the hardships of the dispensary doctor were detailed in bitter words in an article in the *British Medical Journal*:

> Too often he has nothing to look forward to but a life of unceasing toil to the bitter end. For him there is, as a rule, no prospect of an increase in salary or a change of district. He has no chance of getting out of the rut into which he sinks, for he cannot afford to buy books or journals to keep himself abreast of the advance of science; and if he had them he would have no time to read them. His mind becomes subdued to that it works in [*sic*], and he lives without a thought beyond the trivial round of daily drudgery. So he must stagger on under the growing burden of years till he dies under the yoke.[2]

By contrast, in 1912 the nationalist newspaper *The Leader* published this verse on the subject of the Irish doctor:

> When landlords are now swept away by our race
> The doctors, it seems, must step into their place.
> Must dominate Ireland, supreme and alone,
> In wealth, intelligence, culture and tone.
> But they had much better their manners go mend
> The men who broke landlords will not to them bend.
> We'll drink down their medicine, should it be meet
> But never will swallow their pride and conceit.
> Let doctors keep curing diseases and coughs,
> Not trying to strike us as great killing toffs.
> Let them to their powders and poultices stick,
> And not with presumption be making us sick.

---

1 This chapter is based on Greta Jones, '"Strike out Boldly for the Prizes that are Available to You": Medical Emigration from Ireland 1860–1905', *Medical History*, vol. 54, no. 1, January 2010, pp. 55–74.

2 "The Poor Law Medical Service in Ireland", *BMJ*, vol. 1, 26 March 1904, p. 738.

 | DOI:10.1163/9789004324466_004

Alas for our land when from carrot or spud
Come snobs who behave like a prince of the blood
And so they are doctors that trio down there
Who hold their profession with lordliest air?
They must be reminded these bounders of class
Of times when their motor was drawn by an ass.[3]

Were Irish doctors impoverished or basking in new-found prosperity in the years up to the First World War? Anne Digby's work on the medical profession in England and Wales in the late nineteenth century allows some comparisons to be made.[4] In her examination of the incomes of the medical profession in England and Wales for the years 1877, 1899 and 1909, she suggests the following. A 'small' medical income yielded around £300–399 per annum. A 'standard' income was between £400–599 and £600–799. A 'good' living was £800–999. First-class livings were those producing £1,000–1,499 each year. A smaller number were over £1,500.

Digby suggests that in 1877 three-fifths of country practices in England were 'standard practices' (*c.* £400–800) and a remaining fifth divided between small (under £400) and first class (over £1,000). Urban practices, on the whole, provided greater opportunities for average and higher incomes. In the 1890s the proportion of smaller practices increased, but by 1909 the figures had returned to the 1877 configuration. Digby attributes the recovery of medical incomes to a fall in recruitment numbers to medical schools in the 1890s in response to overcrowding in the profession.[5] In Digby's view, the majority of English-based doctors could aspire to a standard income (*c.* £400–800) with, at either end, a small tail of the very successful or struggling doctors, the latter more likely to be found in rural practices. In confirmation, Henry May's book on income tax and the medical profession published in 1903 based his tax advice to doctors on an income averaging £400–700 over three years, falling into Digby's 'standard' income range.[6]

In the 1870s a report on medical incomes in the military was commissioned by the government because of difficulties in recruiting medical officers to the armed forces.[7] The report described the career trajectory of the medical

3 'The Doctors', a poem in *The Leader*, 14 December 1912, p. 489.

4 Digby, *Making a Medical Living*, Table 5.2, p. 144.

5 Ibid., p. 145.

6 Henry J. May, *Medical Practitioner's Accounts* (London: Gee & Co., 1903), pp. 60–62. (Below an annual income of £160, no income tax was due.)

7 'Report of the Committee to inquire into the causes which tend to prevent sufficient eligible candidates from coming forward to the Army Medical Department', PP 1878–9, vol. XLIV C.2200 (44), pp. 304–5 (48–49).

graduate in general practice as one in which a new graduate might expect to obtain an income of £300 per annum (small) "within 5 years of commencing practice" which would rise to £500 (standard) within 10 years and peaked at around £800–1,000 (good to first class) towards the end of a career.[8]

Replies about medical incomes in Ireland were received by the Committee from the medical schools at Queen's College Belfast and in Dublin the Carmichael Medical School, Dr Steevens' Medical School and the Catholic Medical School. None of the advice they gave suggested significant differences between Ireland and England and Wales. The Carmichael School believed, with a few exceptions, that the usual course for a graduate in Ireland was to seek a dispensary medical officer's post. The rate of pay was £90–140 per annum plus fees for acting as registrar of births and deaths, and a further £30–50 per annum for vaccinations. To this a part-time appointment as medical officer of health at around £10–20 per annum was usually added. So the income for a newly graduated doctor in Ireland could be expected to be £120–220 per annum from the public purse.[9]

As for private practice, according to the representative of the Carmichael School, "it would of course be impossible to gauge but it may be stated that there is hardly any district in Ireland where it would not be worth at least £150 a year". This gave an average starting salary for doctors of around £270–370, small but comparable to that in Britain. This might be even higher if one of the more lucrative public appointments was secured. According to the Carmichael School, "The County infirmaries and lunatic asylums are more valuable but they are obtained with more difficulty."[10]

The consensus among the Irish medical schools was that a medical graduate could expect an income of around £270–370 at the commencement of employment. Ten years later they would earn a standard to good income, £800–1,000, according to Dr Steevens' Medical School, and £500 in the opinion of the medical school of Queen's College Belfast. Twenty years into a career, in the view of the Belfast medical school, this would rise to a standard income of £700, a figure surpassed by the calculation of Dr Steevens' Medical School of an income of £800–1,000 (good) after ten years.

Information from the Irish medical schools erred strongly on the side of optimism, and it must be remembered that the schools were keen to recruit

---

8 Digby, *Making a Medical Living*, p. 143. This is calculated for single-handed practices.

9 'Report of the Committee to inquire into the causes which tend to prevent sufficient eligible candidates from coming forward to the Army Medical Department', Appendix D 'Selection from Replies on the Probable Average Earnings of Civil Medical Practitioners', p. 304 (48).

10 ibid.

students. None more so than the medical school of the Catholic University, whose representative claimed "I am frequently astonished at the incomes former pupils enjoy and at the substantial proofs of material prosperity that families and homes present." This included a student who, after ten years, was earning £900.[11]

1 General Practice in Ireland and England

Becoming a general practitioner was the most common outcome for a medical student but, as we shall see, this was by no means an easy option, particularly in Ireland. Building up a practice was often slow and, in some areas of Ireland, very difficult. Even if private practice was assured, the doctor would seek to protect themselves financially in the first years of their practice through part-time appointments, usually in the Poor Law services, the local country infirmary, the police, insurance companies and in whatever part-time work was offered by the local lunatic asylums. Part-time posts increased annual income, and even established general practitioners sought them. They were also, in the early years of a practice, a form of advertising to the local community, because the part-time dispensary or Poor Law infirmary doctor usually became a well-known figure in an area.

Acquiring a practice was not easy. The main route was purchase. This was frequently arranged through a specialised medical agency who facilitated partnerships and transfer of practices. These agencies would also supply locums. An advertisement for one in 1840 in England gives some idea of how these firms operated:

> *Medical Agency Office.* A respectable professional medium for transacting Medical Business requiring a Confidential Agent and for negotiating the transfer of Practices ... Mr Lane's Practices for disposal are too numerous for an advertisement but range from 100L to 300L. Practitioners in the Country requiring a superior Assistant or any of inferior grades may be gratuitously supplied by addressing a letter post-free to Mr Lane...[12]

The dynamics of this is illustrated in a surviving book of correspondence for Lara and Co., a firm which facilitated the sale of practices primarily for England

11 Ibid., p. 304.

12 *Provincial Journal Advertiser*, supplement to the *Provincial Medical and Surgical Journal*, London, 31 October 1840, vol. 1, no. 5, p. 95 (Supplied to me through the kindness of Dr Elizabeth Lake).

and Wales, although they did get inquiries from Ireland. One part of their work was valuation: this was an estimate of the worth of a practice based on the calculation of average turnover, usually over the final three years before sale. There were bargains to be had: bankrupt practices might be cheaper, and agencies would sometimes refer the client to a promising practice on the market which, because of the age and infirmity of the incumbent doctor, had been somewhat neglected and had greater potential than its book price would indicate.

What you bought was the patient list and the goodwill of the previous doctor, although no patient on the list could be absolutely secured. A change-over often led to a fall in patient numbers at the start, in spite of a recommendation by the previous practitioner. Part-time appointments in the Poor Law or elsewhere enjoyed by the previous incumbent were also considered to come with the practice, and although there was no guarantee, it was generally assumed that the new incumbent would most likely succeed to them. Additionally, some equipment might be included in the price; and, if the practice was not conducted from the doctor's home, the opportunity to rent or buy a surgery and sometimes the doctor's house. To take an example:

> A Physician would Dispose of a Country Practice with a Good Introduction averaging about 500L a year with almost certainty of success to a qualified person who would purchase his freehold property consisting of a large and commodious house…To save trouble, the price of the practice is Two Years Purchase and 2500L for the House and grounds part of which might remain on mortgage.[13]

J. Henry May (author of the *Medical Practitioner's Accounts*, an income tax guide for doctors) also gave advice on the valuation of practices.[14] Valuation was based on 'goodwill' and an average of cash takings for the three years preceding sale. Added to this would be stock such as fixtures, fittings and any debts still to be collected. Poor Law, public health and other part-time appointments would be taken into consideration. An example of how this worked was a practice in which takings averaged £432 over the last three years, the stock or fixtures and fitting were worth £150 and appointments outside the practice anticipated at £50 per annum; the total of £632 would be the price of the practice.

Setting up in practice was not cheap. According to May the following sorts of expenditure were involved, although they were eligible for some tax relief. A doctor could claim for rent (one third), rates (two thirds), servants and repairs, all under the category of 'Establishment'. They could also claim surgery

13 Ibid., p. 95.

14 May, *Medical Practitioner's Accounts*, pp. 70–72.

expenses, an assistant, drugs, repairs, fittings, alterations. Some income tax relief could be claimed for housekeeping, coachman, horse or motor car expenses. Stationery was allowed, as were the establishment costs for a branch surgery. Then depreciation of stock, bad debts, doubtful debts and discounted debts could be put against tax. Life assurance was also allowable. This left remaining income to be presented to the Inland Revenue.[15]

Therefore, the needy graduate might have to contemplate measures other than outright purchase. The most easily available was an assistantship to a general practitioner, which could eventually lead to a partnership. Assistantships, however, had their drawbacks. They might not lead to a partnership, and some new graduates moved from assistantship to assistantship in the first years of their professional life. Scottish and Irish assistants were common in England, and in 1867 John Baxter Langley's treatise on the *Laws and Customs of the Medical Profession in Relation especially to Principals and Assistants* advised his brethren to take care when considering applications from the 'sister isle'.[16] He complained that when graduates from Ireland were asked:

> "Who is to do the work in the surgery, make up the medicine, fold up the mixtures and pills or keep up the books?" [They] look puzzled and not infrequently indignant at the suggestion of what they think degrading employment.[16] [Nonetheless] because some assistant from Dublin or Belfast has turned out to be a drunken savage, it is not fair to assume that every graduate from the 'Green Isle' is necessarily a blackguard.[17]

Langley does advise, however, of the possible romantic complications of inviting a young man into a house with daughters, and advises the doctor to keep watch.

There were other methods to gain a practice. A loan coupled with an insurance policy to cover it might start you off in a practice, although this meant that earnings had to cover the cost of repaying the loan. Even the purchase of a modest practice worth £400 to be repaid over five or six years might entail at least £80 payment per annum, not counting the interest. More frequent was the graduate who took a temporary salaried position, which had the advantages of a fixed income, and then saved up for a practice. In the late nineteenth

15 Ibid.

16 John Baxter Langley, *Via Medica: A Treatise on the Laws and Customs of the Medical Profession in Relation Especially to Principals and Assistants with Suggestions to Students on Preliminary Education* (London: R. Hardwicke, 1867), p. 35.

17 Ibid., p. 37.

century a doctor retiring from the army or colonial service after ten years' service would receive an honorarium. This might be around £1,000 and could be used to buy a practice.[18] Or you might become a ship's doctor for a time, hoping to save sufficient from your earnings after a few years of travelling. At any time in the period 1860–1960 there were Irish doctors circulating the globe in ships.

Opinions differed on the merits for an Irish doctor of starting a practice in England. In the view of a writer in the *Journal of the Irish Medical Association* (*JIMA*) in 1868:

> [From] a pecuniary point of view, even an assistant to a general practitioner in England is much better off than a Poor Law Medical Officer in this country; his pay will be at least as good, he will have no expense and a horse will be kept for him when required. Such appointments may easily be obtained by application to a respectable agent in London whose address will be seen in any medical paper. Much better than this, however, is the purchase of a partnership or the transfer of an English practice.[19]

The writer then mentions a pamphlet by Baxter Langley entitled "A Few Words of Advice on the Buying and Selling of Medical Practices". This advised that "a practice in London is expensive and will fetch two years purchase. In Southern Counties a practice paying £500 a year will require a year's purchase especially in a market town". Less was paid for Midlands and less still for Northern practices except in the 'best towns'. So, according to the writer, you needed to invest £300, £500 or £1,000 for a practice, but with the result that "we have known several young medical men who have done so and who are now making a large annual income, much larger than if they had remained in this country".[20]

Rivington's discussion of the kind of practices available in Ireland admitted that their desirability was entirely contingent on their social and economic structure. The writers on medical practices were quite clear that a small, rich town would have more doctors per population than a poor but populous one. He listed fashionable seaside towns having "a migratory constituency or a considerable number from the upper classes of society as ordinary residents or

---

18 D.G. Crawford, *History of the Indian Medical Service 1600–1913* (London: Thacker and Co., 1914), vol. 1, p. 444.

19 'The Existing Professional Prospects of Young Men entering on Practice', *Journal of the Irish Medical Association* (*JIMA*), no. 23, 27 May 1868, p. 90. Published as a supplement to the *Medical Press and Circular.*

20 Loc. cit.

as invalid visitors". Then there were towns comprising "a large manufacturing interest and numerous factories, employing hundreds and thousands of operatives". These, he noted, had only a small proportion of doctors relative to their population and the poverty of their inhabitants was an obstacle to securing a good living. There were also "Decaying towns, out of the way places with a poor and scattered population difficult of access" which again had a small number of practitioners. Then more prosperous rural areas existed where there are "many small farmers and where there is a chance of getting a practice out of neighbouring villages and small towns".[21]

Although practices in large towns with a working-class clientele were not the most sought after, Robert Esler, a graduate of Queen's College's medical school who worked in Peckham, London, told his compatriots in 1890 that a good living could be made by a popular, hard-working doctor even in the poorest areas of London:

> Within the four mile radius [of Peckham] there are mixed practices ... But I am asked what about the 6d men? Some of them do very well indeed. I know of one man whose practice consists mainly of club patients and 6d fees who has two horses and as many carriages.[22]

This situation must have applied in large working-class areas of Belfast and Dublin too.

2 General Practice in Ireland

The dynamics of setting up practice in Ireland are illustrated by the case of Ballinasloe, a country town situated in County Galway in the largely rural, western province of Connaught. Its population in 1871 was 5,052, which by the census of 1891 had declined to 4,642.[23] The total population served by its medical

---

21 Rivington, *The Medical Profession*, p. 4.

22 Robert Esler, 'Some experiences of medical practice in the metropolis', *Transactions of the Ulster Medical Society*, Session 1890–91, p. 69. Sickness clubs, into which members paid a weekly sum which could be drawn on to employ a doctor, were a common form of working-class insurance in the nineteenth century.

23 Population figures from W.E. Vaughan and A.J. Fitzpatrick, *Irish Historical Statistics: Population, 1821–1971* (Dublin: Royal Irish Academy, 1978). The population is given as 3,911 in the *Irish Medical Directory* for 1873, but Vaughan and Fitzpatrick's corrected figures have been used. Ballinasloe is not typical in that only around a third of the population in Ireland was living in towns of over 2,000 people in 1900. The small country town was, however,

practitioners would of course be larger, including villages and rural areas in the surrounding districts. Ballinasloe was relatively prosperous, although rural poverty could be found in the hinterland. In 1875 there were eight doctors recorded as practising in Ballinasloe. In 1895 there were eleven medical practitioners.[24]

In 1875 the medical superintendent of the lunatic asylum, R. Eaton, was replaced by Robert V. Fletcher, who went on to enjoy a long career as Medical Superintendent in charge of Ballinasloe Asylum. It was the most lucrative public appointment in the district, and Fletcher's salary was estimated for 1875 at £450 per annum plus £145 in allowances, giving him a 'standard' income (by Anne Digby's measure) of £595 per annum.[25] Fletcher, a graduate of Edinburgh in 1865 and the Royal College of Surgeons of Ireland in 1869, had been assistant resident physician at Downpatrick and then at Waterford Asylum before taking up the appointment at Ballinasloe. After twenty years at the Ballinasloe Asylum, by 1895 Fletcher's salary had risen to £650 plus £150 allowances, qualifying by Digby's criteria as a good income.

The Lunatic Asylum provided income for the medical fraternity of Ballinasloe, most of whom would also be in general practice. In 1875 Dominick Burke was a visiting and consulting physician there; his salary on 31 December 1873 was £125 per annum. He was also the medical officer of the Ballinasloe Workhouse, from which position he earned £120 per annum. To this he added a further £18 as consulting sanitary officer, £15 for various duties as medical officer of health and £18 for work as executive sanitary officer. This gave a total of £296 from the public purse alone, excluding any income from general practice. By 1895 James J. Delahunt, who graduated in 1879, had succeeded Burke as consulting physician at the Lunatic Asylum. His salary was £120 per annum, with apparently none of the accumulated additions which Dr Burke enjoyed in 1873. However, Dr Delahunt also added dispensary work at £120 per annum plus £14 for vaccination, which made a total of £245 for Delahunt from public appointments. Dr Michael Comerford (graduated 1862) and Dr Eaton, the former

---

important in Ireland's cultural, economic and political history. Ballinasloe had also one of the largest lunatic asylums in Ireland.

24 Names of doctors are taken from the *Irish Medical Directory* published by the Irish Medical Association for 1875 and 1895 and cross-checked with the UK *Medical Directory*, except for 1895 when no local list is published. Some names on one list are missing from the other. In this case the names on the *Irish Medical Directory* are prioritised because their local knowledge is likely to have been more up to date.

25 Figures for remuneration are taken from the *Irish Medical Directory* 1875, p. 203 (Dispensary salaries), p. 236 (Workhouse salaries), p. 273 (Lunatic Asylum salaries); and ibid. 1895, pp. 251 and 314.

superintendent at Ballinasloe (graduated 1855 and 1856) also held positions in the asylum, probably for ad hoc consultations for neither is in the *Irish Medical Directory* as receiving regular salaries. But a Dr Rutherford in 1875 got £50 per year as apothecary for the inmates, a sum which had risen to £125 in 1895.

The dispensary work in 1875 was looked after by Dr Patrick Horne. Ballinasloe Dispensary was one of six in the Ballinasloe Union, and Dr Horne earned £120 for this plus £6.6s for vaccination. This was the highest paid and most populous dispensary district in the Union. Dr Thomas Kearns in Ahascragh earned £50, and Dr E. P. Sharkey, who graduated in 1833 and retired in 1885 due to 'old age', got £100 in 1873 for work in the Creagh Dispensary.[26] In 1891, according to the *Annual Report of the Local Government Board for Ireland*, the six dispensary districts of Ballinasloe between them had an average salary of £121, ranging from £118 to £143.10s.[27] From the study of Ballinasloe doctors, incomes in the range £435–710, which Henry May's income tax advice to doctors regarded as the average medical income, were within reach of all of them. But this would have been on the important assumption that, as the Irish medical schools maintained in 1878–9, a minimum of £150 per year through private practice was available to the new graduate. If this is true of the ten doctors examined, the superintendent of the asylum would have an income of £695 in 1875, rising to £800 in 1895. This would be considered standard to good. Of the others, only two had no part-time appointments (at least from the Poor Law). Of the remainder, three earned £50 per annum each from the public purse. The rest had part time salaries, of £296, £245, £126.6s and £100 respectively, out of the Poor Law and asylum system. If at least £150 might be had in private practice in most dispensary districts at the start of a career, these doctors needed a sum double that from private practice, and in some cases more, in order to reach an eventual standard or good income.[28] However, the opinion of the Irish medical schools was that most doctors reached within ten years a standard general practice.

These were not the only part-time public appointments for Irish doctors or their counterparts in England. In factory districts, posts as certifying surgeons were available; coroner's courts paid doctors' fees for reports on deaths; there were medical officers for military camps and naval bases, appointments at county infirmaries and fever hospitals (a medical officer at an Irish county

26 *Annual Report of the Local Government Board* (*Ireland*), PP 1890–1, vol. XXXV, p. 216.

27 Ibid., p. 269.

28 'Report of the Committee to inquire into the causes which tend to prevent sufficient eligible candidates from coming forward to the Army Medical Department', PP 1878–9, vol. XLIV (44), pp. 259–305.

infirmary could be paid from £40 to £250 per annum in 1875). The pay for medical officers in prisons ranged from £60 to £415, averaging around £150 in 1897.[29] Registration of births and deaths involved fees. Added to this was part-time work for Friendly Societies, insurance companies, and for the Royal Irish Constabulary (RIC). However, the level of prosperity of Irish doctors, unless in a full time public appointment, was clearly dependent on private practice.

3 Private Practice

Generally, the richer the patient, the richer the doctor. Fees were adjusted according to the social status of the patient. This is why wealthy areas sustained more doctors per head of the population than crowded but poorer areas in Belfast and Dublin. A supplement on fees is set out in the *Transactions of the Ulster Medical Society's* 1880–81 session.[30] It produced a table to indicate "the minimum of remuneration to which any Practitioner is entitled whatever be his professional rank or the extent of his practice". The advice accepted that those with substantial practices and reputations were entitled to more than the amounts quoted, so that the fee scale in the table represents the minimum acceptable charge.

The table divided the patients into three classes according to house rental. Class 1 was a rental of £10–25, Class 2 £25–50, Class 3 £50–100. A single visit to a Class 1 patient was quoted as 2s.6d and to a Class 2 patient as 5 shillings. A Class 3 patient could be charged 10s.6d. Any patient above Class 3 might be charged a guinea. The table also gives higher fees for night visits, visits longer than normal, consultations at the practitioner's house, letters of advice, attendance on servants, consultant's fees. Costed separately were lunacy certificates, midwifery (including an extra charge for difficult or protracted labours), certificates of death for insurance companies. These figures accord well with the doctor's fees quoted in Farmar, in his case for the year 1898, so we must assume that their congruence provides a pretty accurate benchmark for calculating the incomes of Irish doctors in the late nineteenth century from private practice.[31]

29 See *Irish Medical Directory* 1897, p. 335.

30 *Transactions of the Ulster Medical Society*, 1880–81 Session (Dublin: John Falconer, 1881), p. 90.

31 Tony Farmar, *Patients, Potions and Physicians: A Social History of Medicine in Ireland* (Dublin: A&A Farmar and the RCPI, 2004), p. 114. Farmar quotes from the *Irish Times Almanac 1898*. They calculated a fee scale of 2s.6d to 3s.6d for a house visit where the annual rental was £25 or less, and from 5s to 10s.6d for a visit to a house whose rental was above £50. A consultation for better-off patients could be 1–2 guineas.

Although the general rule was that a doctor became wealthy by looking after wealthy patients, the fee table in the *Transactions* suggests that a 'small' medical income of £300–400, if sustained entirely by private practice, would require a weekly income of around £6–8 or 30–40 visits per week to Class 1 and 2 patients. Out of those fees, the costs of travel (feeding and stabling a horse and, later, maintaining a motor car) would have to be discounted. A substantial living of around £900 needed a weekly fee income of £18, or at least double the amount of visits. The hard-working doctor was known in Ireland, but it is unlikely that the volume of visits could sustain a practice alone. In reality, extra income from certification for insurance companies and part-time public appointments reduced the number of visits a doctor might have to make, hence the importance of these part-time posts to the medical career. The problem of making a medical living was also compounded by the tardiness or failure of some patients to pay their fees.

There were, of course, extremely wealthy doctors in Ireland in the nineteenth century. But wealthy doctors had wealthy clients. The most prestigious doctors were generally to be found in the precincts of Dublin's Merrion Square or in nearby Monmouth Street. The fee book, for 1858–79 of one of these, Sir Dominic Corrigan, indicates that Corrigan had an annual income of around £4,000. A proportion of this income, around £300 per annum, came from teaching courses at the Richmond Hospital and Maynooth College, but most was from patient visits or consultations. For trips outside Dublin, Corrigan's fee book indicated that he received a £100 for a consultation in Tipperary and £42 for Longford. Corrigan of course represented a small coterie of doctors whose client list was varied, but among which he counted the social and financial elite.[32]

Status came about through hospital posts which, as well an income, conferred prestige and hence advertised the doctor as especially skilled or gifted. The same was true of professorships in medical schools, which were well paid and still allowed private practice and consultancies. A high professional profile could be accrued in a number of ways, including hospital appointments, public appointments, a position in one of the medical colleges or medical organisations, editorship of a journal and participation in government inquiries. Often these positions, it is true, were gained by hard work, scientific publications and philanthropy. Once achieved, they gave the doctor access to a

32 See O'Brien, *Conscience and Conflict*, pp. 173–4. Farmar says that 44 out of 95 houses in Merrion Square were inhabited by doctors, and that they might earn £3,000 a year. Ibid., p. 114.

wealthy and important clientele. Often the position of physician to the King or Queen in Ireland was achievable by these means, and with that a knighthood. This then brought access to the dinner tables of the wealthy and titled. The diaries of Sir Charles Cameron, chief public analyst for Dublin, are full of accounts of the important dinner parties to which he was invited.[33] The other outcome of the process was, of course, that the larger the number of hospitals and medical schools, the more opportunity arose for the ambitious doctors to achieve wealth and social status. This accounts for some of the resistance to reducing the number of hospitals by re-organisation or the number of medical students.

After the disastrous years of the Famine, the Irish economy improved. Ireland in 1900 was a much more prosperous place, according to various measures of economic wealth.[34] Among the beneficiaries of this were the medical practitioners. Nonetheless, the fall in population after the Famine meant that there were parts of Ireland where the problem of securing a medical living was increasingly severe. The situation is illustrated in the table below. Areas of population increase demonstrate a corresponding increase in doctor numbers. This includes industrialising Belfast and the middle-class suburbs of Belfast and Dublin. Nonetheless there were areas of population decline in which the numbers of doctors either fell only slightly or remained static.

Whereas, in most cases, population decline led to a reduction in the number of doctors, in the area of Thurles and Ballina this was not the case. Consequently, in areas of declining population still supporting the same number of doctors, there must have been fierce competition for Poor Law posts and private patients.

Rural practices were generally not as rewarding financially as urban ones, because of greater difficulties in establishing private practice and the increased costs of travel for the doctor. In this respect, Ireland's greater number of rural practices compared with England presented problems for the new graduate setting up in practice. This was aggravated by the fact that, although emigration was experienced in all areas, the rural west, a very poor part of Ireland whose farming was dominated by the small tenant farmer, saw the greatest depopulation in the wake of the Famine. Another factor singled out by the *Journal of the Irish Medical Association* was the land reforms of the 1880s. Whatever their role

33 RCSI Archives, Sir Charles Cameron's Diaries.

34 For a general discussion of these issues, see Cormac Ó Gráda, *Ireland: A New Economic History 1780–1939* (Oxford: Clarendon Press, 1995).

TABLE 8 Ratio of doctors to population in Ireland (an asterisk indicates places of population decline)

Place	Pop. 1871	No. of doctors 1875	Ratio of doctors to pop.	Pop. 1911	No. of doctors 1908	Ratio of doctors to pop.
Belfast Co. Antrim	174,413	108	1614.9	386,947	235	1646.5
*Charleville Co. Cork	2,482	6	413.6	1,925	4	481
*Thurles Co. Tipperary	5,008	5	1001.6	4,549	7	649.8
*Dungarvan Co. Waterford	6,520	5	1304	4,977	3	1659
Athlone Co. Westmeath	6,565	6	1094	7,472	5	1494
Blackrock Co. Dublin	8,089	11	735	9,080	10	908
Sligo Co. Sligo	10,670	7	1524	11,163	8	1395
*Ballina Co. Mayo	5,843	4	1460.7	4,662	5	932.4
*Westport Co. Mayo	4,417	5	883.4	3,674	4	918
Bangor Co. Down	2,560	4	640	7,776	12	648
*Ennis Co. Clare	6,503	10	650	5,472	8	684
*Fethard Co. Tipperary	2,106	4	526.5	1,473	1	1473
Total Pop.	225,176	175	1286.7	439,170	302	1454.2

SOURCES: *IRISH MEDICAL DIRECTORY* (SUPPLEMENT TO THE JOURNAL OF THE IRISH MEDICAL ASSOCIATION), THE *BRITISH MEDICAL DIRECTORY* AND THE *CENSUS FOR IRELAND*

in ameliorating grievances over land, they had made the situation worse with regard to private practice. One doctor wrote:

> the abolition of the old fashioned landlords may diminish agrarian discontent, [but] it will drive from the country districts those comparatively wealthy families on whom the hard worked doctor had to depend, if he is to supplement the income derived from a badly paid dispensary appointment.[35]

The hardships of the western doctor in poor rural areas was graphically illustrated by Thomas Myles, president of the Royal College of Surgeons 1900–2, addressing a group of graduating students at the College in 1900.[36] The western doctor had few private patients, and to reach them he had to travel longer distances, sometimes over difficult terrain. He described: 'one of my pupils on the Western seaboard who was caught in the mist and fog of the mountain side had to pass the night under the shelter of the rocks there and wait for the friendly daylight to appear, lest in the darkness he should stumble over some frightful precipice on the rocks below.'[37]

Consequently, there was a tail of medical practitioners struggling to make a living in poorer rural areas or in areas where the population but not the number of doctors was in decline. This tail of poor medical incomes in Ireland is evidenced by comparing bequests from a sample of Irish-educated doctors probated in Ireland and equivalent English-educated practitioners probated in England as shown in the table below. There is a greater 'tail' of Irish bequests of under £1,000 and £1,000–3,000 than among the English bequests. Fewer English doctors were in the category of bequeathing under £1,000, and a greater proportion had impressive legacies of over £20,000. Nonetheless, the table also draws attention to the fact that there is a solid range of Irish wills showing a greater number of bequests in the middling category of between £3,000 and £20,000. Thus, making a medical living in Ireland could be difficult for many, but not always or for everyone.

35 A.B. Mitchell, "The Poor Law Medical Service", *JIMA*, vol. 2, no. 4, April 1902, p. 30 (read before the Belfast Medical Students Association, 16 February 1902).

36 A sympathetic account of his character and influence on his students is given in E.F. St. John Lyburn, *The Fighting Irish Doctor* (Dublin: Morris & Co., c.1950), p. 59. Lyburn graduated from TCD in 1930.

37 Thomas Myles, "Military and Dispensary Appointments" (given 2 November 1901), *JIMA*, vol. 1, no. 12, December 1901, p. 90. Thomas Myles was president of the Royal College of Surgeons in Ireland, 1900–2.

TABLE 9[38] Bequests of doctors aged 50 and above, 1876–1910, Ireland[39]

Bequests £	No. of doctors	Percentage
Under 999	32	26
1,000–2,900	31	25
3,000–4,999	15	12
5,000–9,999	18	15
10,000–19,999	14	11
20,000–49,999	11	9
50–100,000	2	2
100,000+	–	
Total	123	

SOURCE: OBITUARY LISTS IN THE *BMJ* AND PROBATED WILLS IN IRELAND (PUBLIC RECORD OFFICE OF NORTHERN IRELAND)

TABLE 10 Bequests of doctors aged 50 and above, 1876–1910, England

Bequests £	No. of doctors	Percentage
Under 999	19	15
1,000–2,900	31	25
3,000–4,999	12	9.5
5,000–9,999	15	12
10,000–19,999	22	17
20,000–49,999	20	16
50–100,000	2	2
100,000+	2	2
Total	123	

38 Data from Jones, "'Strike out Boldly'". p. 67, Tables 4a and 4b.

39 Names were compiled at random from obituaries in the *British Medical Journal* from December to November for 1876/7, 1891/2, 1898/9, 1906/7 and 1909/10 and cross-checked with Probate Records for Ireland and England. Where age at death was not available, the date of first medical qualification in the *Medical Directory* was taken and a nominal age of 25 at this point was given. All subsequent years till the date of death were added to this age. This does not give an accurate age at death, but after checking the procedure against instances where age at death is given, it provides a reasonable guide to whether the person falls into the age range of over 50 years at death.

4 The Doctors' Boycott

The ability to obtain a comfortable living from medicine, particularly for a new graduate, was dependent, as shown in Ballinasloe, on securing posts in the Poor Law medical service. The income levels of Poor Law posts in Ireland were on the whole broadly commensurate with England, as shown in Table 11.

TABLE 11 Poor Law vacancies advertised in *The Lancet* and BMJ, 1875

England	Ireland
Bakewell: £25 for Dispensary and fees, £75 for Workhouse	Tipperary Surgeon: *c.*£100
MO Chorlton Union: £250 p.a.	Dispensaries Mufford Union, Donegal: £100 p.a. and fees
Dover MO for Workhouse: £180 p.a.	Kilkenny Union MO Dispensary District no. 2: £100 p.a. and fees
Headington Union MO: £70 p.a.	Killala Union MO for Dispensary District: £110 p.a. and fees, and Workhouse £50
	Naas MO for Clare and Tunahoe North Dispensary District: £125 p.a. and £15 p.a. for Sanitary Officer duties
	Milford Co. Donegal Ramelton Dispensary: £100 and fees

However, it was in the area of remuneration for Poor Law work that a major conflict arose between the doctors and the Local Government Board of Ireland (the LGB). On 13 February 1904 an article appeared in the *Journal of the American Medical Association* (*JAMA*) describing an ongoing boycott by Irish doctors of Poor Law and dispensary posts. Knowledge of this battle had crossed the Atlantic. The boycott to which the article referred had been initiated between 1900 and 1902 when the Irish Medical Association (IMA) had taken the decision to initiate a campaign for better salaries for dispensary and Poor Law medical officers. This had long been the ambition of the Irish medical profession, and there were complaints about Poor Law remuneration going back to the mid-nineteenth century. The overcrowding of the profession both in England and Ireland in the 1890s and early 1900s was, however, an additional factor in pushing the medical profession in Ireland towards increasing militancy.

Adding to these tensions was the problem arising from a decision in 1902 of the LGB. Under the Local Government Act 1898 which democratised local government in Ireland, the LGB was contracted to pay half the expenses of Poor Law medical services, leaving the remainder to be raised through local taxation. In theory at least, councils might set rates of pay and raise the salaries of medical officers without consultation with the LGB, and subsequently demand back 50 per cent of the cost of the increase from them. Alarmed at the possible financial consequences, in 1902 the LGB successfully secured an amendment to the Local Government Act (Clause 6), which limited the ability of the guardians to raise the remuneration of Poor Law medical officers. The LGB now had to approve any additional income raised for dispensary salaries. Even in the cases where councillors wanted to pay more, they were restrained from doing so if they felt that the LGB would not make up the shortfall. The often acrimonious disputes that arose between the Poor Law medical officers, their dispensary committees and Poor Law guardians were not always caused by Clause 6, but it certainly made the situation worse.

Thomas Myles gave an address to the students at the Royal College of Surgeons in 1901 on "Military and Dispensary Appointments" arguing

> I am convinced that if all the graduates qualified in any one year bound themselves together not to accept dispensary appointments until the terms of service were improved, a very real improvement would soon be effected.[40]

In October of the following year, a report of a Committee of the IMA discussed the possibility of a boycott as a means to raise salaries.[41]

It was the County Mayo branch of the Irish Medical Association (formed in 1902 at Ryan's Hotel Claremorris, Mayo) which forced the issue by demanding that all Mayo doctors sign up to a covenant which would oblige them to boycott vacant posts that were, in their view, below the level of remuneration they considered fair.[42] Mayo, a county situated in the poorest part of Ireland, was behind the drive for a boycott, and the propaganda of the IMA emphasised repeatedly the difficult situation of doctors in that part of the world.

The Mayo resolution was adopted by the IMA at Enniskillen on 17 June 1903 during their annual conference. The resolution required that all dispensary

---

40 Myles, "Military and Dispensary Appointments", p. 90.

41 Report of a Committee of the IMA in October 1901 reported in *JIMA*, vol. 2, no. 1, 7 January 1902, pp. 9–11.

42 "The Formation of a County Mayo Association", *JIMA*, vol. 2, no. 1, January 1902, pp. 4–5.

posts advertised below £200 per annum should be boycotted. The boycott should be extended to workhouse appointments at less than £120, while £300 should be the minimum salary acceptable for joint posts. More generally the resolution demanded that quinquennial increments should be instituted, a superannuation scheme on civil service lines be provided, and a month's paid holiday be inserted in contracts.[43]

Much of the boycott was fought out by propaganda largely based upon the situation in the west of Ireland, where the decline in population and the poverty of the small tenant farmer impacted badly, it was claimed, upon the medical profession. According to the *Journal of the Irish Medical Association*:

> The story of the late medical officer of Drumconrath is one of the saddest among many such in the Irish Poor law service. When he was appointed medical officer, more than fifty years ago, the district was a good one for private practice: he was a clever practitioner and was able to live comfortably, and the salary of the dispensary was an item of small importance. By degrees the economic causes referred to deprived him of his private practice, and at 76 years of age … he found himself in bad health, too old to work and with no money saved … With no refuge but the workhouse, as his pathetic letter to the guardians pointed out, this poor old man, victim to the Irish dispensary system, in a moment of despair put an end to his too long life.[44]

Drumconrath dispensary district was part of Ardee Poor Law union in County Louth. The Irish correspondent of the *BMJ* pointed out:

> In former times [it] was a fairly populous rural district, but owing to the depression in agriculture of the last quarter of a century, cultivation has greatly decreased and the land is used for grazing only. As a result the labouring population has greatly decreased, a few herdsmen sufficing for large tracts; and whereas in 1851, when the dispensary districts were formed, the total population was some 27,000, it is now barely half that.[45]

The boycott began in 1902 through to 1904, and all sides observed its progress closely, first in Mayo and then more generally. The *Journal of the Irish Medical Association* regularly published commentary on vacancies in the Poor Law

---

43 For an account of the Enniskillen conference, see *JIMA*, vol. 4, no. 7, July 1904, pp. 202–3.
44 "The Tragedy of the last Medical Officer", *BMJ*, 14 January 1905, vol. 1, p. 91.
45 Ibid., "Local Conditions", p. 91.

system and the impact of the boycott on these. For example, in the case of a post for which the recommendation by IMA was that it should not be accepted for less than £200 per annum, the following events were recorded by the *Journal of the Irish Medical Association*. The post was:

> Repeatedly advertised. Dr W H Delahunt elected but did not take up duty. Removed by L.G.B. Sept. 1903, guardians offered £150 but L.G.B. would not sanction. Advertised for 28/11/03 at £150. Dr Clarke appointed. Expelled from branch.[46]

The boycott was never completely successful. Although it acted as an inducement for dispensary committees to raise salaries, the rise was frequently for less than the minimum demanded by the IMA. Since even more modest increases enhanced the attractiveness of the Poor Law posts, non-IMA members – and sometimes IMA members – accepted vacancies over the heads of those who were elected to the position but had refused to take it up at less than the IMA's recommended £200. They were, in effect, benefiting from the sacrifices made by IMA members.

Because any increase in the pay offered proved too tempting to many doctors, there were calls from members of the IMA to reduce the amount asked for as a minimum salary to overcome this problem. The leadership of the IMA resisted this, as they believed it would amount to a climbdown and seal the fate of the boycott. Instead the IMA used expulsion as a threat to doctors in their organisation who were tempted by the offer of a rise in salary which fell short of the IMA minimum. Certain doctors apologised and backed down under the threat, but some were actually expelled.

The boycott wore away at the resolution of the LGB. Ironically, it raised costs for the councils, as they found themselves employing locums or part-timers at considerably more expense than was normal. They were also forced to advertise posts in Scotland and England, and advertisements raised their costs still further. Thus the LGB felt pressurised by both the doctors and the councils. The first solution it proposed was, given falling population, to amalgamate two small dispensary districts into one, merging two low salaries into one more substantial one; this strategy was strenuously denounced by the IMA since the measure would have reduced opportunities for doctors in the west particularly.

Then in 1904 the LGB capitulated. The breakthrough came in the publication of new scales of salaries for the North Dublin Union sanctioned by the LGB

46 "Vacancies and Appointments", *JIMA*, vol. 4, no. 1, January 1904, p. 31. The appointment was in the Union of Carrickbyrne in the district of New Ross.

and reported in *JIMA* in October 1904. This relaxed the upper limits to salaries. After that date, new more generous pay scales began to spread throughout the system, sanctioned by the LGB. Issue after issue of *JIMA* published evidence of a general rise in salaries in the Poor Law service following the North Dublin settlement. The result was not a rise to the minimum of £200 demanded, but to a level which generally made £150 the norm. However, quinquennial increments were incorporated into the system, some of which were added as backdated payments to the increased salaries. This amounted to a pay rise which, in some instances, brought salaries close to the level demanded by the IMA at the start of the boycott.

In April 1906, the IMA reported that:

> The LGB have, at length after much goading, shown a disposition to do all that in them lies to establish the salaries in their service on a fairer basis wherever they could they have, in conjunction with the Guardians of the particular place, introduced the *scale* [their italics] of salaries. This system is now actually in force in twenty-three of twenty-four Unions throughout this country.[47]

JIMA in 1907 felt that "Now if we can secure for him in the near future a certain pension upon retirement and the redress of some minor grievances, the lot of the dispensary Doctor will not be one to be altogether despised."[48]

The victory was a product of a degree of communal feeling that the IMA encouraged, and of a long tradition of campaigning over the preceding half century frequently focusing on pensions for Poor Law doctors. A poem published in *JIMA* in 1901 urged new candidates for dispensary posts to show solidarity with their elderly colleagues:

> Yet no well assured provision
> For your old age you can make
> So ere you fill the vacancy
> Please pause for others' sake
> Don't rush upon appointments
> So miserably paid
> Don't injure poor old grey beards
> Who have lived and worked and prayed
> For superannuation

---

47 Editorial, *JIMA*, vol. 6, no. 4, April 1906, p. 79.

48 Editorial, *JIMA*, vol. 7, no. 10, October 1907, p. 153.

For some release from care
Take my advice young medico
Just look and go elsewhere.[49]

5 Conclusion

The depiction of the Irish dispensary officer gained a great deal of sympathy from British doctors and the British Medical Association. The BMA were behind the Irish doctors in their struggle, and a resolution in support of the boycott was passed at their conference in Swansea during the summer of 1903. The depiction of the plight of the dispensary doctor touched many. Yet the improvement in the salaries of Poor Law doctors benefited the comfortably off doctor as well as the struggling one, and thus it represents a significant improvement for all Irish doctors, not just the poorest. Moreover, there were critics even in Ireland who felt that the image of the put-upon dispensary doctor was misleading. A letter in the *Journal of the Irish Medical Association* in April 1903 from Dr C.H. Foley, Galway, claimed that the dispensary service was the home of professional failures, a job for life, and attendance on the poor an 'elastic requirement'. The consequence was that the efficient doctor earned less than the inefficient, because the efficient and diligent travelled and boarded away more, incurring more expenses than the lazy one. In addition, Foley argued that the worst cases of hardship were being used to advance the doctor's cause. Some dispensary districts did have private practice and their duties were small and manageable. Given this, the demand for a standardised rate of remuneration would have the effect of rewarding the lazy and hard-working alike.[50]

Certainly all doctors benefited from the increase in remuneration for Poor Law posts. The incomes of prosperous doctors, as well as those of the struggling, were boosted by the capitulation of the LGB to the demands of the IMA in 1904. *The Leader*'s comments on the burgeoning financial and social aspirations of Irish doctors in the satiric poem at the beginning of this chapter were brought closer by the success of the boycott. At the same time, although there was some alleviation of the problems of the doctors of the poor western areas of Ireland, they were not eliminated. Population decline in these areas

---

49 "The Poor Law Vacancy" penned by 'The Man in the Street', *JIMA*, vol. 1, no. 12, December 1901, p. 94.

50 C.H. Foley, "The Moral of Recent Dispensary Vacancies", letter 9 April 1903, *JIMA*, vol. 3, no. 5, May 1903, pp. 68–70.

continued well into the twentieth century and, interestingly, the west was often the leader in doctor militancy in succeeding years.

Among new medical graduates in Ireland, many found it hard to establish themselves. This is illustrated by the fact that, although some graduates emigrated very soon after graduation, others only did so after several years trying to survive in Ireland. The number of Irish graduates unregistered was around 13–15 per cent over the period, and some of them may very well have given up medicine as a profession for financial reasons.[51] A study of graduates from English medical schools who after graduation were unregistered in England after ten years remains to be done. If this category is substantially higher in Ireland, this would, taking other factors into account, be a concrete illustration of the operation of a 'push' factor in the Irish medical profession.

Nonetheless, there were wealthy or comfortable medical practices to be had in Ireland, and when we examine the fate of those who remained in Ireland and those who after ten years were settled in England, a degree of similarity emerges in the structure of their careers. For example, among the cohort of Irish medical graduates of 1875, Charles Emilius Ross graduated from the Royal College of Surgeons in 1875; by 1885 he was practising in Worcester, where he remained throughout his professional life. He worked as a surgeon at St Mary's Cottage Hospital and at Tenbury Dispensary. To these duties he added those of district medical officer of Tenbury Union and surgeon to the Odd Fellows and Foresters Assurance Company. He was still at Tenbury in 1904. His career paralleled that of William James Browne, who graduated the same year as Ross, also from the RCSI via the Ledwich Medical School and Mercer's Hospital. He worked at the Coombe Hospital Dublin and eventually settled in Church Hill, Letterkenny, Donegal, where he was Medical Officer for the Dispensary, district, medical officer attending the Royal Irish Constabulary and resident surgeon for the Londonderry County Infirmary and the Letterkenny Fever Hospital. Also in Donegal was Hugh Thomas Warnock who graduated from the RCSI in 1875. As well as conducting private practice, Warnock was a medical attendant to the Royal Irish Constabulary and consultant surgeon to the Sheil Hospital, Ballyshannon. He was Medical Officer for the Donegal Dispensary District and the Workhouse and Fever Hospital. Gerald Hayden Fitzgerald graduated from Queen's College Galway in 1875 and can be found ten years later in practice at Ponteland, Newcastle upon Tyne. Among the posts he accumulated were Medical Officer and Public Vaccinator for Ponteland District and Workhouse, Medical Officer for the Castle Ward Union and Medical Referee for the Prudential Assurance Society. By 1905 he was retired.

51 See Appendix.

If fewer medical graduates had been produced each year, this would have relieved the pressure upon making a medical living in Ireland for the struggling doctor. Why this did not happen throughout the hundred or so years of this study will be discussed in later chapters, as will the positive benefits financially and professionally of emigration for the Irish doctor. Emigration to English practices was one solution to the numbers of medical graduates produced in Ireland. There was another solution. A substantial minority of medical emigrants, particularly new graduates, either joined the medical services of the army or navy or the British colonial medical services.

CHAPTER 3

The British Empire

The majority of Irish medical emigrants set up practice in Britain, overwhelmingly in England during the period under discussion. But a substantial minority of medical emigrants either joined the armed services or the British colonial medical services. Thomas Myles, President of the Royal College of Surgeons in Ireland and shortly to become Sir Thomas Myles, addressed its medical students in 1901:

> It is our fashion to rail against the British Empire and all that pertains to it. But don't forget that under the flag of that Empire and thanks to the growth of that Empire, thousands of Irish medical men are making a comfortable living and hold posts of honour and emolument in every part of the globe.[1]

Around a third of medical graduates who left Ireland worked in the army, navy or colonial medical services of the British Empire. Among the attractions of a career in the armed or colonial services, even taking into account the year after graduation when they were required to take courses at the army medical college at Netley, were that they could soon expect, in the words of Surgeon General Cleghorn, "a sure and steady income paid monthly".[2]

Salaries in the military and colonial service in the 1870s were considered low, leading to a dip in recruitment.[3] However, a committee of investigation into remuneration of surgeons in the army 1878–9 recommended a rise in rates of pay.[4] Subsequently this meant that an assistant surgeon in the army or colonial service, the lowest rank, received £200 rising to £250 after five years' service and £273.15s after ten years. On top of this were allowances, particularly when on active service, which effectively raised the income to £291, £341.5s

1 Myles, "Military and Dispensary Appointments", p. 90, *op. cit.* fn. 37, p. 55.

2 Writing on a medical career in the armed services in Keetley, *The Student's Guide to the Medical Profession*, p. 98.

3 *Hart's Annual Army Lists 1839–1915*, 1874, p. 381. According to *Hart's List*, in 1874 a new recruit to an assistant surgeon position might earn up to £168 a year and a surgeon around £336. The actual pay would be smaller because of half-pay when not on assignment.

4 'Report of the Committee to inquire into the causes which tend to prevent sufficient eligible candidates from coming forward to the Army Medical Department', PP 1878–9, vol. XLIV, C.2200 (44), pp. 304–5 (48–49).

 | DOI:10.1163/9789004324466_005

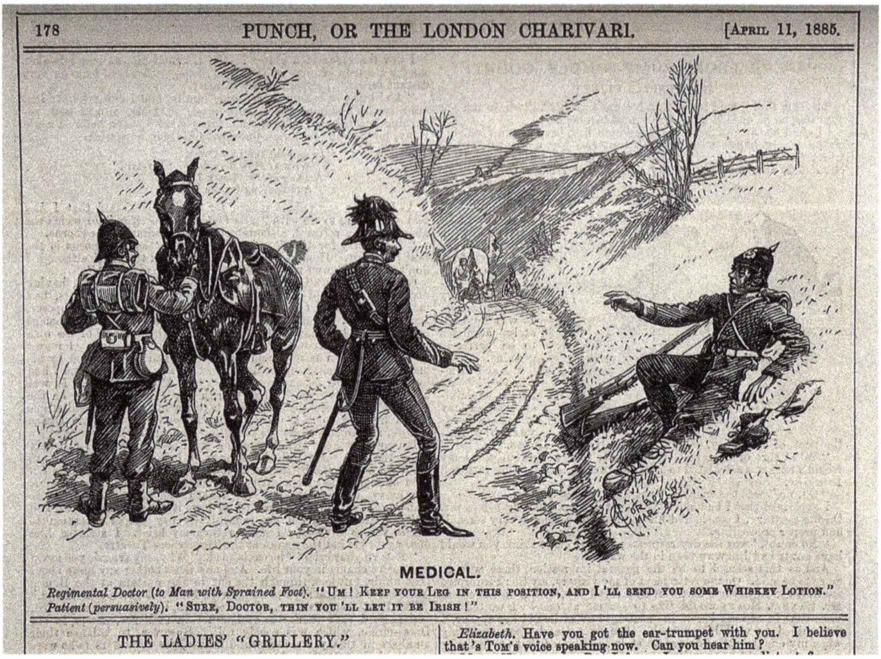
178 PUNCH, OR THE LONDON CHARIVARI. [April 11, 1885.
MEDICAL.
Regimental Doctor (to Man with Sprained Foot). "Um! Keep your Leg in this position, and I 'll send you some Whiskey Lotion."
Patient (persuasively). "Sure, Doctor, thin you 'll let it be Irish!"
THE LADIES' "GRILLERY."
Elizabeth. Have you got the ear-trumpet with you. I believe that 's Tom's voice speaking now. Can you hear him?

FIGURE 2 A military doctor prescribing whiskey lotion for a soldier's sprained foot - his patient requesting Irish. Wood engraving by A.C. Corbould, 1885

and £365 respectively. By 1897 rates of pay had again risen, so that a recruit of five years' service on active duty could expect £450 per annum.[5] A new recruit to the Royal Navy in the mid-nineteenth century could earn a maximum of around £168 per annum for the first five years. However, this was full pay. Half pay, that is for periods when the surgeon was not assigned to full-time duties at sea but was on call, a perennial source of dispute between the Admiralty and doctors, was of course less. A staff surgeon could earn around £500 per annum, varying according to length of service.[6] On top of this, for those who served in the armed forces there was a graduated scale of pensions on retirement, depending on the years served.

The cohorts of Irish medical graduates examined in this study confirm the importance of employment in the colonial and armed services. At five-yearly

5 Crawford, *History of the Indian Medical Service 1600–1913*, vol. 1, p. 385.

6 See Christopher Lloyd and Jack S. Coulter, *Medicine and the Navy 1815–1900*, vol. 4 of J.J. Keevil, *History of the Naval Medical Service* (Edinburgh and London: E.S. Livingston, 1963), p. 20. For a general history of the naval surgeon, see David McLean, *Surgeons of the Fleet: The Royal Navy and its Medics from Trafalgar to Jutland* (London: I.B. Tauris, 2010).

intervals between 1860 and 1895, over a third of the 398 leaving Ireland to seek work went into the army, navy, the Indian Medical Service (IMS) or other colonial medical services.[7] In the 1875 cohort alone, of the 103 graduating that year from the six medical schools, 36 chose these destinations. Overall the IMS recruited slightly more in that year (thirteen), followed by ten for the army, eight for the navy and five for other colonial services in Africa and the British Caribbean. Recruitment tended to be influenced by school. In that year TCD had two army recruits and eight who joined the IMS. The RCSI provided seven naval surgeons compared to five in the army, confirming Nelson Lankford's assertion of the special relationship between the RCSI and the British navy.[8]

Historians have pointed out the high numbers of Irish and Scots in the army, navy and colonial medical services. In the decade 1870–80, the origins of Royal Navy surgeons comprised 103 English, 128 Scots and 251 Irishmen.[9] Although the percentage of both Scots and Irish medical recruits to the navy and army had declined by 1911, Lankford notes that "Scottish and Irish doctors still accounted for one half of the AMD" (Army Medical Department).[10] As Lankford points out, the percentage of Irish medical officers was large compared to Ireland's population and especially impressive given that Ireland's population was declining in the late nineteenth century. Steven O'Connor's book on Irish officers in the British army also notes that 25 per cent of the 1,004 Irish officers in the British army he surveyed from 1922–45 were medical. The figure includes all medical categories – nurses, dentists and veterinary surgeons – but it was "predominantly made up of doctors".[11]

When it comes to the colonial medical services, Mark Harrison records that 26.2 percent of those in the Indian Medical Service during 1837–54 claimed Ireland as their birthplace. This declined during 1855–84 to 10 per cent and rose again during 1885–96 to 12.6 per cent.[12] Of the surgeons employed by the

---

7 Some of the five who went to the colonies were in the service, but one or two who went to the Far East or Africa may also have been in private company employment or serving ex-patriot communities.

8 Nelson D. Lankford, 'The Victorian Medical Profession and Military Practice: Army Doctors and National Origin', *Bulletin of the History of Medicine*, vol. 54, 1989.

9 Lloyd and Coulter, *Medicine and the Navy*, p. 20.

10 Lankford, 'The Victorian Medical Profession', p. 516.

11 Steven O'Connor, *Irish Officers in the British Forces 1922–45* (Basingstoke: Palgrave Macmillan, 2014), p. 84.

12 Mark Harrison, *Public Health in British India: Anglo-Indian preventative medicine 1859–1914* (Cambridge: Cambridge University Press, 1994), Table 1.3, p. 31. Scotland represented 22.7% of the IMS 1837–54, which was then more than the Irish, but it was overtaken by Ireland 1855–84, who then had 26.2% of the total. In the period 1885–96 Ireland had 12.6% compared with 8.3% for Scotland.

colonial service in West Africa and the West Indies during 1840–1909, 45 per cent were Irish, according to Spencer H. Brown, compared to 12.1 percent from Scotland and 32.6 percent from England.[13] In East Africa, Anna Crozier says that the Irish comprised 16 per cent of the colonial medical officers, 29 per cent were Scots and 46 per cent English or Welsh.[14]

Compared with the Indian Medical Service, the other colonial medical services were small during the nineteenth century, but they grew between the end of the nineteenth century and the middle of the twentieth. Thus in the period 1860–95, fifteen of the cohort of graduates studied went to Africa, three to the West Indies and British Guyana and thirty to India. In 1920–40, however, Africa and the West Indies had overtaken service in the IMS. There were fifteen recruits to the IMS for those decades, compared to forty-nine to the African service and six to the British West Indies and British Guyana. This confirms Anna Crozier's view that "More Colonial Service entrants were posted to Africa than to any other colony."[15] Patterns of employment followed colonial expansion in the late nineteenth century; but also, as we shall see below, they were influenced by the vagaries of medical and colonial politics and administrative change.

1 The Indian Medical Service

The IMS was the jewel in the crown as far as colonial medical service was concerned in the late nineteenth and early twentieth centuries. When the First World War broke out, the IMS became even larger by recruitment, transfer from the army and the re-enlistment of retired officers. Until the interwar years, it was the most common encounter between the Irish and the colonial Empire. Recruits were expected to live in India throughout their service, although provision was made for leave back in the British Isles, sometimes for a year or longer depending on the circumstances.[16] Arguably their experience in the IMS took hold of the imagination and destinies of Irish medical graduates more profoundly than even its chief rival in prestige and number of recruits, the army.

---

13 Spencer H. Brown, 'British Army Surgeons 1840–1909', *Medical History*, vol. 37, 1993, Table 2, p. 419.

14 Anna Crozier, *Practising Colonial Medicine: The Colonial Medical Service in British East Africa* (London: I.B. Tauris, 2007), p. 107.

15 Ibid., p. 5.

16 Charles R. Francis, *The Indian Medical Service* (London: Mitchell, 1898), p. 12.

A sample of 104 Irish IMS doctors during 1860–1920 shines some light on their experience. The average age at which they entered the Indian Medical Service was a year or two years after graduation.[17] The youngest age in our sample was 19, the oldest 30. But the usual age was around 22–25. The length of service varied, ranging from four years (although one of the sample left after one year) to around thirty years. In this period the figures are somewhat skewed by those called up or transferred to the IMS or called back from retirement in 1914–18. Although the new recruits of 1914–18 often had a short career, some doctors re-enlisted in the IMS after the First World War.

During 1860–1920 sixty-nine of our sample served thirty years or more, retiring between the ages of fifty and sixty. Thirty-five had shorter careers, but in fourteen of these cases they spent up to twenty years in the service. Those who served relatively briefly sometimes had their careers shortened by the dangers of the service, violent death, or an even more insidious enemy, disease. The high mortality rate of medical officers serving in the army and the colonial services, particularly West Africa, was noted at the time. Rivington claimed that "The chief mortality is not among the older men as in civil life but among the younger men of the Department."[18]

The cohort of thirty graduating from TCD in 1875 illustrates this. Eighteen were practising outside Ireland after ten years. Eight of these joined the IMS.[19] Excluding Allan Nesbitt Fox who was already a veteran of the IMS and returned in 1875 to TCD to enhance his medical qualifications, they were Peter Joseph Farrell, Robert Taaffe, James Joseph Moran, Charles Fetherston, William Beatty Smith, Nicholas John Halpin and Bernard Doyle.[20]

Three of them met violent or premature deaths. Farrell joined in 1876 but died in service two years later in 1878 at Guntur, Pradesh, aged 25. Halpin served six years before being killed by a fall from a horse at Arrah (Bihar, India), aged 31. William Beatty Smith, the son of a Church of Ireland clergyman, was murdered at Chapru Thal in the Kurram Valley in 1879, aged 29, after only two years' service.

The remaining three had typical IMS careers. Bernard Doyle joined the IMS in 1876, aged 26. Doyle served in the Afghan war of 1878–80 and was decorated. By 1895 he had risen to the rank of Surgeon Major in the Bengal Division. He retired in 1902 and died in London in 1921, aged 71. James Joseph Moran, born

---

17 The figures are based on a sample of 104 graduates who joined the IMS during 1860–1920.

18 Rivington, *The Medical Profession*, pp. 210–11.

19 Allan Nesbitt Fox, who is cited in the graduation lists in that year, was already in the IMS having become a licentiate of the RCSI in 1860 via the Ledwich. He returned in 1875 for a medical degree, MB. He retired as Brigade surgeon and died in Dublin in 1896.

20 Biographies of those who served in the IMS can be found in D.G. Crawford, ed., *Roll of the Indian Medical Service 1615–1930* (London: Thacker and Co., 1930)

in 1848 in Cork, served in Bengal, becoming Lieutenant Colonel in 1895 and receiving the Afghanistan medal for his role in the Afghan campaign of 1878–80. He died in Dublin in 1917. The remaining two of the cohort, Robert Taaffe and Charles Fetherston, eventually went into practice. Taaffe joined the IMS in 1876 but served only ten years. Retiring with his honorarium at age 35 he set up as a general practitioner in Ireland at Kingstown near Dublin, where he died in 1925. By the 1890s Fetherston had also left the IMS and set up practice in Melbourne, Australia where he was still active in 1907.

Most recruits in the IMS ascended to the rank of surgeon major. Pay differed according to the period studied, but it rose in the late nineteenth century. When Rivington wrote about medical careers in 1878, this meant an income of £529.5s after fifteen years and £629.12s.6d after twenty years for surgeon majors. By 1897 their pay had increased to £640.14s after twelve years' service and £677.6s.11d after fifteen. But this was by no means the limit. Pay rose when on active service or if special duties were assigned.[21] It also increased with longevity. Salaries rose to over £1,000 after twenty to twenty-five years' service.

There was a pension on retirement, graduated according to the length of service. In 1888 the pension could be in the region of £700, almost double what it had been in 1860.[22] If you retired early there was an honorarium, the size of which depended upon the length of service. Walter Rivington's guide to the medical profession observed in 1878 that "At the end of ten years a surgeon may retire or be informed that his services are no longer required, and be handed £1,000 in lieu of all pension and retirement."[23] This was sufficient, if the doctor had been prudent or had some private income, to contemplate the purchase of a practice on their discharge, as Taaffe did. In the IMS doctors were also allowed, after a number of years and without prejudice to their duties, to take on some private practice. For European trained doctors this could be lucrative.[24] In the 1930s it was estimated that an IMS doctor could earn from £150-£1,000 per annum from private practice.[25]

---

21 Crawford, *History of the Indian Medical Service*, vol. 1, pp. 384–5.

22 Ibid., p. 444.

23 Rivington, *The Medical Profession*, p. 210. At five years the sum would be £400, six years £500, eight years £700 and nine years £800.

24 Mary Ann Scharlieb, a pioneering woman doctor, trained in India and had a private practice there. She returned to England and had a distinguished career becoming one of the first women to achieve a hospital consultancy. Although her motivation for pursuing a medical career was largely religious and philanthropic, the money she earned in private practice also helped her family to escape financial difficulties. In 1930 she died and left over £33,000. See *New DNB* and Greta Jones, 'Women and Eugenics in Britain: The Case of Mary Scharlieb, Elizabeth Sloan Chesser, and Stella Browne', *Annals of Science*, vol. 51, 1995, pp. 481–502.

25 *The Medical Practitioners' Handbook* (London: British Medical Association, 1935), p. 61.

Weighed against these advantages, recruits to the colonial service would be expected to spend considerable time abroad; and in the case of the Indian Medical Service, apart from leave, they were stationed in India permanently until retirement. All army medical officers were expected to spend some time in military campaigns, and this was also true of doctors in the Indian Medical Service. They also had to adjust to climatic and health problems.[26]

One task of the IMS doctor was to follow his regiment into battle, providing help to the injured and on the spot attention in field hospitals. His other duty was to maintain the health of the troops and the garrison in peacetime. Most IMS doctors were expected to spend time with their regiment, and many experienced fighting. The North West Frontier adjacent to Afghanistan was in a constant state of turmoil in the late nineteenth century. Though much of the regimental duty was policing and maintenance of health, medical officers might be engaged in serious wars. Two major wars were fought after 1860 in Afghanistan, in 1878–1880 and in 1919. But the Afghan border was in constant turmoil and there were many skirmishes and military expeditions to impose order on the Afghan–Indian border throughout the late nineteenth century. IMS doctors could also be called up for wars fought in the Sudan, Burma, South Africa and the Boxer Rebellion in China. A number received the China medal for service there.

There were certain battle-hardened medical veterans who saw as much action as the regular soldiers and their officers. They included William Henry Banner Robinson, born 7 December 1865 and educated at the Carmichael School of Medicine and Meath Hospital. In 1884 he became a licentiate of the RCSI and RCPI and in 1893 gained a Diploma of Public Health. He was gazetted as a Major General in 1918 and died aged 57 at Calcutta in 1922. Robinson served in Waziristan 1894–5, Chitral 1895, Tirah 1897, and saw operations in the Bara valley, all on the India–Afghanistan border. Robinson also served in Burma 1885–9 and received a medal with two clasps. He was then awarded the Order of Philip the Magnanimous 1st Class (Hesse) in 1904.

Several Irish doctors in the IMS won the Victoria Cross. They include John Crimmin, born 19 March 1859, who won his VC during the Karen-Ni expedition in Burma in 1889, aged 29. Crimmin died at Woodward House, Wells, Somerset on 20 February 1945. During the First World War John Alexander Sinton, a captain in the IMS, won the VC. He was born 2 December 1884 in British Columbia, but his family moved back to the north of Ireland where he was educated. He graduated in 1908 from the medical school of Queen's College

26 Surgeon General Charles R. Francis, *On the Best Means of Preserving Health in India* (Bristol: J.W. Arrowsmith, 1889).

Belfast. After gaining a Diploma in Tropical Medicine at Liverpool University in 1911 he joined the army. His VC was awarded on 21 June 1916 in Mesopotamia. After retirement he settled near Cookstown, County Tyrone, and died there on 25 March 1956.[27]

The other function of the IMS was its involvement in public health work. There were three regional authorities in which an IMS doctor might work in this capacity: Bengal, Madras and Bombay. The posts varied in importance and status. The chief administrative officer for each region was the surgeon general, but even more important posts might be available for the ambitious doctor in the government of India. Positions in permanent hospitals that served military personnel and their families in India were sought after as a route to income and status. The most prestigious were those with a medical college attached.

Added to these were a wide range of public health positions which grew out of the need to control plague and infection, including overseeing prison health and asylums. The posts could be applied for after several years with a regiment, but the individual would still be under the authority of the army and could be called up for active service if necessary. Although the IMS was initially developed to protect the health of British troops in India, of necessity it extended its operations to the civilian population in the towns and cities of India, thereby creating the first administrative structures for public health.

There was a bewildering medical bureaucracy in India, comprising both civil and military appointments. They included medical storekeeping, supervision of a stud depot or remount agency, examiner of medical accounts, chemical examiner in various provinces, Inspector of Emigrants, hospital staff jobs of various seniority, British regimental and native regimental surgeons, sanitary commissioners, the staff of medical colleges, medical officers in lunatic asylums, prisons and asylums for the mentally defective, male and female superintendents of vaccination and many more.[28] This underlined the dictum attributed to James Mill that India constituted a vast system of 'outdoor relief' to the British and also the Irish middle classes.[29] Each position carried more or less opportunity for the ambitious. Those looking for advancement were advised to seek a position in Bengal, the largest of the three administrative districts, the seat of government and also reputedly the healthiest of the administrative regions.[30] It was the opinion of Surgeon General Charles R. Francis that

27 Richard Doherty and David Truesdale, *Irish Winners of the Victoria Cross* (Dublin: Four Courts Press, 2000).

28 Crawford *The Indian Medical Service*, vol. 1, pp. 380–83.

29 James Mill, *History of British India* (London: Baldwin, Craddock and Joy, 1817).

30 Francis, *The Indian Medical Service*, p. 10.

> The medical charge of a native regiment ... offers but little scope for professional occupation, and men of energy and ambition endeavour to get into civil employ as soon as possible after the necessary two years regimental duty they have performed. [Of these,] I know of no appointment more suitable for an able young man than that of resident house physician or house surgeon in the hospital attached to a medical college. They may be made the starting points for a distinguished career.[31]

India served as a ladder to distinction for many Irish medical graduates. Lankford comments that Irish medical recruits were not, at the point of joining the armed and colonial services, high up on the ladder of social status compared with English graduates in fashionable regiments who had been educated in the more prestigious medical schools. But he also says that, once in position, their advance in the army was largely unaffected. To confirm the point, many Irish medical graduates made a distinguished career in the administrative and educational institutions in India. *Crawford's Roll*, a mine of information for all those interested in the IMS, gives lists of senior medical figures. These show that two Irish educated medical men were Surgeon General and Director General of the IMS between 1871 and 1918: B. Simpson (Trinity College Dublin) and W.R. Rice (Queen's College Belfast). Other senior posts occupied by Irish graduates would undoubtedly be turned up by the assiduous researcher of the Irish in India.[32] Deans of Irish medical schools might very well be able to point to the illustrious IMS careers of their graduates.

They include Sir Charles Sibthorpe (1847–1906), a graduate of the Meath and the RCSI, who joined the IMS in 1870. The bulk of his career was spent as resident surgeon at the General Hospital Madras, and he was Professor of Pathology at the Madras Medical College 1875–90. Afterwards he was Surgeon General for the Government of Madras. Sibthorpe was also on active service in 1878 and 1885. He left the IMS after 30 years' service aged 53, was rewarded with a knighthood, retired to Dublin and died there in 1906, aged 59.[33]

Richard William Havelock Charles, born in Cookstown in 1858, also used his IMS career to propel him up the social ladder. The son of a general practitioner in County Tyrone, he was educated at Cork's medical school, graduating in 1881. He was "elected to the Bengal Presidency, served two years on the Afghan Boundary Commission" and was appointed Professor of Surgery in the

---

31 Ibid., p. 8.

32 Crawford, *Roll of the Indian Medical Service 1615–1930*, Appendix A, pp. 237–41.

33 Sibthorpe's casebooks survive and are now housed in the Library of the Royal College of Physicians in Ireland. See RCPI Archives CS/181873–1906.

Calcutta Medical College. Although he retired in 1908, he subsequently went on to be President of the Medical Board at the India Office 1913–23 and Dean of the London School of Tropical Medicine in 1910–29. He was sergeant surgeon to George V and given a baronetcy. Assiduous work, medical scholarship and a talent for administration secured Charles a distinguished career. The death of another IMS knight was recorded in 1924 in the *Irish Times*. Sir Walter James Buchanan, who died in Dublin, was born in Londonderry. He was a graduate of TCD and entered the Indian Medical Service in 1887. He specialised in prison health and edited the *Indian Medical Gazette*. In contrast a career in general practice for the Irish medical graduate in the provinces of Ireland or Britain, though honourable and sometimes lucrative, would not often propel them up the social ladder. But the Indian Medical Service, pre-eminently, could provide a ladder of social advancement.

2 Far-Flung Shores

Only 2–3 per cent of the cohorts of medical graduates from Irish schools went to destinations other than Britain and the Empire.[34] They were usually emigrants who settled in the country of their destination. Australia and New Zealand were the most important recipients of emigrants among Irish doctors, and Laurence Geary has described the opportunities which settlement in Australia opened up to the Irish medical graduate.[35] A much smaller number in the period before 1945 settled in North America.[36] Anne Digby has pointed out that Cape Colony in South Africa was also a recipient of emigrant doctors in the late nineteenth and early twentieth centuries.[37] An even smaller number went to South America, China and the Far East, and Europe.

---

34 A number of others, around 2 to 6 per cent, posted only a bank as their address. The main reason was that the individuals were travelling or in transit. This is confirmed by the rise in banks given as addresses in the period 1900–15, covering the first year of the Great War. The banks were typically Grindlay's and Glynn and Mills. The author tried and failed to access information on these, but archives do exist at the Royal Bank of Scotland (RBS) on those who used the bank as a *poste restante*. It was not possible to trace the medical cohort as such, but the archives contain fascinating information on other groups and on the customers in general. Thanks to RBS for allowing access.

35 Geary, 'Australia Felix', pp. 162–79.

36 Figures from our cohorts 1860–1940 produced 5.63 per cent who went to destinations outside Britain and the British Empire.

37 Digby, 'Shaping New Identities: General Practitioners in Britain and South Africa', pp. 14–35.

One motivation for travel was health. The climate in Australia and parts of the USA was considered palliative for a 'weak chest', often a euphemism for tuberculosis.[38] Gerald Garry who graduated from Galway in 1883 made a number of trips to America, Italy and West Africa, partly for his own health. But in every place he practised as a doctor. In the years leading up to the First World War he ended up in Egypt, where he found a lucrative practice among the expatriate community. He described Egypt as an 'El Dorado' for the medical profession because of the number of health tourists it attracted.[39]

The small number who went to South America, China and the Far East, and Europe reveal interesting aspects of the peregrinating doctor. In our cohort of medical students graduating in 1875, William Richard Huggard, a graduate of Galway and Queen's College Belfast, worked in London before he settled in Davos, Switzerland. Davos was famous for its tuberculosis sanatoria and was of course the setting for Thomas Mann's novel of sanatorium life, *The Magic Mountain*. Huggard may have gone there himself for treatment, but after, studying on the Continent, he settled there as a medical practitioner in 1885, obtaining a Swiss Federal Diploma which allowed him to practise. He served as British consul in Davos. Huggard wrote on tuberculosis and also on mental science, having worked earlier in his career in London asylums.[40] He published in English and remained part of the British medical network, becoming a fellow of the English Royal College of Physicians in London. Given the large number of British and Irish visitors to Davos, his practice almost certainly catered to British and Irish tuberculosis patients.[41]

The countries outside the British Empire which absorbed Irish migrant doctors were generally those with an expatriate community who wanted to access a British or Irish-trained doctor. British and Irish settlement followed trade. Arthur Pageitt Greene was educated at the RCSI and the College of Physicians in Edinburgh, from which he graduated in 1872. For most of his life he worked as a doctor in Argentina. There he joined a small group of medical men who catered for the British, Irish and Welsh communities in South America.[42] The British trading and construction companies around which expatriate commu-

38 Linda Bryder, '"A Health Resort for Consumptives": Tuberculosis and Immigration to New Zealand, 1880–1914', *Medical History*, vol. 40, no. 4, 1996, pp. 453–71.

39 Dr Gerald T. Garry, *An African Doctor* (London: John Gifford, 1939). He worked as a private doctor in Egypt until 1914, when he was commissioned by the RAMC.

40 William Richard Huggard, *A Handbook of Climatic Treatment: Including Balneology* (London: Macmillan, 1906).

41 See Jones, *"Captain of all these Men of Death"*, ch. 6.

42 Susan Wilkinson (ed.), *Recollections of an Irish Born Doctor in Nineteenth-Century Argentina: The Diaries of Arthur Pageitt Greene, 1848–1933* (privately printed, 2016).

nities grew up, whether railways in Argentina or in the China trade, would also directly hire doctors to look after their employees or, if there was already a doctor practising among the expatriate community, hire them for that purpose.

These opportunities could stimulate the taste for travel and adventure. Henry Lionel Smith, who graduated from the RCSI via the Coombe and Ledwich in 1866, made a career across three continents, spanning trade, emigration and colonial service respectively. He first became a surgeon for the Hudson's Bay Company based at Moose Fort, Canada. After that he was a district surgeon in Albany, Australia, and finally a police surgeon in Mashonaland in East Africa. Subsequently he worked in Rhodesia. He was awarded a medal for his activities during the Mashona Rising in 1893. This eventful career was rounded up by a practice in the more peaceful English district of Teddington, Middlesex.[43]

Peregrination by means of different types of medical employment abroad was not common, but it did occur.[44] Charles Stewart Parnell Hamilton joined the Royal Army Medical Corps (RAMC) at the outbreak of the 1914–18 war. At its end he was seconded as a medical officer by the British military mission to the White Russian, General Deniken, whose army was leading the resistance to the Bolshevik Revolution. This took Hamilton in 1919 from France to the Balkans and Turkey, where he met and married a Russian nurse working with Deniken's army. After the collapse of Deniken's army, he served in India 1922–9 and then took a post in north India as a medical officer for a company which owned tea plantations in Assam. He re-joined the British army in 1939 at the outbreak of war, serving yet again in France for the first few months of the war. After the war he returned to his post in Assam, but in 1947 when the Indian continent was in turmoil over its imminent independence, he retired to Ireland.[45]

European settlement linked to trade in China and Malaysia in the late nineteenth century also offered opportunities for medical practitioners to work abroad. Africa too became an exemplar of both the colonial medical expansion and also a limited but significant degree of European settlement, particularly in East Africa. By the late nineteenth century South Africa in particular was combining both European settlement and British industrial and trade operations, and employed Irish doctors. Shipping companies also took on doctors

---

43 *Medical Directory*, 1914.

44 The career patterns of doctors in the Cape of Good Hope Colony up to 1910 are discussed in Anne Digby, '"A Medical El Dorado?": Colonial Medical Incomes and Practice at the Cape', *Social History of Medicine*, vol. 8, no. 3, 1995, pp. 463–79.

45 Charles Stewart Parnell Hamilton, *East, West: An Irish Doctor's Memories* (London: Christopher Johnson, 1955). Although Hamilton considered himself Irish, he was born and educated in Britain. The paradoxes of identity for Irish migrant doctors are examined in Chapter 5.

and a few appear in the *Medical Register* as working for the Peninsular and Orient Company (P & O) for nearly all of their professional life.

Medical missionaries also migrated. Importantly they sent back students from the countries in which they worked to train as doctors in Europe and North America. Missionaries therefore brought the first inward migration to Irish medical schools, which, though small was of considerable significance in the long run. This was because the outcome of medical missionary work was the creation of hospitals and medical schools in the places in the world where they settled. According to G.H. Choa, 166 hospitals and 241 dispensaries in China were created by nineteenth-century European missionaries between 1807 and 1905.[46] Some of the medical colleges created in the missionary period in China remained important and were eventually absorbed into the university system of the Chinese Communist state after 1949. In 1944 the General Medical Council recognised attendance at four Chinese medical colleges as permitting entry to the United Kingdom *Medical Register*.[47] The institutions created by missionary work or by colonial medicine often survived independence, although they underwent significant change during the years following. Nonetheless, these historical connections played a part even in countries only partially under the influence of European imperial powers. They eventually facilitated a reciprocal flow of doctors into the United Kingdom from schools that had been the product of either the colonial regimes or, in the case of China, medical missionaries.

3 Those Who Returned

Did the Irish IMS and colonial medical officers return to Ireland on retirement? The place of death could only be identified for 74 of a sample of 104. Of these, sixteen died in Ireland and three more can be identified by the 1911 Irish Census as living after retirement in Ireland where presumably they died. This makes a total of nineteen who returned out of the 74. Thirty died in Britain and twenty-five in other places, although in one case of a death at the Majestic Hotel, Bombay, an address is given in Britain. The sample is too small to be representative and is particularly hampered by the difficulty of identifying

46 Gerald H. Choa, *'Heal the Sick was their motto': The Protestant Medical Missionaries in China* (Hong Kong: Chinese University Press, *c.*1990), Table 1, p. 220.

47 They were the Shanghai Medical College and the colleges at Hsiang-Ya, Cheeloo University and Lingnan University.

place of death in Ireland.[48] In some cases it was only possible to do so because the person concerned probated their will in England. Thus it is likely that the number returning to Ireland is an underestimate.

In addition, the deaths in 'other places' were usually premature or of individuals still on active service: eight were aged 35 or under.[49] What is clear is that a good proportion did not return to Ireland: sometimes they retired to seaside towns in England, or a few with the shortest service set up in practice again, mainly in England. Nonetheless there was a stream of Irish practitioners back in Ireland after their service in the armed services and the IMS. In that respect these could be regarded as temporary emigrants, although they might have served thirty years outside Ireland. This again contrasts with general Irish emigration, where the rate of return is much lower.

It was rare in the latter part of the nineteenth or early twentieth centuries for an individual with thirty years' service to retire in their fifties and then pursue their medical career after retirement. Many of those retiring felt the lack of opportunities after they left the IMS or the army. Certainly this was the case with Charles Francis, who retired aged 55 after thirty years' service. In his 1898 treatise on the IMS, he discussed the problems of those who still felt the need for an active role in medicine. Joining the India Medical Board after retirement or on the staff at Netley was rare and highly competitive. Smaller part-time jobs existed, such as medical examiner for recruits to the service, a role which in Ireland was generally carried out by retirees from the armed services. But the opportunities were few and far between. The likelihood was that only those who left after twenty years, aged around 45, would pursue a career back in the British Isles.

Of two examples, the first is James Moorhead, born in 1850 and graduating from Queen's College Belfast in 1875, who joined the IMS in 1876 and left aged 48 after 22 years' service. After a spell back at his old college (he was a first class honours and gold medal student) lecturing on tropical diseases, by 1911 he was settled in London where he set up practice. James Kelly, born in

48 In England and Wales, the information is available online through various search engines. In Ireland, however, although the Irish Registry Office provides information in book form, the process is very time-consuming and frequently inconclusive. The Irish online Census was used, but retirees after 1911 are not yet traceable. More useful were probate and the *Irish Times* obituaries, which often record deaths of IMS officers.

49 The 'other' places of death with age (in brackets) are: Flanders (26); Dinapur (39); Madras (29); Chinsura Hugli (45); Chinsura Hugli (45); Guntai (25); Karachi (34); Arrah, North West Frontier (31); Melbourne (54); Calcutta (52); Calcutta (35); Calcutta (52); Calcutta (57); Mount Abu (51); Majestic Hotel, Bombay (56); Sialkot (56); Port Blair, a seaside town in India (25); Naini Tal (39); Ranchi (55); Montreux (34); Quetta (50); Innsbruck (55); Bombay (61); Bombay (60); Burma (69).

1841 and graduating in 1864, left after twenty years in the IMS age 45 to set up practice in Kingstown, Dublin. After the 1920s and routinely in the 1950s, probably in the light of increasing expectation of life and greater opportunities post 1945, the pattern of moving from army or colonial service into practice became more common.

4 The IMS and the Scientific Mind

This section will propose the importance of the Indian Medical Service as a contributor to science in Ireland. Scientific advancement was not of course the main purpose of the general medical degree, and as medical education reformed and expanded putting increased pressure on the medical curriculum, Laura Kelly points out that "there were persistent pleas for the subjects of botany and zoology to be removed from the medical curriculum from both professors and students".[50] This was less the case for the IMS, where knowledge of the terrain, strange animals and languages was considered to enhance a career.

The list of optional subjects in the exam for the IMS included Comparative Anatomy, Zoology, Natural Philosophy, Physical Geography, Botany and Hindustani. These subjects, though adjuncts to the main medical curriculum, might nonetheless prove useful for a career in India, as Charles R. Francis's description of the IMS in 1898 argued:

> A mere superficial acquaintance with the natural sciences may develop a genuine taste for one or the other of them, and so possibly lead to a valuable appointment *necessitating* an *accurate* knowledge of the one chosen. A good knowledge of chemistry may lead to a professorship of that subject in a medical college or school. A botanist may become, in addition to his professorship of botany or *material medica*, a superintendent of botanical gardens, a post offering a wide scope for the cultivation of vegetable physiology and the development of indigenous products: whilst in the formation of zoological gardens, of scientific institutions and the general advance of scientific knowledge, the zoologist, the natural philosopher, and the student of physical geography will assuredly find instructive and remunerative occupation.[51]

Advancement in India, particularly a position in the medical colleges, required research. There is a considerable literature on the diseases of India authored

50 Kelly, *Irish Medical Education and Student Culture c.1850–1950*, p. 106.
51 Francis, *The Indian Medical Service*, p. 7.

by Irish recruits to the IMS which testify to this. Alexander Porter, a licentiate of the RCSI who joined the IMS in 1865 and became Principal of Madras Medical College, published *Notes on the Pathology of Famine Diseases* (1878) and *The Diseases of the Madras Famine of 1877–88* (1889). William Samuel Jagoe Shaw who graduated from the RUI in 1897 was the author of *A Handbook of Mental Diseases for the use of Students and Medical Practitioners in India* (1925). John Wallace Dick Megaw, a graduate of Queen's College Belfast's medical school in 1899, who became Director of the Calcutta School of Tropical Medicine, was among the most prolific of IMS authors. Among his works was a co-authored book, *Tropical Medicine* with Sir Leonard Rogers, a major pioneer in the subject. It was published in 1930 and went into five editions. Megaw also published another major work, *Public Health in India* (1936). He went on to receive a knighthood for his work in India.

A distinguished scientific career in India could lead to a national profile in Britain. Robert McCarrison (1878–1960) graduated from Queen's College Belfast's medical school in 1900 and joined the IMS in 1901. His career followed the usual progression for a newly recruited assistant surgeon: in 1902–4 he served as a regimental medical officer at Chitral in north India near Afghanistan, and then as an agency surgeon at Gilgit until 1911. Medical investigations in India tended to concentrate on fevers, malaria and plagues, and the effect of famine, and McCarrison mentions Manson's pioneering book on *Tropical Diseases* (1898) as influential in turning his attention in this direction. Whilst surgeon to the regiment at Chitral, he began systematic observations on the incidence of disease among the Indian populations around him; and at Gilgit he investigated links between nutritional deficiency and disease, particularly goitre, on which he produced a number of papers between 1906 and 1916.

War and military duties intervened and in 1920 McCarrison was invalided out of the IMS and returned to Britain. However, he participated in the Deficiency Disease Inquiry 1925–9 and then was sent back to India to take charge of the Nutrition Research Laboratory at Coonoor in south India 1929–35.[52] By 1918 he had turned his attention to beri-beri, a serious nutritional disease caused by the absence of thiamine in the diet. His medical research in India was supported by the Research Fund Association of India. McCarrison was knighted in 1933. By the time he retired from the IMS and returned to Britain in 1935, he was internationally renowned as a specialist in nutrition and disease.

His subsequent fame in England was because nutritional deficiency was an important topic in 1920s and 1930s Britain. Large-scale investigations on

52 Arnold, *Science, Technology and Medicine in Colonial India*, pp. 201–2.

nutritional standards among the poor were being conducted from the late 1920s through the 1930s.[53] McCarrison became one among a distinguished group of nutritionists in the 1930s who had a social as well as a medical mission to improve nutrition among the population. McCarrison entered the national debate in 1936 in the Cantor Lectures,[54] which included summaries of the state of nutritional science in general and moved his concerns away from India. He became an expert on the importance of nutrition to European societies in general, not just India.

But McCarrison was cautious about entering the full-blown debate about poverty, food and ill health. In 1938 he wrote a foreword to a book edited by F. Le Gros Clark on *National Fitness*, lending the authority of his name but cautiously dissociating himself from some of the stronger political positions on poverty and ill health taken up by fellow nutritionists in the 1930s. Fitness did not require war "as the only measure of communal health and stamina". The vision of the authors of the book, he concluded, was not that. But, "with the (other) political questions" in the book about the distribution of income and housing "I have no concern".[55]

With war in 1939 came further opportunities to enhance his national profile. As the consequence of the debates of the 1930s, and with the prospect of the introduction of rationing, the government was moving towards a food policy which discriminated in favour of vulnerable groups. This mobilised McCarrison again to patriotic interventions. In May and June 1940 he contributed, together with the leading nutritionists of the day, to lectures on *The Nation's Larder and the Housewife's Part Therein*.[56]

Other IMS officers found India the springboard for stretching their imagination towards broader ideas. One of these was Richard William George Hingston, who was born in 1887 in England and died in 1966 at his home in Cork, a home in which he had lived for many years. Hingston graduated from Cork medical school in 1910 and entered the Indian Medical Service shortly thereafter. He was awarded the Military Cross during the First World War. In India he served as surgeon naturalist on many geographic expeditions, the culmination of which was the Mount Everest expedition of 1924.

---

53 See Greta Jones, *Social Hygiene in Twentieth Century Britain* (London: Croom Helm, 1986).

54 Robert McCarrison, *Nutrition and National Health: The Cantor Lectures* (London: Royal Society of Arts, 1936).

55 Robert McCarrison, 'Foreword' to *National Fitness: A Brief Essay on Contemporary Britain*, ed. F. Le Gros Clark (London: Macmillan, 1938).

56 Robert McCarrison, *The Nation's Larder and the Housewife's Part Therein: A Series of Lectures at the Royal Institution* (London: G. Bell & Sons, 1940).

Geographical mapping and exploration was an adjunct of military intelligence. Knowledge of the terrain and its people were important to military expeditions, and the information gained by surveying and exploration was filed away to be made available when the time came. But those in the IMS seconded from their regimental duties for exploration often immersed themselves in scientific pursuits where it was possible. Hingston was a doctor, but much of his intellectual life was taken up by the insect ecology of the places he visited on the expeditions. In Ireland, where pure science degrees were rare, medical school was the place where a few keen but frustrated would-be scientists might be found.

Hingston produced a string of popular accounts of his travels whilst an IMS doctor, including *A Naturalist in Hindustan* in 1923 and *Nature at the Desert's Edge: studies and observations in the Baghdad Oasis* in 1925.[57] After his retirement from the IMS in 1927 he continued to travel, usually on joint expeditions funded by charities or universities. The Oxford University Exploration Club assisted in one venture.[58] By the 1920s Hingston was a serious entomologist specialising in the Asiatic black ant. Although he followed a tradition of amateur natural history whose roots were in collecting, observing and recording and which flowered in Ireland in the first decade of the twentieth century, he rightly saw himself as a serious practitioner of science.

Darwin was an inspiration. In 1934 Hingston published a panegyric to Darwin in the *Great Lives* series for Duckworth Press, and in *Nature at the Desert's Edge* in 1925 he described his own work as drawing on Darwin: "My record is largely one of battles and struggles and of methods adopted by the different creatures to maintain their own in the contest for life."[59] Field naturalists had generally remained the most Darwinian among the biological sciences, and Hingston's work was one of the many studies of animal and plant ecology that investigated environment, modification and population change in the animal world.[60]

---

57 R.W.G. Hingston, *A Naturalist in Hindustan* (London: H.F. & G. Witherby, 1923), and idem, *Nature at the Desert's Edge: Studies and Observations in the Baghdad Oasis* (London: H.F. & G. Witherby, 1925).

58 R.W.G. Hingston, *A Naturalist in the Himalayas*, London, H.F. & G. Witherby, 1920 (observations done on active service 1914–16.). Idem, *A Naturalist in the Guiana Forest* (London: Arnold and Co., 1932).

59 Hingston, *Nature at the Desert's Edge*, p. 9.

60 But, in certain respects he was a critic of Darwin's theory. He regarded sexual selection as playing only a minor part in evolutionary change, and he remained sceptical about the role of instinct in animal behaviour. Whilst he admitted its importance in *Problems of Instinct and Intelligence*, published in 1928 shortly after his discharge from the IMS, Hingston argued that rational and learned behaviour played a far greater part in determining animal behaviour than the theory of instinct allowed. In this view he followed an illustrious Darwinian predecessor, Alfred Russel Wallace.

5 The Decline of the Colonial Medical Services

The colonial medical services and the armed services became a less important destination for the Irish medical graduate over time. Between 1860 and 1915 around 37 per cent of those who left Ireland to make a medical living joined the army, navy or colonial medical services, particularly the IMS. In the period 1920–40 this fell to 17 per cent of the total, making Britain an even more important destination for the Irish medical graduate. In the interwar period Africa overtook India as the most important place for Irish graduates seeking a job in the colonial services, a situation which persisted after the Second World War.[61] The war years saw recruitment to the services rise, including to the IMS, but peacetime meant the discharge of many in the armed forces, and India's independence in 1947 ended IMS recruitment. The African colonies had to wait till the 1960s to gain independence, and recruitment was more buoyant there at least during the 1950s. Recruitment to Africa and Mauritius rose in 1945-50 causing a slight overall increase in recruits to the colonial medical services compared to the interwar years.[62]

Two factors were influential in diminishing the attraction of colonial service. Anna Crozier suggests that increased opportunities for medical practice in Britain in the 1920s and 1930s may have deterred graduates who might otherwise have gone into the colonial medical service. There were still attractive places in Africa for European settlement, in South Africa and Rhodesia for example, and some emigration there was taking place even in the 1950s. But most of those in the colonial and medical service in the 1950s were sent in anticipation of preparing a country for independence.[63] In the case of India, increased use of indigenous doctors in the IMS also played a part in the decline in recruitment from Britain and Ireland.

A Commission of Inquiry in 1928 had advocated an acceleration of 'Indianisation' of the medical service of the IMS, and in 1933 J.W.D. Megaw, a graduate of the Royal University of Ireland in 1899, issued a pamphlet on the subject in response. His view was that pressure was on the civilian wing of the IMS to admit more indigenous doctors to the service, but he argued that, given the

61 In our cohort, 49 graduates left for Africa during 1920–40 and only 15 for India.

62 In 1945–60, Africa (including Mauritius) had 43 recruits, the West Indies and Guyana 16, and India only 7. Some among the number of recruits to Africa may have been 'settlers' or employed by companies, but the majority went into colonial service. This meant that the percentage in the colonial medical services 1945–60 was 29 per cent higher than in the interwar years.

63 Crozier, *Practising Colonial Medicine*, p. 49. For histories of medicine in colonial Africa, in addition to Crozier, see Ann Beck, *A History of the British Medical Administration of East Africa* (Cambridge Mass.: Harvard University Press, 1970); Vaughan, *Curing their Ills*.

original role of the civilian service as an adjunct to the Indian army, the process might weaken the army in India significantly. However, Megaw accepted that the process would go on. In 1922 there had been 35 Indians in civil posts in the IMS; by 1932 this had risen to 97, and the number of Europeans had declined from 326 to 195.[64] In addition, many other civilian appointments in the IMS were coming under pressure to be filled by individuals outside the IMS altogether, a process which Megaw claimed actually discriminated against Indian officers of the IMS as well as shrinking the military reserve which might be better maintained by permitting temporary secondment of medical officers to the civilian side of IMS work. He complained that as far as European recruits to the IMS were concerned, "An impression was created that it was unsafe to enter a service in which the conditions and prospects were liable to sudden and dangerous change."[65] Concerns about the future of the IMS were voiced in Ireland. The opinion of the *Irish Times* in 1933 was that the reorganisation of the Indian Medical Service would "put an end to the careers of hundreds of capable Englishmen and Irishmen", including the "physicians and surgeons of the Indian Medical Service".[66]

Gradually, as former colonies became independent, the role of the colonial medical services in general declined. Some post-war work in ex-colonial countries, or soon to be independent countries, became relocated in international organisations operating under trans-national bodies. The medical agencies of the United Nations, began, after the Second World War, to put together programmes of systematic disease eradication in many colonial and ex-colonial nations. The migration of doctors continued, including Irish doctors, to the ex-colonial world, but in a diminished form and in very different political and structural circumstances.

6 Conclusion

Anna Crozier talks about national tensions within the colonial service in Africa between the Irish and English, and Lankford agrees that they also existed in the armed services. Army doctors in general suffered from a degree of social insecurity in the late nineteenth century. This abated in face of improvements in their conditions of service towards the end of the nineteenth century, and as Lankford points out, more English medical graduates were joining the service

64 J.W.D. Megaw, 'Note on the Future of the IMS' (pamphlet), 28 July 1933, p. 9.

65 Ibid., p. 4.

66 *Irish Times*, 2 November 1933, p. 6.

towards the end of the nineteenth century. Nonetheless, social distinctions by school, social background or private wealth generally existed, with nationality sometimes added. As Lankford points out, the Guards (the most socially prestigious regiment) had few Irish members and most of their medical officers were English.[67] This led to a degree of mobilisation by Irish MPs and political leaders on behalf of the Irish medical profession in defence of the professional opportunities of the Irish doctor.

But both Crozier and Lankford agree that, once in the service, the Irish grasped the opportunity for promotion and advancement. In the opinion of Lankford, the effect of service in the army, navy or colonies was also to create a level playing field for the Irish medical professional. Lankford says:

> among Irish born doctors, those who graduated from Irish universities with more pronounced Anglican ties, those who held degrees from universities that appealed more to Catholics and Non-Conformists, and those who held medical licenses but no university degrees, differed little in promotion patterns.[68]

Lankford also comments on the remarkable fact that as Ireland's population fell in the late nineteenth century, her share of medical posts in the armed services still remained high. But was this because of poverty, as Lankford asserts? He quotes Thomas Longmore, professor of surgery at Netley, in 1864, "that it was mostly the poorer students of Ireland and Scotland who sought medical commissions".[69] In explanation for their strong presence in the armed and colonial services, Lankford felt that English graduates benefited from the wider availability of medical practices in England, until the overcrowding in the medical profession in Britain in the 1890s led to rising numbers of English graduates applying to the armed services. He believes that the heavy involvement of the Irish in the army and naval services in particular was caused by Ireland's relative poverty.

In the late nineteenth century, however, with the revival of the Irish economy after the Famine years and greater disposable income, the number of doctors who could be supported in practices in Ireland rose. But at the same time so too did the numbers educated in Irish graduate schools. It could be a long and arduous search for these to find a practice in the British medical marketplace.

---

67 Lankford, 'The Victorian Medical Profession and Military Practice', p. 521.

68 Ibid., p. 523. Among the successful Irishmen in the RAMC that he singles out is the Dubliner Alfred Keogh, 1857–1937, whom he describes as a great administrator.

69 Ibid., p. 517.

The armed and colonial services were a quick route to solvency. But they did not necessarily always attract the poorest graduates. Trinity College Dublin, the oldest and most prestigious medical school in Ireland, was more expensive than its rivals because all aspirant medical students had to take an additional year to acquire a BA before studying medicine. Added to this, living in Dublin was more expensive than elsewhere, and Lankford talks of the additional expense for Netley students of taking a year of training before being on full salary. Yet Trinity College provided a significant number of recruits to the army, more than other medical colleges in the years leading up to the First World War. TCD sent 57 of its graduates into the army or navy, only exceeded among the medical schools by the RCSI with 65. The army had perhaps more social cachet than the navy, very much the preserve of the RCSI, but this suggests an important point. Migration was not necessarily the last resort of the impecunious Irish medical graduate. As the next chapter will show, medical emigration helped consolidate and improve the prospects of both doctors and the Irish middle classes.

CHAPTER 4

Medicine, Migration and the Making of the Irish Middle Class

Training a son or daughter to become a doctor in the late nineteenth century required money, and, therefore, it was the middle-class family that bore the brunt of the costs. There were exceptions but a working-class entrant to medical school was very rare. Why therefore would a middle-class family expend money on a son or daughter who might leave to practise outside Ireland permanently?[1]

The argument of this chapter is this. First to expend money on educating a potentially migrating doctor was still an important gain for the middle-class family. It preserved their social status and sometimes, as we shall see, enhanced family wealth. Second medicine in the late nineteenth century was particularly important for the Catholic middle class. It was an important means of upward social mobility into professions for the aspirant Catholic family. However, professional labour was not the only means of accumulating wealth and enhancing social position. This chapter will show how, as well as the large incomes from medical labour open to the most distinguished doctors, family connection, accumulated wealth from other sources, inherited wealth and sheer opportunity played a part. Two generations of Darwins, Erasmus and Robert, were successful doctors. Nonetheless much of their wealth derived from their connections to commerce and industry. Ireland too has examples of the integration of a section of the medical profession with wider wealth generating schemes some of which came from migration.[2]

1 The Costs of Medical Education in Ireland

Acquiring a medical education took around five years, and even longer if students had to retake exams or were required, as in Trinity College Dublin, to

1 To get an idea of the current value of doctors' incomes in the nineteenth and early twentieth centuries, a multiple of 80 should be used before 1914, with a little extra added to take into account the cheapness of labour at that period. After the First World War and due to inflation, a multiple of 40 should be used. There are some differences in the costs of living between Ireland and England during this period, but they are not large.

2 Janet Browne, *Charles Darwin: Voyaging*, vol. 1 (London: Jonathan Cape, 1995), pp. 7–9.

 | DOI:10.1163/9789004324466_006

spend a year matriculating with a BA before they commenced their medical studies. More cost ensued if, after graduating, a specialist qualification was acquired.[3] Families bore the brunt of these costs. They included certain fixed fees for mandatory courses, and further fees for dissection practice and hospital attendance. Added to these were a whole plethora of charges: registration fees, fees for entry to examinations and for licensing. There were also a range of variable charges which differed between medical schools, including entrance fees or library fees.

Estimating the comparative costs of a medical education is therefore a very slippery science. This was particularly so since the prospectus of a medical school would sometimes try to gain an advantage over its competitors by highlighting relatively low charges for some components of their course, only to recoup the difference in other less publicised areas. However, the *British Medical Journal* and *Lancet* considered that one of their functions was to give the prospective medical student or their parents a clearer idea of the ultimate cost of enrolling in British and Irish medical schools. At the end of the nineteenth century, in around September in anticipation of the academic year, they produced a comparative analysis of the costs of a medical education.

Medical schools can be grouped according to cost. The most expensive were in London, where five years' study could cost around £600.[4] Acquiring a medical degree by apprenticeship to a famous consultant was even more expensive. Peterson mentions 'signing on' fees of 500 guineas in the first year.[5] A medical education might also be completed by "a visit to one of the great Continental medical schools, especially those of Vienna and Berlin".[6] Both routes, apprenticeships and visits to European centres of excellence for further qualifications, were familiar in Ireland.[7]

Added to the costs of education were those of subsistence. London was an expensive place to maintain a student. An education in an English provincial school was cheaper, and a medical education in Ireland cheaper still, though in some cases only marginally so. Based on a comparison of the costs of a medical degree using the *BMJ* prospectus for 1891, a medical education in a provincial

3 The Diploma in Midwifery was useful for those intending to set up in general practice, and a Diploma in Mental Science eased the graduate's path towards the posts of assistant superintendent or superintendent in mental asylums. Candidates for the army or the Indian Medical Service were also required from 1863 to attend the training school at Netley for a year, a requirement which was put aside in 1915 under the pressure of the First World War.

4 Peterson, *The Medical Profession in Mid-Victorian London*, pp. 68–76.

5 Ibid.

6 Keetley, *The Student's Guide to the Medical Profession*, p. 87.

7 See the discussion of George Johnston's career below *passim*.

English school required fees of £300–450 over five years and maintenance of £140–180, a sum total of £440–630. Using figures for comparability and not as indices of the full costs of a medical education, Birmingham Medical School in 1891 charged £63 for its lectures, £3.3s for its library fees and £24 for a hospital attendance of nine months, a total of £90.3s for a year's study and £400–500 for five years. Over five years the rates for different courses changed, however, and in the fifth year some of the fees would be paid direct to the hospital in which the final training took place. This would mean that the Birmingham Medical School charged a total of £450–500.[8] By comparison the Catholic School of Medicine charged £84 for an equivalent year or £420 for five years, and TCD charged £87.13s.6d or £438.7s.6d in total.[9]

Some Irish medical schools were even cheaper. The view of Keetley, author of *The Student's Guide to the Medical Profession*, was:

> [at Cork] the fees at the college and hospitals, as well as the University fees for examinations, are extremely low and the student who is not of extravagant habits will find Cork a cheap place to live in.[10] … [And] a degree can be got from Belfast in a very economical way.[11]

Galway, which struggled to attract medical students in the nineteenth century, charged marginally less than all the Irish schools.[12] If medical education could be accessed near home, the costs of subsistence might also be reduced further. Sometimes relatives and family friends helped out. Joseph Marshall Lynn of the RAMC died aged 93 in Armagh in 1899 leaving £33,025.5s.9d. Childless he bequeathed "all my medical books and instruments to Reverend E. Hazelton for the use and benefit of any of his sons whom he shall bring up to the medical profession".[13] If we attribute a more frugal rate of subsistence in general for the Irish medical student, with fees at £300–450 and subsistence at £125–250, the total cost of a medical education in pre-1914 Ireland was in the range £425–£700.

Irish families continued paying fees for the medical education of their children well into the twentieth century. In 1937 William Doolin, in an article on

8 *BMJ*, 5 September 1891, vol. 2, p. 553.

9 Ibid., p. 549 (Catholic Medical School) and p. 548 (TCD).

10 Keetley, *The Student's Guide to the Medical Profession*, p. 86.

11 Ibid., p. 85.

12 In Galway, six months' clinical instruction was provided at 4 guineas; courses in the first year at £3, and £2 in subsequent years. *BMJ*, 5 September 1891, vol. 2, p. 551.

13 Probate Calendars UK, Northern Ireland (PRONI) Calendar of Wills, Will of Joseph Marshall Lynn, died 10 October 1899, probate granted 24 November 1899.

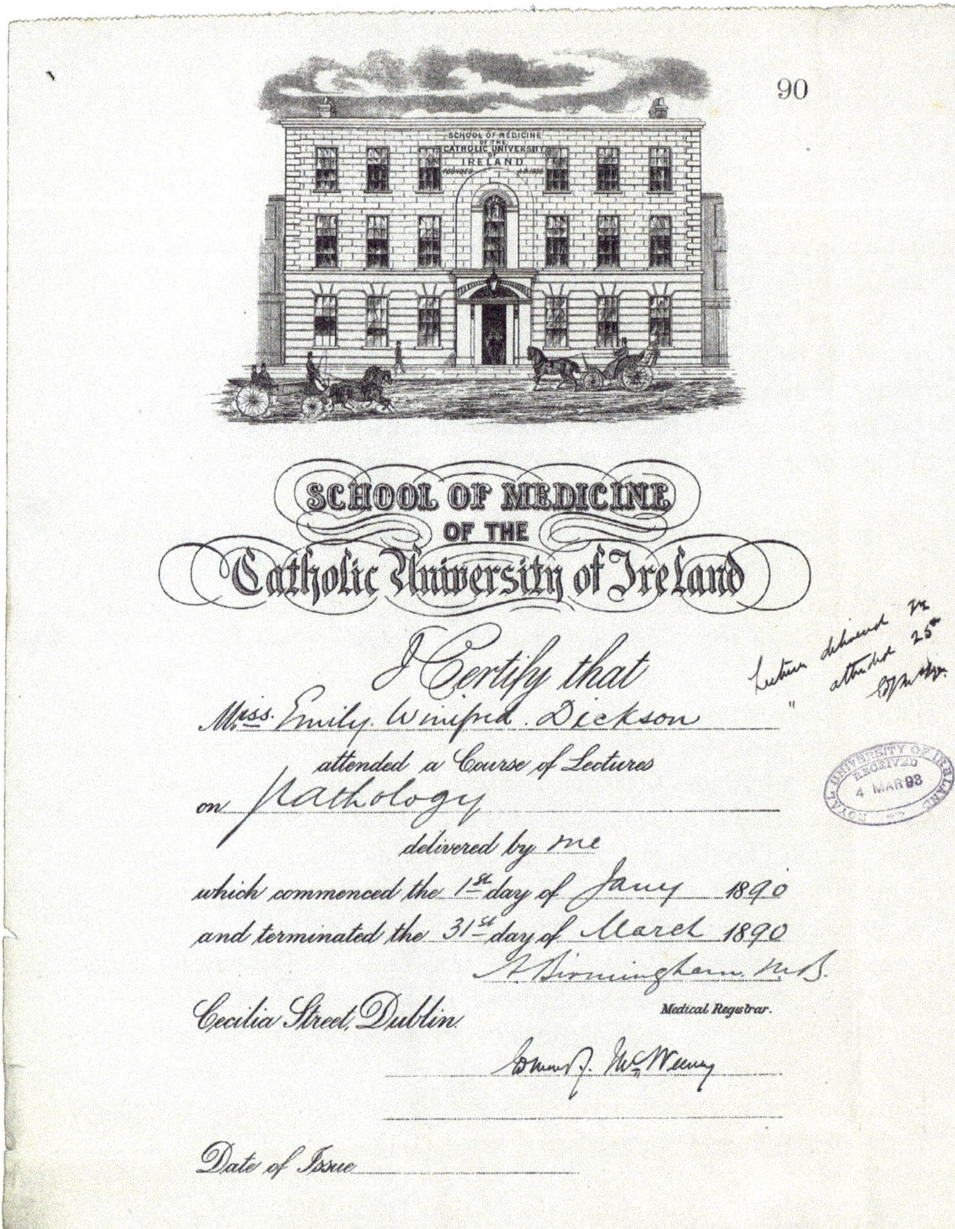

90

SCHOOL OF MEDICINE OF THE CATHOLIC UNIVERSITY OF IRELAND

SCHOOL OF MEDICINE OF THE Catholic University of Ireland

I Certify that

Miss. Emily Winifred Dickson

attended a Course of Lectures

on Pathology

delivered by me

which commenced the 1st day of Jany 1890

and terminated the 31st day of March 1890

A. Birmingham, M.B.

Medical Registrar.

Cecilia Street, Dublin.

Edmund J. McWeeney

Date of Issue

Royal University of Ireland Received 4 MAR 93

FIGURE 3 School of Medicine of the Catholic University of Ireland Pathology attendance certificate of Emily Winifred Dickson

HTTP://DIGITALHERITAGECOLLECTIONS.RCSI.IE/DICKSON/ITEMS/SHOW/22

ACCESSED NOVEMBER 24, 2020

medical education in the Irish Free State, gave comparative figures for the yearly cost of a medical education in Trinity College and the National University of Ireland. Calculating over a five year period this was £730.15s at Trinity College and, with an extra £101 for the pre- medical school BA, a total of £831.15s. At University College Dublin (UCD) five years at £158.14s per year amounted to £834.10s. The figures are not absolutely accurate; some fees were paid direct to the hospital at which the student would train on the wards.[14]

Putting aside familial affection, a major motive for the expenditure on medical education was to preserve the class position of family members. This is graphically illustrated by the preparedness of some families to go on paying fees for their children to retake failed medical exams. However, this chapter will argue that the benefit to the family and to the middle class as a whole of educating even an emigrant doctor was significant.

2 Catholics, Medicine and Social Mobility

In 1873 R.S.D. Lyons, Professor of Pathology at the Catholic Medical School, made a plea for more government assistance to the University system in Ireland.[15] Although his argument was directed at securing government help for the Catholic University in particular, it was more wide-ranging. Lyons argued that the demand for education in Ireland was more buoyant than elsewhere in the British Isles. In fact he quoted figures which suggested that there was one graduate to every 3,095 persons in Ireland, compared to one per 6,486 in England. This was partly due to the slower pace of industrialisation in Ireland, which meant that the professions were more important for the Irish middle class. His view seems to be borne out by the fact that, anecdotally, demand for university places in Belfast was observed to rise in years of industrial depression and fall when trade picked up.

In Lyons' view, the young men who entered commerce at sixteen or eighteen could be persuaded to enter university instead to acquire a wider set of skills than just medicine or law, although Lyons admitted that law and medicine at university would continue to be the dominant faculties. If the universities

14 William Doolin, 'Medical Education in the Irish Free State', in *Irish State Hospital Year Book* (Dublin: O'Neill Publications, 1937), pp. 36–9. Fees for medical school were abolished in NI in 1962 and in the Republic of Ireland in 1996.

15 Lyons (1826–86) taught at the Catholic University of Ireland 1856–86. He had served with distinction in the British army as a doctor particularly interested in the pathology of plague. He became Liberal MP for Dublin 1880–85.

were expanded, they could both serve the wider ambitions of the middle class and enhance the intellectual resources of Ireland overall. Lyons' argument was that demand for more university education arose chiefly from the changing condition of the Irish Catholic middle class. This stratum was thirsty for higher education and had the means to pay for it.[16]

Trinity College was a predominantly Protestant school. R.B. McDowell charts an average of around 10 per cent Catholic students at the start of the twentieth century, which then climbed till it reached "well over 20 percent in the years from 1923 to 1930". It then fell to less than 10 per cent by the mid-1930s, but expanded again post-war to 23 per cent by 1950.[17] Queen's College Belfast medical school had Catholic students, but similarly it was predominantly Protestant. The Catholic medical student was therefore much more likely to be found at the Catholic University medical school, the RCSI or the Queen's Colleges of Cork and Galway.

Trinity had a reputation as genteel and upper-class as well as Protestant. However, the records of 'father's occupation' at the medical school support the contention of the historian of Trinity, R.B. McDowell, that Trinity educated the sons of the professional middle class. Under 'father's occupation', 25 per cent recorded 'professional', 23 per cent commercial and industrial sector, and only 23 per cent 'land', independent means or 'gentleman'. The remainder were salaried employees, teachers, librarians or clerks, a proportion which was growing towards the end of the nineteenth century.[18]

Nineteenth-century censuses show that Protestants were over-represented in medicine in Ireland, as they were in the professions as a whole in relation to their numbers in the Irish population. According to John Hutchinson's calculations, Catholics made up 77.69 per cent of the Irish population in 1861, but only 35 per cent of doctors were Catholic. During 1901–11, the percentage of Catholics in the medical profession increased from 35 to 48 per cent, although there was a slight drop in ratio of Catholics in the overall population to 73.86 percent in 1911.[19]

Recruitment to medical schools in the late nineteenth century was fed by increasing numbers of Catholic students. By 1911 the successor to the medical

---

16 Robert Spencer Dyer Lyons, *Intellectual Resources of Ireland: Supply and Demand for an Enlarged System of Irish University Education* (London: Smith, Elder and Co., 1873). The original paper was presented at the Catholic University in 1857.

17 McDowell and Webb, *Trinity College Dublin 1592–1952*, Appendix 2, p. 504.

18 The TCD admission registers to the medical school for 1870 and 1895 were examined and a total of 144 entries identified; 10 more were identified in each of the admission registers for 1865, 1880, 1885, 1890 and 8 from 1868. The total sample was 192.

19 John Hutchinson, *The Dynamics of Cultural Nationalism: The Gaelic Revival and the Creation of the Irish Nation State* (London: Allen & Unwin, 1987), Table 8.2, p. 262.

school of the Catholic University, the medical school of University College Dublin, was the largest in Ireland. In other schools, there was a substantial proportion of Catholics.[20] In 1902–3 in the Queen's Colleges of Galway and Cork it was 38 per cent and 63 per cent respectively; and in 1908–9 65 per cent and 67 per cent.[21]

The increase in the number of Catholics in the medical profession accelerated in the Free State after partition. In 1926, 92 per cent of the population in the new state were Catholic and in 1946 over 94 per cent. Over this time the numbers of Catholics in the medical profession in the south increased. In 1948 the President of UCD, Michael Tierney, claimed that of the 2,300 doctors he estimated were practising in the Republic of Ireland, the majority were graduates of UCD and the NUI Colleges in Cork and Galway.[22] This left 330 from the College of Surgeons which was denominationally mixed, and 300 from TCD which was still predominantly Protestant.

TABLE 12 Percentage of Catholic medical students and doctors after 1922 in Southern Ireland[23]

Date	% Catholics in the 26 counties	% Medical students who were Catholic	% Doctors who were Catholic
1926	92.6	68.4	78.2
1936	93	90	82
1946	94.2	–	84

The medical profession proved more amenable to the entry of Catholics than, for example, law. Catholics comprised around 72 per cent of solicitors and 70 per cent of barristers in the Free State in 1936, as opposed to the figure

20 Two schools in Ireland – Queen's College Belfast and TCD – were predominantly Protestant. However, at QCB between 1902–3 and 1908–9 the percentage of Catholics rose from around 4.6 per cent to 8.5, whilst in TCD it was 10 per cent 1908–9. For Belfast see tables on 'Numbers and Religious Persuasions of Students entering each year since its opening', in 'Final Report of the Queen's Colleges', PP 1908–9, vol. XX. Cd.4831, p. 24. For TCD see McDowell and Webb, *Trinity College Dublin 1592–1952*.

21 Tables on "Numbers and Religious Persuasions of Students entering each Year since its opening" in 'Final Report of the Queen's Colleges', PP 1908–9, vol. XX, Cd. 4825, p. 13 (Cork) and Cd. 4883, p. 10 (Galway).

22 National Archives Dublin, S14402 A. Memorandum from Michael Tierney to the Irish Government.

23 Source: *Census of Ireland* 1926, 1936, 1946.

of around 82 per cent in medicine. In business and banking the proportion of Catholics was only around 60 per cent.[24]

Medicine was therefore an important route into the professions for Catholic families. Who were the Catholic middle classes who invested in a medical education?

3 The Catholic Middle Classes and Medicine

To give an idea of the social origins of medical students, particularly Catholic medical students, four cohorts of graduates, from 1910, 1915, 1920 and 1925, were cross-referenced against census material. The students were from the two Queen's Colleges in Cork and Galway (part of the National University of Ireland), University College Dublin (the former Catholic University and also part of the National University), the medical school of Queen's University Belfast and the Royal College of Surgeons.[25] Among the 108 studied, 31 were Protestant: 6 at Cork, 5 at the RCSI and the remainder at Queen's University Belfast medical school. The remaining 77 were Catholic. Census material can tell you (among other things) the occupation of the father of the student and the religion of the household. The numbers used are relatively small and spread across six medical schools. Nonetheless, together with other characteristics of the medical school – vicinity, cost, reputation and denominational character – the study establishes certain parameters for a more extensive study of social class origin in relation to medical education.

Overall figures show that land was contributing to the education of a new generation of Catholic doctors. Farmers were the largest occupation of the group as a whole, comprising a third of the total.[26] The numbers were largest in UCD, which had as many farmers' offspring as Cork and the RCSI put together. Children of farmers were also being sent into medicine in Ulster, but Belfast was a large industrial and commercial centre and this is reflected in recruitment to its medical school. At Queen's the recruitment of just three farmer's sons and daughters was lower than other medical schools. The six students at Galway had two farmer's sons among them.

24 *Census of Ireland* 1936.

25 The numbers of students were 18 at RCSI, 25 at Cork, 6 at Galway, 26 at Queen's Medical School Belfast and 33 at UCD.

26 Laura Kelly's study of students from the north of Ireland studying in Glasgow reported around a third from farming families; see 'Migration and Medical Education: Irish Medical Students at the University of Glasgow, 1859–1900', *Irish Economic and Social History*, vol. 39, no. 1, 2012, pp. 39–55.

The term 'farmer' in Ireland covers a wide range of economic positions. There was a transfer of land from landlords to tenants from the late nineteenth century, brought about by a series of Land Acts. Nonetheless 'farmers' could include the small farmer of the west barely scraping a living, to affluent ranchers and mixed farmers on good agricultural land who hired wage labour. Poorer farming areas were spread across the country but were concentrated in Mayo, Galway, Roscommon and Kerry, and no farmer from those areas in our sample sent a student to medical school in the period under examination. The areas from which farming families did send medical students were Kilkenny, Clare, Cork, Limerick, Meath and Westmeath, Carlow, Tipperary and Tyrone, all areas with stretches of good land and larger farms. The title 'farmer' also often disguised other business interests adjunct to agriculture. One Meath farmer whose son was at UCD is described as a 'miller and farmer', and in 1901 the household contained a governess and nursemaid. Another in Tipperary ran an auctioneer's business from his farm premises, employing two clerks as well as a farm servant and a domestic servant. A farmer from Limerick who boarded his son at Cork is described as a 'shopkeeper' as well as farmer and employed a manager. Another father with a son at the RCSI is described as a 'farmer and publican'.

It was unusual for a farmer to have two offspring studying medicine. A viable family business in addition to land, whether a shop or a public house, meant that funds were available for a medical education; but it also brought the possibility of gainful employment for other members of the family in the business or the farm. Therefore, it was generally the second, third or fourth child in a farming family who was put to medicine. Some of these families had, through farming, reached a stage of gentility quite as impressive as some Trinity students. An indication of this is that several families had to be traced back from the boarding school in which the future medical graduate was described in the census as resident and before he or she took up their medical studies. *The Leader*, in its vendetta against doctors, deplored the transformation that these patterns of middle-class social ambition had brought about, claiming that the ideals of simple, frugal and modest Ireland were being lost.[27]

Even outside industrial Belfast, the improvement in the financial situation of the middle classes in Ireland in the late nineteenth century spread beyond farming. A third of our samples were from the commercial and business sector. For example, in Cork's medical school there was a strong representation of the retail classes. Seven fall into this category, including three draper's sons. In Bantry, a small seaside town in County Cork, a draper's son and a doctor's son with, respectively, a shop and a surgery on Main Street, both graduated

27 'The Doctors', a poem in *The Leader*, 13 December 1912, p. 489.

together from Cork's medical school in 1910. Only Belfast had more sons of retailers, though in Belfast's case this is skewed towards large- scale merchandising, to be expected in a town of its size and industrial prosperity.

Finally, 16 per cent of parents were in government employment. Apart from a few civil servants – 'first class' or 'second class' – they comprised customs and excise officials, members of the Royal Irish Constabulary, a coroner's registrar and a postman. But the strongest representation among government employees by a small margin were National School teachers. Their influence is greater than the bare numbers. Frequently a household where the father's occupation was not teaching might have a wife or daughter described as a teacher in a National School.[28]

Very few from working-class backgrounds made it into medicine. Those few were in occupations which involved skilled manual labour. In our sample three described themselves as cooper, hackle maker (the maker of instruments for combing flax) and tailor. However, they may very well have owned the businesses rather than being employed as wage earners by others. There is no information from the census which can throw light on this. However, in one household in Cork the father is described as a bricklayer with three sons. His two eldest sons, both in their twenties, were a carpenter and bricklayer. These were skilled occupations, relatively well paid in Ireland. In the expansion of and improvement in rural housing in the late nineteenth century, the household income for five people, three of whom were working in these trades, was sufficient to support the youngest son, aged nineteen, at medical school. He is described as a student at the University of Cork and becomes in 1915 one of our cohort of medical graduates.

Another case was Moira Elizabeth Connolly, a graduate of the RCSI in 1925. In the census of 1911 she is recorded as living in Dublin, aged twelve, with her father James described as the National Organiser of the Socialist Party. James Connolly was later executed in 1916 for his part in the Easter Rising, and during his imprisonment he was attended by Surgeon Francis Tobin, a licentiate of the RCSI. Tobin reputedly promised Connolly that he would assist in the education of one of his children, and Moira Elizabeth was most likely the beneficiary of that promise. The existence of a wealthy patron was also important for the future Minister of Health Noel Browne, the son of an Inspector for the National Society

28 See Monica Nevin's study of social class origins of university students in 1967, including medical students: 'A Study of the Social Background of Students in the Irish Universities', *Statistical and Social Inquiry Society of Ireland*, vol. XX1, Part V, 1967, pp. 62–95 (Read before the Society 1968). It showed that medicine had a larger proportion from the higher professional and managerial classes and also a continued influx of farmer's sons and daughters into the profession.

for the Prevention of Cruelty to Children (NSPCC) in Ireland. Browne's family was in dire financial straits due to the premature death of his father. He was helped in the 1930s through Trinity Medical School by the wealthy Chase family.[29]

The other area of significant social change was, however, in the recruitment of women, who by 1910 were beginning to appear more routinely in the lists of graduating medical students.[30] Elizabeth Kiely and Máire Leane have pointed out that medicine was an important means of mobility for women. They accounted for 10 per cent of doctors in the census of 1926 and for 17 per cent in 1951, compared to 1 per cent of the legal profession in 1926 and 4 per cent in 1951.[31] Nonetheless Moira Connolly was in this respect unusual. She was both from a working-class family and a woman.

By the beginning of the twentieth century, prosperity was lifting up the sons and daughters of Catholic farmers and shopkeepers into the professions and medicine was the greatest beneficiary. The farmer's son at the Catholic Medical School and its successor UCD was by the 1900s rivalling his Trinity counterpart in expectations and style of life. The shopkeeper in Cork who settled for a more modest education nearer to home for his son or daughter in rural Ireland was accessing a marginally less expensive education but also with the expectation that gentility and upward mobility was within the grasp of his family.[32]

4 Income, Class and Migration

What role did migration play in the process? Over-production of medical graduates, given a market for doctors in Britain, the British Empire and the wider

29 In post-war Northern Ireland, which from 1945 abolished university fees and instituted means-tested subsistence grants, the record of social mobility improved, but was still not impressive. In 1951/2 around 72 per cent of the fathers of entrants to the medical schools were from the higher professional and managerial classes, while 29 per cent were from clerical, skilled, semi-skilled and unskilled occupations. In 1963/4 the proportions were largely unchanged. "Analysis of full-time entrants by faculty and social class of father 1951–2 and 1962–3", *Committee on Higher Education*, 1963–5, Belfast, HMSO, 1965, Table 93 p. 304 and Table 94 p. 305.

30 See Laura Kelly, *Irish Women in Medicine c.1880s–1920s: Origins, Education and Careers* (Manchester: Manchester University Press, 2015).

31 Elizabeth Kiely and Máire Leane, *Irish Women at Work 1930–1960* (Dublin: Irish Academic Press, 2012), pp. 64–5. My figures roughly correspond. During 1915–30, 13 per cent of my cohorts were women; and during 1950–60, 18 per cent. See the Appendix.

32 In the South, social mobility from working-class households remained low. See National Archives Dublin, TAOIS 2006/133/216. The studies referred to there are by Monica Nevin and Bertram Hutchinson, the latter demonstrating in 1968 that of 2,500 individuals from Dublin attending university, only 3 per cent were from skilled manual or routine non-manual occupations.

world, increased opportunities for the Irish middle class as a whole, including the aspirant Catholic middle class. It reduced pressure within Ireland, if not immediately, for the new Irish graduate. Although some graduates struggled to gain a foothold in a practice in Ireland, left and came back within ten years after graduation, most who moved to Britain settled there. Without migration, the route into the professions for the new graduate would have been slower and more arduous, or possibly even unachievable.

How did working outside Ireland impact on the prosperity of Irish-educated doctors? The contrast between British-educated doctors working in England and Wales and Irish-educated doctors in Ireland was pointed out in Chapter 2. They were measured by looking at the bequests in the wills of doctors in the probate calendars. Judged by bequests, Ireland had a higher proportion of doctors in modest to standard incomes (26 per cent) than in Britain, and fewer in the high earning capacity which comprised 22 per cent of the British sample. But it also had a solid middle of doctors on standard to good incomes. Around 52 per cent of doctors practising in Ireland left bequests in the range £1,000–10,000, more than in Britain.

Did migration improve the prospects of the Irish medical doctor? A sample was compiled from the bequests of Irish medical graduates to compare those who worked outside Ireland in general practice and their compatriots in the armed and colonial services.[33] The effects of working outside Ireland in whatever sphere produced a comparable pattern of distribution of bequests to that of working within Ireland, as evidenced by the Tables in Chapter 2. If no appreciable gain could be detected for those working outside Ireland, there was certainly no appreciable decline. The benefits of emigration were primarily in securing a range of opportunities which would otherwise be unavailable to many Irish graduates.

Among the sample there is still only a small percentage of very wealthy, and a long tail of those leaving under £1000, but a solid middle range of wealth measured by bequest. Whilst the rewards for those working in the army, navy and colonial services seem overall more insecure, it must be remembered that among those attracted to work in the armed service and colonies were often medical graduates without the resources to purchase a practice and in need of ready income.

---

33 The sample was compiled using different names from those in the tables in Chapter 2. The 1911–12 list of obituaries in the *BMJ* was used, together with names from the cohorts from 1860 to the early twentieth century and Irish-educated doctors whose deaths appear in *Crawford's Roll*.

TABLE 13 Bequests of doctors aged 50 and above from Ireland, making a medical living outside Ireland

Bequests £	Bequests of doctors outside Ireland in army, navy, IMS, colonies, shipping companies, missionaries	Bequests of Irish doctors in general practice in Britain	Total	Percentage
Under 999	11	17	28	25
1,000-2,999	15	15	30	26
3,000-4,999	11	9	20	17
5,000-9,999	6	7	13	11
10,000-19,999	5	7	12	10
20,000-49,999	2	6	8	7
50,000-100,000	–	3	3	3
100,000+				
Total	50	64	114	

SOURCE: CALENDAR OF WILLS FROM PRONI, NATIONAL ARCHIVES, KEW AND NATIONAL ARCHIVES DUBLIN

Bequests are not of course an infallible guide to wealth or actual earnings.[34] It is probable that some doctors in practices who earned below £1,000 nonetheless accumulated sufficient over their lifetime to leave bequests above their annual earnings. Their bequests may indicate modest remuneration but a thrifty lifestyle. The opposite is also true. Money can also be distributed among the family before death. One relatively wealthy doctor in his will probated in Ireland in 1941 referred to the sums of money he had already given to two of his sons, both doctors, during his lifetime, which effectively diminished the wealth he left in his will.[35] So wills can give clues to wealth, but they are not the absolute definitive measure of it.

5 Migration, Money and the Middle-Class Family

Money came back into Ireland from migration. This happened by various means. Robert Taaffe left the IMS after a relatively short career and used his

34 See the discussion in the Appendix.

35 Calendar of Wills, National Archives, Dublin, Will of William McDowell Aikin Wright MD, died 1932, probated 1941.

honorarium to set up a practice in Dublin. He left a legacy of £10,937.9s on his death in 1925.[36] William Richard Huggard, a graduate of Queen's College Belfast in 1875 who practised in Davos, Switzerland, probated in Ireland, Scotland and England on his death in 1911. In addition to the £4,403.6s.1d he left in England, £1,147.10s was left to his brother, Martin Huggard, a Dublin solicitor.[37]

One particular route for money returning to Ireland was through veterans of the army, navy or IMS retiring back to their native land. Many did not retire to Ireland, but even these sometimes probated back in Ireland, or in both England and Ireland, reflecting family and friendships in both countries. It was less common for those in general practice in Britain. They had often set up house, married and had children and this had implications for the distribution of their money after death. However, a general practitioner in East London, who died in 1932 back in retirement in County Down, left £19,168.0s.3d to relatives there. In his case there was family money moving between Ireland and Britain, including a bequest to him during his lifetime of £800 by his Irish aunt. The highest amount bequeathed from our sample was James Joseph Moran of the Indian Medical Service who died in Dublin in 1917 and left £34,519.17s.10d to his relatives.[38] The expansion of Empire was often an important aid to the accumulation of wealth. This is illustrated by two careers.

Robert Reid, born around 1827, gained licentiates from the RCSI in 1857 and the RCPI in 1865.[39] He joined the Indian Medical Service shortly after his first licence in 1857 and is recorded in the IMS lists up until 1890; then, in his sixties, he returned to Ireland and settled in the north. Reid left over £21,000 on his death in 1907. Of this, £13,950 of his estate was in securities: he had stocks and bonds mainly in banks and railways in China, Japan, New Zealand, Russia, Australia, Uruguay and Chile. He left £5,044.7s.2d in deposits in Grindlays Bank. Grindlays, originally set up to support travellers to India, had interests in the Far East as well as India, and may very well have steered Reid's deposits in that direction. Reid also had money in the Hong Kong and Shanghai Banking

36 Taaffe probated in both England and Ireland. The figure of £10,937.9s is taken from the Calendar of Wills, National Archives, Dublin. Taaffe died 20 December 1925, probated Dublin and London 1926.

37 See Calendar of Wills for England and Wales. William Huggard died 9 October 1911 in Zurich, probated in England November 1911 and in Scotland 1912. It is not clear to whom, apart from his brother, his estate was distributed.

38 National Archives, Dublin, Will of James Joseph Moran, died 9 April 1919, probated 2 June 1917.

39 It is likely that Reid returned to Dublin on leave from the IMS for the RCPI qualification.

Company.[40] Reid's wealth reflected British imperial expansion and the trajectory of global capitalism in the nineteenth century.

So did that of Alexander Sharp Deane. A graduate of the Royal College of Surgeons in Ireland in 1875, he started his career as a ship's doctor for the Peninsular and Orient Shipping Company in the Far East. By 1911 he was recorded as an employee of the Chinese Imperial Maritime Customs Service. This was a tax collection agency for the Chinese government employing mainly foreign and British staff. On his death in Dublin in 1922, Deane left over £30,931.12s.8d.[41] Some was probated in England, where he left a legacy to his brother-in-law Cecil B. Harmsworth, Under Secretary of State for War 1919–22. These substantial incomes from practice in the Empire support Anne Digby's findings for the Cape of Good Hope Colony, that better incomes and opportunities for doctors were available in parts of the Empire, but "the risks of professional failure were often greater".[42]

Belfast's industrial and urban growth also provided opportunities. John Frederick Hodges MD, who died in 1899, left over £37,000.[43] Medically qualified at the RCSI, Apothecaries Hall, TCD and in Glasgow, he practised for a while in Newcastle, County Down, Ireland. Hodges' interests gradually moved towards chemical analysis, agriculture and public health. He was professor at Queen's College Belfast and, in addition to his salary from the College, was paid by the Belfast Corporation for whom he acted as a public analyst.[44] Hodges also received fees from work as a medical officer for the Belfast, Omagh and Tyrone Poor Law unions.

Hodges' investment income was considerable, and in a very direct way it mirrored the history of Belfast itself in the nineteenth century. Mostly it was in companies based in the North of Ireland and arising from its growing population. He had £500 invested in bonds issued by the Belfast Water Company, a private company contracted for certain water supply services by the Corporation. There were shares in Dunville & Co., which distilled whisky and imported tea, and in Forster Green and Co., tea and coffee importers. He also had shares in the Ulster Bank and in tramways and railway companies.

---

40 PRONI, Calendar of Wills, Will of Robert Reid, died 26 March 1907, grant of probate 13 May 1907.

41 Calendar of Wills, England and Wales, Alexander Sharp Deane, probated 1922.

42 Digby, '"A Medical El Dorado?": Colonial Medical Incomes and Practice at the Cape', p. 463.

43 PRONI, Calendar of Wills, Will of John Frederick Hodges, died 13 December 1899, probated 26 January 1900.

44 "Death of Professor J.F. Hodges", *Belfast Newsletter*, 14 December 1899, p. 7, col. 3.

6 Migration and a Medical Dynasty

The Dublin medical dynasty of the Johnstons illustrates the importance of inheritance, broader connections and opportunities, including migration when amassing wealth. Andrew Johnston (1770–1833), who became a licentiate of the Royal College of Surgeons in Ireland in 1803, was a ship's surgeon during the Napoleonic Wars. The family hailed originally from Armagh in the North of Ireland, but Andrew settled in Dublin where he practised medicine.[45] George Johnston (1814–1889), Andrew's son, also became a doctor and Master of the Lying-in Hospital at the Rotunda Dublin 1868–75, a prestigious post in Irish medicine.[46] The useful family connections were through Francis Johnston (1760–1829), Andrew Johnston's elder half-brother and a famous architect.[47] Francis died a wealthy man in 1829 but childless, and some of his wealth passed to his brother Andrew, and on Andrew's death to Andrew's children.[48]

Andrew's son George benefited from his uncle Francis's business connections in other ways. He married Henrietta Williamson, the daughter of Francis's colleague John Williamson, a family with Armagh connections, who was a Dublin property developer. There were subsequent bequests from the Williamson family to George Johnston and his family.[49] Nonetheless, professional labours were still important to George, the future master of the Rotunda. His father Andrew Johnston died leaving a large family behind. George was aged around twenty at that point and training to be a doctor. Andrew's estate at his death in 1833 was substantial. Some of his large family were still very young.[50] At his death, Andrew's six sons were given the rents from a considerable num-

45 PRONI D4540.8/5, Family History of the Johnstons.

46 PRONI D4540/5/4/2, George Johnston's application for the mastership of the Rotunda Lying-in Hospital, October 1868.

47 Francis Johnston built the General Post Office and Nelson's column in Dublin.

48 PRONI D4540/2/5/27, Will of Andrew Johnston. Francis died in 1829. The will of Andrew Johnston, who died four years after Francis in 1833, included a property in Eccles Street, Dublin, where Francis had lived 1809–20, probably number 34, which Francis had remodelled whilst living there. It is not easy to calculate the exact amount of his legacy, but the cash and government bonds amounted to around £9,500.

49 PRONI D4540/2/9/1, Will of Anna Williamson. In the will of Henrietta's unmarried sister Anna, in 1873 George was bequeathed £1,000 and his wife Henrietta left five shares of £50 each in the Waterford and Limerick Railway.

50 PRONI D4540/2/5/27, Will of Andrew Johnston. His daughter Henrietta was to receive £3,400 in government bonds at 3½% interest together with £600 in cash, provided her mother consented to any marriage she contracted. If she remained unmarried she was to receive the interest only from the government bonds. Andrew's wife and George's mother Sophia were bequeathed a cash sum of £1,500, a further £4,000 in government bonds and the family house in Upper Temple Street and all its contents.

ber of properties that Andrew had either purchased outright or for which he had bought the leasehold.[51] With rents from the properties he was left, George enjoyed a modest income.[52] The sum was insufficient to generate a middle-class income in the upper regions of comfort, but enough to remove some of the pecuniary pressure on a newly minted graduate and ease his transition into his profession. Legacies might, of course, increase on the death of the surviving parent or of siblings, a not uncommon occurrence at that time.[53] Andrew Johnston in his will counselled his six sons to banish such thoughts from their minds:

> I remind my children that maternal love and brotherly affection living in unity and the bond of peace is pleasing to God who giveth all things and unless guided by his holy word in all pursuits, evil thoughts and actions will possess our minds.[54]

Andrew's son George, born in 1814, therefore had some capital and his family wealth permitted an expensive education. This included apprenticeship to two surgeons at the Richmond and Hardwicke Hospitals in Dublin; then a period in Paris taking courses in midwifery under Dubois and Cazeaux on the diseases of women; plus courses on diseases of children under Trousseau and the Guersins. George then entered a period of life from 1840 in which he made his income as a doctor in the post of surgeon to the Emigration Commission for South Australia. This was not on convict ships, but on a scheme devised by Edward Wakefield to populate South Australia with fit and respectable citizens who would form the nucleus of a thriving British colony.[55] Their passage was assisted by an Emigration Commission, and this included medical superintendence. The post of surgeon was relatively well paid compared to the first

---

51 PRONI D4540/2/5/27, Will of Andrew Johnston. This included a house in Scotch Street and Thomas Street in Armagh, the town of his birth, and houses and land in College Green, Foster Place and Sackville Street in central Dublin. Andrew also bequeathed the house in Eccles Street, Dublin. There was land in Balinteer County Dublin, again a suburb of Dublin; two houses in Johnston's Court off Grafton Street; and land in Milltown, County Kildare.

52 The yearly income of the house in Scotch Street, Armagh was given as £26.8s.9d, and since there were quite a few freehold properties in their possession it is likely that the three elder sons enjoyed around £100 or more per annum between them.

53 Of Andrew's twelve children, only seven survived to be included in his will of 1833.

54 PRONI D4540/2/5/27, Will of Andrew Johnston.

55 Reginald Hamilton, *Colony: Strange Origins of One of the Earliest Modern Democracies* (Kent Town: Wakefield Press, 2010).

years of private practice.[56] It required frequent trips for George back and forth between Ireland and Adelaide, Dublin being one of the ports from which Irish emigrants to the South Australian colony embarked.[57] In 1843 he married Henrietta Williamson, at which point he took up a position as assistant physician in the Rotunda under Dr Shekleton, eventually becoming Master 1868–75.[58]

The Mastership of the Rotunda paid well. Exactly how well is difficult to estimate, since the salary was by negotiation. It included student fees which in the Rotunda, the leading centre for midwifery and obstetrics in Ireland, would be considerable.[59] Again a private practice would be considerably enhanced by this position.[60] On George's death on 7 March 1889, he left assets of £19,642.13s.10d and, like his father, property. This included houses in Adelaide, South Australia which, when George was travelling there, was undergoing rapid expansion. There was a land boom, and the purchase of plots of land by the emigrants was encouraged by the government. George invested in three houses, and on 10 June 1847, probably in anticipation of a move back to Ireland, documents were drawn up giving power of attorney to an agent in Adelaide to manage his properties there and collect rent on his behalf.[61] He certainly remained a Dublin landlord, often using a William Johnston, possibly his elder brother, as his solicitor in his land transactions. In 1862 George was leasing out two houses in Wood Quay to tenants.[62]

What Andrew and George achieved was a very solid and wealthy position in the Dublin upper middle classes. Medical labour added to this, although it was not the only factor. It gave George a regular income and, with a first-rate medical education behind him, the Mastership of the Rotunda, a prestigious social position as well as a medical prize which would increase his client list. Family wealth and connections consolidated his position in Dublin's upper middle

---

56 Derek Whitelock, *Adelaide 1836–1976: A History of Difference* (St Lucia: University of Queensland Press, 1977).

57 See 'Ninth Annual Report of the Colonial, Land and Emigration Commissioners', Reports from the Commissioners, 1 Feb.–1 Aug. 1849, vol. XXII, Cmd 1082, pp. 1–97.

58 He wrote a textbook on midwifery with Dr Edward Burrows Sinclair: Edward B. Sinclair AB, TCD and George Johnston MD, Edinburgh, *Practical Midwifery: ... an account of 13,748 deliveries ... in the Dublin Lying-in Hospital during ... seven years, commencing November 1847* (Dublin: M'Glashan & Gill, 1858).

59 Thanks to Anne M. Byrne, head librarian of the Rotunda, for help with the query. In the 1840s the government recommended that a putative Master should be given an annual salary of £350 plus a third of students' fees, but this was rejected by the governors.

60 For example, as well as the professor's salary, a considerable income from private consultancy would accrue to a medical position of that prestige.

61 PRONI D4540/2/2/1.

62 PRONI D4540/1/1/1.

class; but so too did the opportunities arising from leaving Ireland to work, in this case in Australia. For those with fewer connections at home and no established position in the profession, migration could, especially in parts of the Empire, create a sudden flow of wealth and of desirable contacts.

However, some doctors in Merrion Square, the hub of Ireland's best-known doctors, left more modest legacies than colleagues with less illustrious careers. Sir Philip Crampton Smyly of 4 Merrion Square died in 1904 leaving £7,621.16s.11d. Sir James Craig of 18 Merrion Square died on 12 July 1933 bequeathing £4,123.13s to his family.[63] Sir Charles Cameron left £2,046.3s.6d in 1921. However, Sir Christopher Nixon at 2 Merrion Square left £41,081.13s.4d on his death in 1914.[64] An illustrious career in medicine or in the administration of medicine in the Empire had the potential to push one up the social ladder. But the accumulation of wealth, whilst often a consequence of these factors, was a much more complex process.

7 Migration and Poverty

There were always medical graduates who could look no further than the costs of their education from their families and who had minimal contacts among the wealthy. These had to rely on their own efforts. Migration abroad or to England might very well bring them contact with financial opportunities or at the very least supply them with a decent respectable living. Even 'a penny doctor,' as described by Robert Esler to his compatriots, might aspire to a carriage. A doctor in the army or colonial service, by his efforts and resourcefulness could hope to improve his status or be presented in far-flung lands with opportunities which would not cross his path at home.

However, migration was also a risk and some migrant doctors struggled. Although there are exceptions, wealth generally leaves more traces than failure or poverty. Nonetheless, it would be interesting to see how the dropout rate of British-educated doctors, that is their absence from the *Medical Register* after ten years, complicates the picture.[65] For the Irish-educated doctor, the dropout

63 For Smyly and Craig who died 8 April 1904, see Calendar of Wills online, National Archives, Dublin.

64 Ibid. Christopher Nixon died 19 July 1914.

65 See the discussion in the Appendix. Crowther and Dupree looked at 1,288 graduates of Edinburgh and Glasgow medical schools in the 1880s and found that around 29 of the cohort were untraceable after five years. They conclude that some, though not in the UK *Medical Register*, were probably in practice in places where registration was not required. See Crowther and Dupree, *Medical Lives in the Age of Surgical Revolution*, pp. 123–5.

figure averaged 13–15 percent during 1860–1960, a remarkably stable figure for the whole period. In Ireland, Britain or elsewhere, to drop out of the register was usually the outcome of a variety of factors, amongst which professional failure must have played at least some part. If the number of unregistered doctors was higher for the Irish-educated doctor than for those educated in England, Wales or Scotland, it might indicate greater wastage due to lack of opportunities. But there are no comparative figures for absence from the *Medical Register* of graduates from England, Wales or Scotland to allow us to make definite statements.

Nonetheless, there were those who struggled to establish themselves in both Ireland and Britain. A failure to secure a practice or Poor Law position in Ireland might lead to a succession of unsatisfactory assistantships in England and an eventual practice in a place unfavourable to a decent medical income. In the age of tuberculosis, health problems might dog a career. On the whole the lowest bequests in wills were among those who died soon after the cut-off age of fifty used in the survey, indicating that for most doctors it required time to secure an ample income and also in some cases premature death interrupted the accumulation of wealth. The lowest bequest in our sample was £78.17s.6d for a doctor who had worked in Liverpool and who died at 53 in 1906. However, one army veteran who graduated in 1875 from the RCS died near Manchester in 1927 in his seventies. He left £104.5s.6d to his brother, an electrician, around £4,000 in today's money. A family with fewer resources, a long period subsisting on a pension and perhaps other problems may have been at work. The study did not examine those who were intestate, for they do not appear in the will calendars, but there must have been some in this position due to financial problems.

On the whole, however, medicine was a relatively sure route to a reasonable income, both for those who remained in Ireland and for the migrant doctor. Of our cohorts of doctors traced in the Irish census, one from Cork, the son of a draper who graduated in 1915, left £4,050.7s on his death in West Ham in 1937. The bricklayer's son, graduating in the same year, died prematurely in 1935. After practising in Yorkshire for most of his professional career, he left £12,157.4s.8d. A GP's son, who graduated in 1925 from Cork followed by a career in the IMS, died in 1962 back in County Cork; he probated in England, but left the bulk of his estate of £9,679.8s.6d to an Irish relation.[66]

Some historians have argued that doctors in the mid-nineteenth century did not enjoy high status, because they were seen as recruited predominantly from

66 Calculated using the graduate list of Cork Medical School for these years, cross-referenced with the Irish Census 1901 and 1911 and Calendar of Wills for England and Ireland.

the 'middling ranks'.[67] By the end of the nineteenth century, however, medicine offered a route to gentlemanly social position, even allowing for the hierarchy in the profession. Entry to the *Medical Register*, in addition to its other benefits, put a mark of professional competence upon doctors. Nonetheless, it still remained the case that doctors had to negotiate the social distinctions characteristic of their times. A wealthy practice required the doctor to mingle with rich patients. A knowledge of drawing room etiquette might be required, and a show of wealth in their houses and carriages which would impress their patients. The houses of the wealthy doctors in Merrion Square were places "where at times royalty itself rubbed shoulders with the lawyers and the doctors, the clergy, the academics, the writers, the artists and the officers of the army".[68] Moreover, the successful doctor had to be able to exercise a degree of authority over rich and sometimes obstreperous patients through the medium of manners and personality as well as knowledge and skill. This did not go unnoticed by the colleagues of the 'great' doctors, who are described critically by one commentator as "fashionable, dogmatic, patronising and overly ambitious" and arriving at a diagnosis by guesswork and speculation, though with an "impressive rapidity and an air of authority which inspired confidence".[69]

To gain that position, the medical practitioner had to put behind him the taint of selling cures as opposed to treating the sick by his professional skill. Social sensitivities about the interface between the doctor and the representatives of Irish local democracy were also in evidence particularly in the years leading up to the strike in 1902. Dispensary and workhouse posts were never abandoned even by the doctors in the higher earning brackets, as can be seen from Hodges' financial profile. But those who were more dependent upon such employment often chafed at the encounter with the elected Poor Law official. Public representatives on Boards of Guardians and dispensary committees were by the 1890s drawn largely from small farmers and businessmen. One bitter letter, reprinted in *JIMA* in 1902 from the newspaper the *Cork Constitution*, complained:

> How long are educated men dealing with matters relative to the well-being of the community at large to be the abject slaves of Rural District Councillors? Who are these Rural District Councillors? Men who, for the most part, of the class who would actually apply for dispensary relief and

67 M. Jeanne Peterson, 'Gentlemen and Medical Men: The Problem of Professional Recruitment', *Bulletin of the History of Medicine*, vol. 58, 1984, pp. 457–73.

68 O'Brien, *Conscience and Conflict*, p. 176.

69 Richard Mulcahy, *Memoirs of a Medical Maverick* (Dublin: Liberties Press, 2010), p. 67.

> what, in all common sense, can be expected in regard to fair treatment from these self- constituted "Employers" or better word "Slave Drivers" to the unfortunate Dispensary Medical Officer.[70]

Laura Kelly and others have noted that sensitivity about the social position of the doctor pervaded the medical schools from the mid- nineteenth century.[71] The medical school laid increasing emphasis on encouraging behaviour held to be suitable for a gentleman and on controlling, if not eliminating, much of the rowdy behaviour which had been characteristic of the early-nineteenth-century medical student. Doctors themselves laid emphasis on the importance of this in the conduct of their profession, and especially the avoidance of subordination and the taint of trade.

For the average, modestly rewarded doctor, part of their education in the age of the fee-paying patient was etiquette. The 1880–1 edition of the *Transactions of the Ulster Medical Society* published a table of 'fees' from which it urged the doctor never to depart. Part of the reason was to discourage doctors from accepting 'tips'. Tipping the doctor, usually by a present such as a new shirt or scarf, was ironically common at interments. In the view of the *Transactions of the Ulster Medical Society*, this put the doctor on the same social level as the gravedigger and was considered a demeaning practice which undermined the doctor's professional status and dignity.[72]

8 Ireland's Intellectual Resources

There was another important way in which medical migration contributed to the consolidation of the Irish middle class. Lyons was perspicacious in identifying the intellectual importance of the Irish university to the country's culture and society, and the number of medical students was the key to the survival of the university. Most universities, not just the Catholic University who would not have survived without its medical school, were dependent on medical

70 "Cork Council and Poor Law Officials", letter from Philip G. Lee, 10 April 1902, *JIMA*, vol. 2, no. 5, May 1902.

71 For a fuller discussion of the culture of the medical student, see Laura Kelly, 'Irish Medical Student Culture and the Performance of Masculinity c.1880–1930', *History of Education*, online May 2016; and eadem, *Irish Medical Education and Student Culture c.1850–1950*, 2017.

72 Robert Esler, "On the Disposal of the Dead" (Paper given January 1878), *Transactions of the Ulster Medical Society*, Session 1877–8, pp. 50–2.

school students in the nineteenth century.[73] An obituary of Sir Bertram Windle, appointed President of University College Cork in 1911, described Cork as "little more than an excellent medical school which manufactured doctors for export".[74] The figures for Queen's College Cork certainly bear this out: in 1894–6 medical students accounted for around 84 per cent of the total number of its students. Although this proportion dropped in the next two decades, in 1906–7 medical students were still 70 per cent of the student body. Queen's College Galway was less dependent on medical students, a fact which was occasionally felt to threaten its survival, but in 1880, 57.6 per cent of the students were studying medicine, a figure which fluctuated but was still around a third in 1905–6. TCD as an old established foundation had a wider range of faculties, including a large theological department as well as teaching the natural sciences, so the proportion of medical students compared with the student body as a whole was less. However, in the period 1860–95, TCD was still producing more medical graduates than any other school except for the RCSI.[75]

Student fees were an important part of the economy of universities, and that meant medical student fees. Although the Queen's Colleges had been built with government grants and received an annual subvention, the RCSI depended wholly upon fees, as did the Catholic University until it was incorporated into the Royal University in 1880. So that for all Irish universities fees were critical and in some cases vital. This meant that the integrity of the universities and all their faculties, including the scientific and literary culture to which they gave rise, were indirect beneficiaries of the medical school. The medical school was often the place where, in the absence of science faculties, many putative scientists found a niche.[76] Zoology, botany and chemistry were all adjuncts to medical education. In the later nineteenth century anthropology emerged in Trinity as a product of the anatomy department.[77]

A much larger medical culture than otherwise would have existed was maintained by the over-production of doctors. This was to the advantage

---

73 F.O.C. Meenan, *Cecilia Street: The Catholic University School of Medicine* (Dublin: Gill and Macmillan, 1987).

74 John J. Horgan, 'Sir Bertram Windle: An Appreciation', *University College Cork Sessional Lists 1928–9*, pp. 119–28. Windle died in Canada in 1929.

75 See the tables in the Appendix.

76 Natural philosophy had several important practitioners and, by the end of the nineteenth century, science faculties and laboratories were beginning to emerge in Irish universities. But compared with medicine and the attractions of a degree which would lead to a professional career, they remained relatively weak.

77 See Greta Jones, 'Contested Territories: Alfred Cort Haddon, Progressive Evolutionism and Ireland', *History of European Ideas*, vol. 24, no. 3, 1997, pp. 195–212.

of the professors in the hospitals, ancillary staff and medical schools themselves. In Cork in 1906–7 the professor of anatomy, through whose hands all the students passed, had a salary worth £978, composed of the basic wage and class fees. This income was extra to his private practice. Teaching students was an important source of income for some of the top medical doctors in Ireland.

Medicine was the largest professional grouping in Ireland throughout most of the nineteenth and twentieth centuries. There were more teachers and clerical staff in the population but, compared with lawyers and engineers, medicine was the leading profession in Ireland. Accountancy and engineering showed substantial growth after the Second World War, but only in 1971 did engineers overtake medicine by a small margin. Medicine was still 42 per cent of all the higher professions in 1926; 32.7 in 1951; and 23.9 in 1971.[78] This compares with England and Wales where, according to Perkin's work on the growth of the middle class in the nineteenth century, medicine accounted for only 20 per cent of the higher professions in 1911.[79] In Ireland, however, its importance was much greater: a leading vector in the creation of the Irish middle class.

9 Conclusion

The Leader observed in 1905 that "Even as it is the ambition of every Irish family to count a priest amongst its members, there is also very frequently a desire in most middle-class homes to devote a son to the medical profession." Although *The Leader* thundered against the 'West Briton' attitude of many Irish doctors, it admitted that "It is noteworthy that, though we often speak of the revival of Irish industries, one never hears of the necessity for the revival of the doctor making industry." This was a pity, since "it is very doubtful if the natural genius of the Irish will ever find its best development in the mechanical arts. Their best opportunity would always be therefore Law, Medicine and Theology and at the administrative arts, or in the army."[80]

The 'doctor making industry' was important to the middle classes for income and social status. It had especial value for those families who, in the

78 Farmar, *Patients, Potions and Physicians*, Table 9.1: The Growth of the Professions in Ireland 1926–71, p. 190.

79 Harold J. Perkin, 'Middle Class Education and Employment', *Economic History Review*, vol. 14, 1961, pp. 122–130. Calculated from Table 3, p, 129, using the seven 'higher' professional categories.

80 'The General Medical Council', *The Leader*, 13 May 1905, p. 187.

late nineteenth century, found they now had the resources to educate a son or daughter in medicine and hence propel them to professional status. Medicine remained, however, a largely middle-class profession. Ciaran O'Neill has studied Irish Catholic elites in the nineteenth century, measured by those families who could afford to send their sons and daughters to the most exclusive Catholic boarding schools in Ireland and England and, particularly their daughters, to schools abroad.[81] These families were often the Catholic landed gentry or the most wealthy Catholics in society. O'Neill examined the occupational destination of a sample (around 1,307) of Catholic boys educated in exclusive Catholic schools, and came up with some interesting observations.[82] During 1850–99 38 per cent of Catholics from these schools went into the military, compared with 19 per cent of boys from the English public school, Winchester. The next occupational category for Catholic boys was landowner or gentlemen (21 per cent as opposed to 11 per cent for Winchester), and 12 per cent went into government service or politics (compared with 8 per cent for Winchester). The figures for medicine were low, around 6 per cent.[83]

Medicine was not, therefore, quite the most elite or socially sought after occupation for the wealthiest Catholic families. Nonetheless it played a role even here. O'Neill points to the Meldons, a wealthy Catholic family of property owners. They increased their wealth by adding to it a portfolio of occupations and interests, among which they counted, law, business and also medicine.[84] As the example of the Johnstons shows, medicine might not be the first choice for the most socially exclusive among Irish families (Protestant and Catholic alike), but it was not uncommon for a member of a wealthy family to take up medicine and to use it to acquire further prosperity and influence in the world at large.

81 Ciaran O'Neill, *Catholics of Consequence: Transnational Education, Social Mobility and the Irish Catholic Elite 1850–1900* (Oxford: Oxford University Press, 2014).

82 In Ireland the schools were Clongowes Wood, St Stanislaus, Castlerock, Blackrock; and in England Stoneyhurst, Ampleforth, Radcliffe, the Birmingham Oratory, Oscott, St Augustine's, Ushaw, Sedgley, Downside and Beaumont.

83 O'Neill, *Catholics of Consequence*, pp. 119 and 120–21.

84 Ibid., p. 120.

CHAPTER 5

Partition

After the Easter Rising by Sinn Féin, the more radical wing of Irish nationalism, the days of British rule in Ireland were numbered. Partition in 1922 created two states on the island of Ireland. This affected medicine in several ways. In Northern Ireland, six largely Protestant counties remained part of the United Kingdom but were given a devolved parliament to deal with social questions including health. The new state was called Northern Ireland, though known colloquially as Ulster, and it retained all the monarchical symbols of the British constitution and allegiance to the Crown. Hence when the United Kingdom went to war in 1939, so did Ulster. The medical school of Queen's University Belfast was within its jurisdiction.

In the newly independent state in the South, the twenty-six counties were known officially as Saorstát Éireann but also as the 'South of Ireland', 'Éire' or the 'Free State'. Although all descriptions of the twenty-six counties are redolent with political overtones, for the purposes of this study it will be generally referred to as the Free State or Éire, and from 1949 as the Republic of Ireland. Nominally the Free State was a dominion and part of the British Commonwealth, but these constitutional arrangements were effectively ignored and in 1949 Southern Ireland officially became a republic severing all remaining ties to the Commonwealth.

Some participants in the War of Independence on the extreme wing of Irish nationalism never accepted the legitimacy of partition. This was signalled by their refusal to call either state by their official name, referring instead to the twenty-six counties and the six counties. Civil war over the terms of the Treaty of 1922 which brought about partition, broke out in the South during 1922–3. A government was formed in 1922 by the Fine Gael party who accepted the treaty creating partition. Eventually Fianna Fáil, the virulent opponents of the Treaty became the government of the Free State in 1932. This action signalled its *de facto* acceptance of partition, even though the new constitution drawn up by Fianna Fáil for Saorstát Éireann in 1937 claimed sovereignty over Northern Ireland.

The tensions arising from the Civil War dogged Irish politics in the South, including medical politics. Robert Collis described this in his autobiography.[1]

1 Robert Collis, *To Be A Pilgrim: The Autobiography of Robert Collis* (London: Secker and Warburg, 1975). Collis was reputedly one of the figures who persuaded the Rockefeller Foundation to visit Ireland in the 1920s.

 | DOI:10.1163/9789004324466_007

The conflict revolved around the position of Trinity College Dublin, which was regarded, somewhat unfairly, as catering predominantly for the education of the Protestant Irish and as an institution which had been supportive of British rule. Collis, a Protestant Irish nationalist, described Trinity College Dublin as "conservative medically and politically". The medical school of University College Dublin, the successor to the Catholic University, was "divided inside itself after the Irish civil war". Henry Moore, Professor of Medicine at UCD, was in favour of the Treaty. The new Irish Minister of Health, according to Collis, though knowing nothing about medicine, was a friend of Moore. They shared hostility towards Trinity and "between them they managed to pour cold water onto the RF proposal of a Dublin medical school run by TCD and UCD".[2]

The question of replacing one elite with another and the nature of the new ruling class in the Free State has absorbed historians. Various theories have been advanced on the subject, including whether the Rising of 1916 and the Civil War that followed the Treaty represented more than just a Catholic nationalist and Protestant unionist conflict, and was effectively a struggle for supremacy between rival Catholic nationalist groups.[3] But one thing should be noted. The development of the Catholic medical school and the Catholic hospitals in the nineteenth century had already created parallel medical structures in Ireland along denominational lines. Even so, as we shall see, joint cooperation and collegiality were still strong in Irish medical circles, even whilst political tensions existed.

There was already a Catholic medical elite waiting to take up positions of medical influence. Take, for example, one of the cohort of 1875 graduates from the RCSI, the Rt. Hon. Michael Francis Cox. He was educated at the Catholic University, St Vincent's and the Richmond Hospital. He rose to be consulting physician at St Vincent's, examiner in medical jurisprudence at the Royal University of Ireland and Demonstrator of Anatomy at the Catholic University. A practice and address at 45 St Stephen's Green East showed that he had reached the elevated ranks of fashionable and prominent doctors grouped around that square. In 1922 Cox replaced Sir James Craig as president of the Royal College of Physicians of Ireland (of which Cox had been a member since 1892). Cox was a luminary of sorts in the old system, a member of the Privy Council in Ireland. But he also, according to his own words, qualified for the new order

---

2 Ibid., pp. 56–7.

3 See Fergus Campbell's discussion of the period 1916–23 as a war between the relatively Anglicised Catholic middle-class elite and the more radical and less secure newly emerging Catholic middle and lower middle class: Fergus Campbell, *The Irish Establishment 1879–1914* (Oxford: Oxford University Press, 2009).

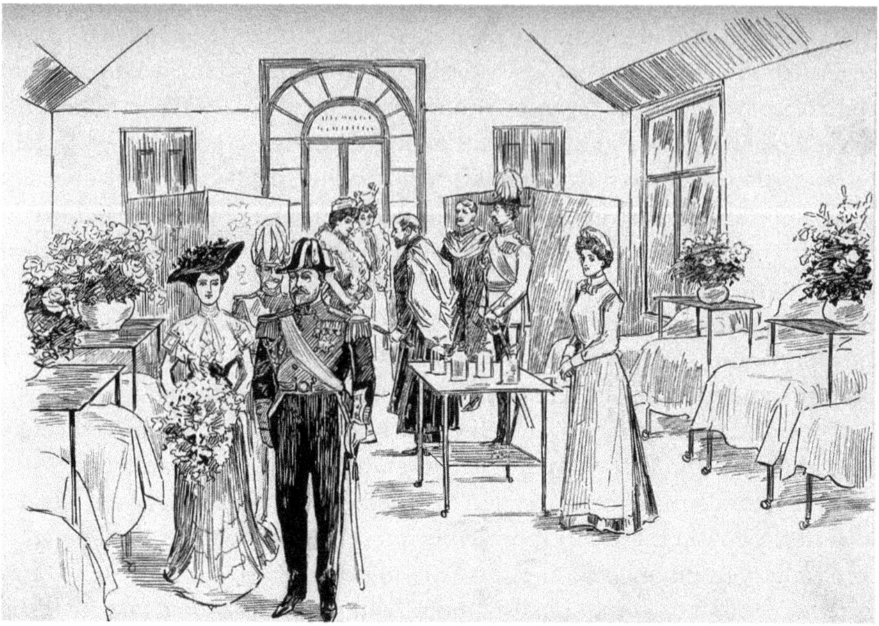

FIGURE 4 A visit by the King and Queen to the Clarence ward of the Royal Victoria Hospital in Belfast. Pen and ink drawing, 1903
SOURCE: WELLCOME COLLECTION. ATTRIBUTION 4.0 INTERNATIONAL (CC BY 4.0)

since "feeling himself out of sympathy with the government he resigned his membership of the Privy Council two years ago".[4]

In 1922 the Royal College of Physicians of Ireland put forward three names and the Royal College of Surgeons in Ireland two as medical representatives to the newly constituted Irish Senate. But they were "puzzled and disappointed that none of the persons recommended by the Royal Colleges have been accepted". Instead the appointees were George Sigerson, H.L. Barniville and Oliver St John Gogarty.[5] All three were qualified medical professionals with long-standing connections to the nationalist movement and, importantly for the incoming government in 1922, pro Treaty.

4 *The Lancet*, 12 April 1922, vol. 1, p. 353.

5 *The Lancet*, 16 December 1922, vol. 2, p. 1299. George Sigerson (1836–1925) had taught zoology at the Catholic University, but his main scientific interest was in neurology. He was a cultural nationalist and is largely remembered for his contribution to the revival of the Irish language and Gaelic games. H. L. Barniville (*c*.1887–1960) was Professor of Surgery at UCD from 1928. Oliver St John Gogarty (1878–1957) was a specialist in otolaryngology and worked at the Richmond and Meath Hospital. He was well known in the 1920s among the educated public primarily as a controversialist and writer. He was originally a member of Sinn Féin but accepted the Treaty of 1922 which involved him in relocating to London for a short time because of fears for his safety.

1 The Settlement in Health

There were several planning committees which met 1919–20 to consider the path of future health development in a Home Rule Ireland, but they were overtaken by events on the ground.[6] The health infrastructure in the South of Ireland was damaged during both the War of Independence against the British and the Civil War that followed. The workhouses, in many cases abandoned or destroyed in the fighting, were abolished by the new government. Some of the remaining ones became county-run homes for the elderly. The headquarters of the Local Government Board for Ireland (LGB), located in the Customs House on the Dublin Quays, went up in flames in 1921. But the authority of the LGB was being flouted anyway in many provincial areas of Ireland. Local councils under Sinn Féin control rejected its authority. In practice this meant refusal to surrender their books for audit to the LGB, to allow LGB inspections or to take any instruction from them. The LGB's authority over the administration of workhouses and dispensaries was effectively disappearing. In certain areas the Sinn Féin dominated councils were pursuing a policy of sacking district nurses who were policemen's wives and rejecting the medical expenses of policemen who were injured in the fighting.[7] In retaliation the Westminster government held back its grants to local councils, regarding any other policy as subsidising revolution. This meant that dispensary doctors in certain areas reported a drop in their income. It also led to cases where wages did not appear at all. For example, it was reported in 1921 that the staff at Ballinasloe Asylum had been without salaries for two months, and £25,000 was owed.[8]

There were more immediate dangers to doctors because they travelled sometimes in places which were not safe or after curfew. This put them inadvertently at risk of being caught in crossfire or encountering roadblocks put up by government or rebels. Those with motor cars found themselves a particular target of insurgents, who would attempt to take their car. More common and damaging in the long run, however, was the implied threat of being singled out

---

6 An Irish Public Health Council was created and overseen by the Local Government Board in 1919. It comprised E. Coey Bigger, medical commissioner to the Local Government Board, Sir John Moore, President of the Royal Academy of Medicine in Ireland and chairman of the Public Health Committee of the GMC, and the Insurance Commissioner and Registrar General, Dr Robert J. Rowlette. Representatives from the IMA and Dr Alice Barry of the Women's National Health Association were appointed. Among the non-medical representatives were two from the insurance industry, a veterinary surgeon and, from Dublin, Sir James M. Gallagher ex-Lord Mayor and Mrs J. McMordie of Belfast's TB and Insurance Committees. The Council did not survive the events of 1922.

7 *The Lancet*, 'Ireland', 21 August 1920, vol. 2, pp. 416–17.

8 *The Lancet*, 9 April 1921, vol. 1, pp. 767–8.

as insufficiently enthusiastic about one side or the other. By spring 1921 around 250 local councils had switched their allegiance to the new Irish parliament formed by the insurgents and had been refused subsidy by the LGB. In April Dáil Éireann, the newly constituted Irish parliament, issued this statement:

> Where a local authority has, by resolution, declared allegiance to Dáil Éireann and has severed all relationships with the English Government Board [sic], instructing its officials to cease communication, written or verbal, direct or indirect with that institution, any of its officials, or any persons acting on behalf of any of its officials, will be deemed to be a treasonable offence and dealt with accordingly.[9]

As the Irish correspondent in *The Lancet* commented, "I do not pretend to interpret the threat in the closing words of this warning, but to a man living in a country district in Ireland it is not to be taken lightly."[10] The medical profession found themselves protesting against dismissals of dispensary or workhouse medical officers consequent upon their attendance upon an injured policeman and or treatment of discharged soldiers (from the Great War) – a category of people unpopular with Sinn Féin. By November of 1921 in areas of insurgent strength, and this was most of the twenty-six counties, the workhouse system had been effectively abolished. The county councils took over the functions of the boards of guardians, and dispensary committees and the LGB no longer supervised the system. It was replaced by a committee of Dáil Éireann.

In the North there was also an escalation of conflict in the form of individual attacks on Protestant unionists and by Protestant unionists on nationalist Catholics. In some cases this evolved into full-scale civil disorder. Certain areas of Northern Ireland in which the minority Catholic population lived felt, justifiably, under considerable threat. When partition was finally agreed, the Catholic nationalists in the North felt disappointed, bitter and unprotected in the new state – feelings mirrored among many Protestants in the South. The impact of this was to survive in the politics of Northern Ireland for a long time.

Two medical systems emerged from the events of the early 1920s, linked historically but diverging over successive decades. In Northern Ireland the Ministry of Home Affairs took over administration of the workhouse and dispensary system. The Local Government Act of 1929 in Britain finally abolished the workhouse system, but it was not enacted in Northern Ireland and the workhouse system continued there until the eve of the Second World War. On the

9 *The Lancet*, 23 April 1921, vol. 1, p. 877.
10 Ibid., p. 877.

whole until 1939 Northern Ireland remained a rather conservative part of the United Kingdom in regard to its social and medical systems. The Insurance system set up in the United Kingdom in 1911 continued both North and South. In the North, however, the benefits were kept in line with Britain and, because of the rise in unemployment in Northern Ireland in the interwar period, this effectively constituted a significant subsidy from Westminster to Northern Ireland.[11]

In the Free State health became the responsibility of the re-named Department of Local Government and Public Health. In 1925 the Local Government Act created county boards of health to subsume the medical functions which had been carried out under the old Poor Law. The county councils were given the task of organising health, including the employment of doctors in the dispensaries, county hospitals and in public health. An act of the new Dáil, however, created a public appointments board. The Appointment Board was widely welcomed as mitigating some of the cronyism disfiguring public appointments in dispensaries and elsewhere in Ireland. But it did not altogether dispel these, although frequently it was personal or political animosities (often originating in the Civil War period) which fuelled conflict. This was demonstrated by the events at Loughrea in 1933 in Éire, where one hundred police were drafted to facilitate the appointment of a new dispensary medical officer, an appointment bitterly disputed by another faction in the town.[12]

Although the Appointments Board and the takeover of health by county councils were generally welcomed, there was unease among the medical profession at other changes. In 1926, the Irish language was made compulsory for some public appointments. This covered the medical posts of dispensary doctor, tuberculosis officer, medical officer of health, the medical staffs of publicly run hospitals, sanatoria and asylums. In reality there were never enough Irish speakers to fill these posts. However, the pressure arising from the Irish language requirements irritated much of the medical community, Catholic and Protestant alike. Given that learning the Irish language had been strongly linked to nationalist politics in the preceding decades, the provision acted as a ladder of opportunity for a relatively small coterie of Irish-speaking medical doctors associated with the Irish revolution.

The secretary of the BMA, Dr Thomas Hennessy, complained about this during a discussion in the Irish Senate in 1928 of a bill to bring another

---

11 For a discussion of the issues around welfare and the Northern Ireland government, see John Privilege, 'The Northern Ireland Government and the Welfare State 1942–8: The Case of Health Provision', *Irish Historical Studies*, vol. 39, no. 155, 2015, pp. 439–59.

12 See *Irish Times*, 9 September 1933, p. 7. In this case it seems like political rather than religious rivalry.

profession – the law – within the purview of the language measures. He considered that the bill had "something of the jackboot about it". He warned that as a consequence of the Irish language provisions:

> he could quite understand medical students and lawyers for that matter, but especially medical students, going to England and spending their £1,500 to get qualified there, and at the same time cultivating the customs and business habits of the country in which they expected to live.[13]

In 1931 *The Lancet* complained about an advertisement for a consultant in ophthalmology, arguing that "Knowledge of Gaelic on the part of the ophthalmologist will (not) hasten by a moment the revival of the Gaelic tongue."[14]

At the end of this period of change, what had been achieved? First, as in any revolution, power passed from some hands to others. Early in 1922 W.T. Cosgrave became Minister for Local Government and Public Health; and Michael Collins, the former guerrilla leader, was made head of the new Insurance Commission. The Insurance Commission dealt with the provisions of the National Insurance Act of 1911, parts of which applied to Ireland. Those medical men and women who had a nationalist history were, in some cases, advanced to become the voices of the new regime. There was an exodus of some of the leading voices from pre-revolution Ireland. Henry Robinson, who had headed the LGB since 1898, resigned and went to England.[15] The master of the Rotunda, Henry Jellett, emigrated to New Zealand where he continued his illustrious career. In 1926 the Registrar General, Sir William Thompson, left the post he had held from 1909.[16] The office of Registrar General was abolished and its statistical functions absorbed into a new department. As for the broader community, there is evidence of a move of Protestants to the North; and the position of Catholics in Northern Ireland, unhappy about the political settlement which put them in a largely Protestant state, became considerably more difficult. There was a palpable feeling among them that the best jobs in medicine particularly in the public health sector were now out of their reach.

13 'A Waste of Time and Money', *Irish Times*, 8 November 1928, p. 5.

14 *The Lancet*, 23 May 1931, vol. 1, pp. 1154–5.

15 See entries in the *Dictionary of Irish Biography*. Robinson (1857–1927) resigned and went to England on the advice, so it is said, of Michael Collins, the leader who lost his life at the hands of anti-Treaty forces. Robinson, a Catholic, received a baronetcy on his resignation.

16 Ibid. Sir William John Thompson (1861–1929) was President of the Statistical and Social Inquiry Society of Ireland 1918–20 and worked with Lady Aberdeen in her anti-tuberculosis research in the first decade of the twentieth century. His main medical career was spent at St Vincent's Hospital and the RCSI.

2 The Registration Crisis

The right to be admitted to the *Medical Register* of the United Kingdom had been indispensable to the migrating Irish doctor. In August 1923, however, the Executive Council of the Irish Free State convened a conference of representatives of the medical colleges to discuss the question of medical registration.[17] In 1924 the colleges advised the new government against changes, but a year later the government signalled its intention to set forth a bill creating a separate Irish *Medical Register* to be administered within Ireland. W.T. Cosgrave, the President of the Executive Council, stated:

> That such an important profession within our State should have its centre of gravity and its disciplinary headquarters in the capital of another country is held to be so incompatible with our constitutional status that we must be prepared to accept and face whatever minor and temporary disadvantage may accrue from the cessation of this previous arrangement.[18]

The minor and temporary disadvantage to which Cosgrave referred was the possibility that Irish medical graduates would not be automatically accepted on to the United Kingdom *Medical Register* and therefore lose their right to practise in Britain.

Alan Gregg was a representative of the RF who was visiting Ireland at that time to investigate the possibility of grants to the new county health boards and to medical education. He wrote to Rockefeller headquarters to observe that 'O'Higgins remarked also "I know the profession will suffer, that its schools will lose students but you must be satisfied to suffer something for the status and dignity of the country."'[19] In 1925 Gregg also sent a telegraph about the effect of this initiative to Richard M. Pearce, director of the medical sciences division at the RF in New York:

> Barry tells me neither in London nor Irish 'Times' was there any reference to exception being made of Trinity College Dublin in respect to

17 For a full discussion of the Rockefeller visit to Ireland, see Greta Jones, 'The Rockefeller Foundation and Medical Education in Ireland in the 1920s', *Irish Historical Studies*, vol. XXX, no. 120, 1997, pp. 1–17.

18 Rockefeller Foundation R.F.1.1 403A, Box 1, folder 4, Newspaper Clippings, *New York Herald*, 10 September 1925.

19 Rockefeller Foundation R.F.1.1 403A, Box 1, folder 6, Medical Education, Communication: Irish Free State Programme, 3 September 1925. The O'Higgins refers to Kevin O'Higgins, Minister for Justice.

> severing connection with General Medical Council. He and his colleague Pringle of Trinity were thunderstruck on reading declaration of Free State Government.[20]

However, Trinity was not the only medical school alarmed. The qualifying bodies in Ireland, the RCPI and RCSI, had also come out against the measure when consulted in 1923, and so did the President of University College Dublin, Denis J. Coffey, who warned that "if the Irish student does not get the opportunities he has been accustomed to he will rapidly seek medical education in England or Scotland".[21] This might result in a significant diminution of students in Free State medical schools, and even the possibility of their potential students crossing the border to Northern Ireland whose arrangements for registration on the United Kingdom list remained unchanged. There were voices in support. This included periodicals such as *The Leader*. In *The Leader*'s view:

> With the inevitable exceptions, we never thought much of the medical doctors in Ireland from an Irish point of view or those that Ireland produced for exportation. In the lump they are a poor Anglicised shoneen lot, mostly recruited from the first generation of gombeen or other parents who wanted a doctor in the family. The Irish nation is in no humour to be wagged by a crowd, particularly when we suspect that the mob of medicals are led by a string pulled by the Ascendancy gang.[22]

The Leader also pointed to what they saw as Coffey's reluctance to come out publicly against the move to create a separate Irish *Medical Register*. It was true that he had allowed his name to go forward on lists of those opposed, but "he probably knows that the change will do to his medical school no appreciable harm, he and his colleagues do not want to come out against the Ascendancy crowd who may really be hit by the change".[23]

In fact, Coffey's alarm was genuine, and in less public forums, for example to Rockefeller, he fully endorsed the campaign against a separate Irish register. In 1930 TCD sent twenty-five graduates to Britain; but during 1920–40 the percentage of UCD graduates practising in Britain was larger than TCD (32 per cent to 25 per cent). Thus, UCD had a considerable investment in access to the

---

20 Rockefeller Foundation R.F.1.1 403A, Boxes 5–7, Medical Education (Development Aid) 1923–7, Gregg to Pearce, 28 August 1925.

21 R.F.1.1. 403A, Box 1, Folder 4, Coffey to Greg, 18 September 1925.

22 'Surgeon's Knife', *The Leader*, 19 September 1925, p. 155.

23 *The Leader*, 19 September 1925, p. 152.

UK *Medical Register*. This meant that pressure behind the scenes was applied by Coffey, whatever his reluctance to speak out on an issue on which he might be accused of being insufficiently nationalist.

The battle against the proposal was fierce. Mr D. L. O'Gorman was reported sarcastically by *The Leader* as having "dilated on the fact that Irish doctors were 'scattered all over the globe'". And further, this poor down-trodden farmer, one of the class who carries the country on their shoulders, said:

> Whatever the faults of the Irish farmer, whether he was the small farmer or the middle-class man, he had always endeavoured to give a good education to his sons and daughters, and if the government's proposals were adhered to, it would render it more difficult for Irish parents to do so as they could not afford to send their sons to Belfast, Edinburgh or London.[24]

A compromise was finally achieved. The Medical Practitioner's Act of 1927 created a separate Irish *Medical Register* in the Free State, administered by Irish authorities. But the crux was that Irish doctors would still be automatically entered onto the UK register and graduates from British schools, on application, onto the Irish register, thus preserving the status quo to all intents and purposes. This continued the situation where medical schools in Ireland were inspected by the General Medical Council of the United Kingdom. Visitation and accreditation by the General Medical Council went on. Practically all Irish medical graduates maintained their listing on the UK register, given the access it offered to jobs in Britain and the British Empire. For Irish medical schools the compromise was essential for their survival at their existing size, although the view of Pearce at the headquarters of the RF in New York, among whose aims was the reduction of what they regarded as the wasteful proliferation of medical schools in Ireland, was that "personally I hope that the Irish government stands by its program. Undoubtedly, the carrying out of this program will automatically wipe out several schools and simplify the problem."[25]

3 Connections Maintained

After partition, not only did the graduates of Irish medical schools continue to be entered on the *Medical Register* of the United Kingdom, but Ireland retained representatives on the General Medical Council which carried out the

24 Quoted in *The Leader*, 29 August 1925, p. 80.
25 R.F. 403A, Box I, Folder 4, Dr. R.M. Pearce to Gregg, 24 September 1925.

periodic inspections of Ireland's schools. Irish representation on the GMC set up by the 1858 Act was generous, and in 1905 there were seven representatives from Ireland. Three were from the Royal College of Physicians of Ireland, the Royal College of Surgeons in Ireland and the Apothecaries Hall. Added to this were university representatives from the University of Dublin (Trinity College Dublin) and one from the Royal University of Ireland (representing the medical schools of the Queen's Colleges of Cork, Galway and Belfast). Additionally there was a crown appointee and one directly elected representative. This compared with seventeen representatives from England and nine from Scotland.

The Lancet pointed out in 1906 that Ireland with only 2,632 medics compared to 24,351 in England and 3,733 in Scotland was relatively well served by its representation on the GMC.[26] In 1908, following the Irish Universities Act, the Catholic Medical School became the medical school of the newly inaugurated University College Dublin and was awarded its own GMC representative. Irish representation on the GMC continued after partition, which helped maintain collegiality between British and Irish doctors.

Doctors in Ireland both North and South remained members of the British Medical Association. The BMA had an Irish committee, and from 1914 an office in Dublin and a full-time secretary, Dr Thomas Hennessy. Membership of the IMA and BMA overlapped, and cooperation continued after partition. In 1933 the annual conference of the BMA took place in Dublin, attended by delegates from both jurisdictions in Ireland and from the British Isles. In 1936 the IMA and BMA established an Irish Free State Medical Union, which in 1941 became the Medical Association of Éire. This basically combined the branches of the BMA in Southern Ireland together with those of the IMA. The members were assured that there would be no effect upon registration on the UK register and that the Free State Medical Union would continue to have rights of attendance at BMA meetings, could use the BMA library, receive the *British Medical Journal* and their IMA membership would entitle them to automatic membership of the BMA if practising in Britain.[27]

However, differences were emerging. *The Lancet* and *British Medical Journal* remained staple reading for Irish doctors, but the *Dublin Quarterly Journal of Medical Science*, the chief Irish periodical for medical science, was renamed the *Irish Journal of Medical Science* in 1925. In 1932 in Northern Ireland the *Ulster Medical Journal*, a descendant of the *Transactions of the Ulster Medical Society*, was founded to cater for the specific interests of doctors in Ulster.

26 *The Lancet*, 8 April 1905, vol. 1, p. 963. The Census of Ireland 1901 quoted a smaller figure for medical practitioners (1,331), and *The Lancet*'s figure is probably taken from the *Medical Register* for that year.

27 See 'An Irish Medical Union', *Irish Times*, 15 June 1935, p. 9.

But ties remained based on mutual professional interests, and the fact that a considerable proportion of Irish doctors continued to pursue careers in Britain. The peculiar dynamic of this can be seen in various medical organisations. Ireland had had a system of locally funded district lunatic asylums since the nineteenth century. Access to these posts was more likely for those who, after their degree, acquired a Diploma in Psychological Medicine (DPM). Again there were differences between Ireland and Britain. The Irish Board of Lunacy was separate and based in Dublin. In Ireland there was no Mental Deficiency Act (1913), which in Britain led to the growth of institutions certified by the Ministry of Health as suitable for the referral of the mentally deficient from local authorities.

Nonetheless, Irish graduates had a significant investment in seeking posts in mental institutions in Britain, as had British institutions in employing them. This meant a commonality of educational and professional interests, demonstrated by the Medico-Psychological Association of Great Britain and Ireland. In 1922 out of 676 members of the Association, 94 or 14 per cent were Irish-educated. Of the 94, one had a private address in Ireland, one a central role in the inspection system in Dublin, another was employed in an asylum in India and one was a barrister at law in England.[28] That left 90 Irish educated members attached to lunatic or mental deficiency institutions, of which 40 worked in institutions in Ireland and 50 in institutions in Britain.

Partition in 1922 did not rupture these relationships, but it would also be naïve to ignore the political consequences. Take for example the Right Hon. Michael Francis Cox, a graduate of the medical school of the Catholic University, who became president of the Royal College of Physicians of Ireland in 1922. He was also a member of the Medico-Psychological Association of Great Britain and Ireland. Cox was a Visiting Inspector of Lunacy for Ireland in Dublin. William R. Dawson, a graduate of Trinity College Dublin, had also been Inspector of Lunatic Asylums working from Dublin Castle. He was President of the Medico-Psychological Association 1911–12 and co-editor of its journal, the *Journal of Mental Science* 1920–21. He took an opposite political path to Cox, becoming Chief Medical Officer for the new Ministry of Home Affairs established in Northern Ireland in 1922. Nonetheless, presidents of the Association continued to be appointed from both parts of Ireland, including Michael J. Nolan, Medical Superintendent of Downpatrick Asylum in 1924 and Richard R. Leeper of St Patrick's Hospital Dublin in 1931.[29]

---

28 Probably dealing with cases of committal.

29 See Greta Jones, 'Eugenics in Ireland: The Belfast Eugenics Society', *Irish Historical Studies*, vol. XXVIII, no. 109, May 1992, pp. 81–95. Both Leeper and Nolan took part in the debate on whether the provisions of the Mental Deficiency Act 1913 should be enacted in Ireland.

4 The Border in Ireland

Arguably the most significant consequences for medicine were the borders not between Britain and Ireland but within Ireland. Religious segregation in medical education increased throughout the nineteenth century, and partition strengthened the process.[30] In 1908–9, 94.5 percent of all students at Queen's Belfast's medical school were from Ireland, of which 89.9 percent were from the historic nine counties of Ulster.[31] In 1937–8 the proportion from Ulster had risen to 96.5 per cent. During that session, only 25 students from outside Ulster were among the 724 recorded as attending. There was a greater likelihood, at least in that year, of being from the British West Indies (3) than from other parts of Ireland (2), and certainly more chance of being from Britain than the twenty-six counties of independent Ireland.[32]

The other effect was that Queen's medical school grew, reflecting the greater reluctance of Northern students to cross the border in search of a medical education. In 1860 Queen's medical students accounted for only 11 per cent of the total of first-year students in Ireland, but by 1935 it was 25 per cent or a quarter of all students. The connection between this and the troubled politics of the country is indicated by the figure of 34 per cent of first-year students which it recorded in 1930 at the end of a period of unprecedented upheaval and rapid change in the South. UCD's figure for first year students in Ireland was around a quarter.[33]

Trinity medical school still educated around 18 per cent of first- year medical students in 1935, and 16 per cent 1945–60. This was far more than the falling population of Protestants in the South, and it shows that TCD was still able to attract some Catholics, students from the North and, due to its historic reputation, from outside Ireland. In fact 48 per cent of all foreign students, that is from outside Ireland, in the Southern university system were in Trinity in 1964–5, compared with 20 per cent in UCD.[34] However, a cold wind blew through Trinity after 1922 and 'the Trinity-educated doctor' entered the demonology of the Irish Catholic Church. This led in 1944 to the stipulation by the Archbishop of Dublin John McQuaid that Catholics attending Trinity required a special dispensation from the Church. It was not wholly effective, but nonetheless symptomatic of the Catholic Church's hostility.[35]

---

30 Kelly, *Irish Medical Education and Student Culture c.1850–1950*, pp. 214–18.

31 *QUB Calendar for 1910*, Table IV, p. 25.

32 *QUB Calendar for 1938–9*, Students in Attendance Faculty of Medicine, pp. 513–25.

33 See the tables in the Appendix.

34 'Report of the Commission on Higher Education 1960–7', vol. 2, Table 170, p. 793.

35 J.H. Whyte, *Church and State in Modern Ireland, 1923–1970* (Dublin: Gill and Macmillan, 1971), pp. 305–6.

In a more religiously segregated system, the legislative framework for practising medicine became more Catholic in the Free State. In 1929 a Censorship Act was passed banning the dissemination of information on birth control. This demand would, one doctor stated, "take many back" because of "the virtual branding of propaganda in favour of birth control as indecent".[36] To the protest of members of the RCPI in 1929, and to the consternation of some members of the Irish legislature, even discussion of contraception was no longer possible, at least publicly, in the South.[37]

The banning of advocacy of birth control was followed in 1935 by a provision in the Criminal Law Amendment Act stopping the import and sale of contraceptives. Although Ireland as a whole was no beacon of contraceptive practice, its demographic history has shown that some form of birth control was beginning to take root, at least among the urban middle classes.[38] In the socially conservative North, the Stormont government did not publicly embrace contraception either, and it refused Marie Stopes' demand that local government in Ireland follow their counterparts in Britain in 1930 and provide limited access to birth control information. Nonetheless, a Marie Stopes Birth Control Clinic with support among some doctors in Northern Ireland was set up there in 1936.[39]

Relationships between North and South often became acrimonious. Although after partition the free movement of people and their right of residence in both parts of Ireland and Britain was maintained, this did not preclude attempts on the part of the Northern Ireland government to restrict the flow of labour into the North from the South. Behind this was alarm that migration from the South might alter the religious balance of the North. This hostility affected medical appointments, particularly in the public sector. In 1935 a circular from the Northern Ministry of Home Affairs required medical officers appointed to dispensary posts in Northern Ireland to be of British parentage and have lived for five years in Great Britain or Northern Ireland. This was condemned by Newry Council, a largely nationalist town in Northern Ireland. In 1935 they had appointed a Monaghan doctor from across the border to

36 *The Lancet*, 18 August 1928, vol. 2, p. 889.

37 For a discussion of these issues, see Greta Jones, 'Marie Stopes in Ireland: The Belfast Mother's Clinic 1936–4', *Social History of Medicine*, vol. 5, no. 2, August 1992, pp. 255–7.

38 Cormac Ó Gráda, 'New Evidence on the Fertility Transition in Ireland 1880–1911', *Demography*, vol. 28, no. 4, 1991, pp. 535–48.

39 For a discussion of the issues, see Jones, 'Marie Stopes in Ireland'1992, pp. 255–77. See also Lyndsey Earner-Byrne, *Mother and Child: Maternity and Child Welfare in Dublin 1920s–1960s* (Manchester: Manchester University Press, 2007); and Leanne McCormick, '"The Scarlet Woman in Person": The Establishment of a Family Planning Service in Northern Ireland 1950–1974', *Social History of Medicine*, vol. 21, no. 2, 2008, pp. 345–60.

the post of Mullaghglass Dispensary in defiance of the ban. The unfortunate doctor, now resident in Armagh in Northern Ireland, contested his exclusion. He claimed to be a British citizen of British parentage, and in fact had been appointed on 14 November 1935 twelve days before the order was issued. But his claim was dismissed in 1937 by a court in Belfast.[40]

Northern Ireland certainly exhibited a closed and defensive attitude to perceived incursion from the Free State. The introduction of the National Health Service into Northern Ireland in 1949 increased fears of further immigration from the South. The Safeguarding of Employment Act of 1948 was an attempt by the Northern Ireland government to control the flow of labour into Northern Ireland from the South. Discussion took place about applying it to medical personnel. The National Health Service had effectively created a significant increase in jobs and practices in Northern Ireland, thereby leading some Southern doctors, at least according to anecdote, to move North.[41] The topic was discussed by the Ulster Unionist Council in the early 1950s.[42] On 5 January 1951 the executive committee of the Ulster Unionist Council considered a resolution from Mid and West Tyrone Unionist Association:

> That the Parliament of Northern Ireland be requested to carry into effect legislation to ensure that only professional men born in Northern Ireland and GB will be employed under the NHS of Northern Ireland and that doctors, dentists, chiropodists and other professional born in Eire be precluded from taking advantage of the higher [sic] Health Service in NI.

One of the Tyrone members of the executive, Mr Allen, argued that this was “a very dangerous resolution to be discussed at conference”. Brian Faulkner, a future Prime Minister of Northern Ireland, commented that “the people of Tyrone have great feeling about it”. The Executive Committee decided to write to Tyrone pointing out that “if this resolution was discussed publicly at the conference it would only be used against us by our enemies”. In fact the provisions of the Safeguarding of Employment Act were not extended to public medical appointments.[43]

40 ‘Free State Doctor Banned’, *Irish Times*, 29 April 1937, p. 13.

41 The existence of a large Catholic minority in the North meant that it was accepted that Catholic doctors should be educated at Queen’s so that Catholic areas could have access to Catholic doctors. The issue was to do with publicly funded posts.

42 PRONI D/1327/6/23, Papers of the Ulster Unionist Council, Meeting of the Executive Committee, 5 January 1951 and January 1952. (Thanks to Professor Henry Patterson who supplied this reference.)

43 PRONI D/1327/6/23, Papers of the Ulster Unionist Council, Meeting of the Executive Committee, 5 January 1951 and January 1952.

Catholics in Queen's University Belfast (all faculties) constituted around 25 per cent of the students in 1915, lower than the Catholic population in the six counties of Northern Ireland as a whole. In 1926 the percentage of Catholics in the population of Northern Ireland was 33.5 per cent. But Catholic students at Queen's dropped in subsequent years to around 20 per cent, rising again to between 22 and 25 per cent in 1960.[44] Relative economic disadvantage among the Catholic population might account for this, but also a sense among the Catholic middle class of the North that the short journey to a medical school in Dublin or elsewhere in the Free State might be more professionally advantageous in the long run.

The medical school at Queen's always expected to educate a proportion of Catholics in anticipation of the needs of the Catholic population of Northern Ireland, although entry into the medical school was the most competitive among the faculties. However, the religious composition of the two major hospitals in Northern Ireland – the Royal Victoria largely Protestant and the Mater largely Catholic – was felt by some Catholics to reduce their opportunities after graduation. Catholics were expected train in the Mater and Protestants in the other hospitals, particularly the Royal Victoria. Also affecting opportunity were networks of referral and patronage in medicine. Inevitably the unrest of the early 1920s in the North affected these and Catholics suspected, correctly in many cases, that Protestant co-religionists would be favoured over Catholics.[45]

5 The Future of Medicine in Ireland

Opinion in Ireland differed on the likely future of Irish medicine after the border was erected. Surgeon McArdle believed in 1922: "There can be no doubt but that new found liberty will cause a rejuvenescence (sic) all round and that our profession should be foremost in taking advantage of the heartening

44 The Catholic population in 1961 was about 34.9 per cent. Figures from Vaughan and Fitzpatrick, *Irish Historical Statistics: Population 1821–1971*, Table 15, p. 50. Figures for Catholics at Queen's are from the Catholic Chaplaincy and supplied to me courtesy of Professor Leslie Clarkson.

45 On the first point, a Catholic doctor returning to celebrate his graduation from Queen's after a distinguished career in the United States confided after graduation his disappointment when it was expected that he would naturally gravitate to the Mater for postgraduate training and posts. He felt that this was unnecessarily restrictive and militated against his advancement in medicine. Subsequently, on arrival in the USA he sat the Examination for Foreign Medical Graduates as the means to establish a right to practise in the USA. He considered the EFMG to be extremely undemanding compared with the undergraduate education he had received. (Personal communication.) See Chapter 7 for the position of Irish medical migrants to the USA.

conditions that are sure to prevail."[46] Others were not so sure. An editorial on the registration question in the *Irish Times* in 1925 claimed:

> Two ideals are at war in this country. One is the idea of international culture which admits no barrier to the march of science and seeks to keep Ireland in the forefront of the ever advancing movement of human thought. The other is the parochial ideal which would put on our country a double bereavement of brain and soul. By the accident of fate Ireland missed the blessings of the Roman civilisation; and now some of her sons seek to isolate her from the civilisation of the twentieth century.[47]

Which of these two predictions was true? Dr Thomas Hennessy, the Irish secretary to the BMA, reminded his colleagues that "medical science like all other sciences acknowledges no territorial or national limitations".[48] It is true that preoccupation with revival of language in the Free State caused some interruptions to the progress of medical science. The RF complained that the public health officials they had sent to the USA for training to help develop the new County Health Boards in the Free State found it hard to get jobs back in Ireland and had decamped to Britain for employment, a situation they partly blamed on the preference for Irish language speakers. There was also reluctance to engage with British research institutions. The First World War had seen the development in Britain of a Ministry of Health and a concomitant research organisation, the Medical Research Council (MRC). In a reply to a query in a letter of 11 April 1922 asking for a transfer of a portion of the MRC's funds to the Provisional government in the South, they were told there was nothing to stop applications for research money from Ireland so long as Ireland retained Dominion status, a constitutional position already enshrined in the Treaty of 1922.[49] But there was very low take-up of the offer.

J.W. Bigger, who ran the bacteriology department at TCD, approached the MRC in the late 1930s and was successful in obtaining funding.[50] In the 1950s, when the RF was considering a grant for genetics research at Trinity, he was described by them as being very active and the bacteriological tradition he

---

46 *BMJ*, 4 February 1922, vol. 1, p. 206.

47 "Science at Bay", a leading article in the *Irish Times*, quoted in *The Leader*, 29 August 1925, p. 78. *The Leader* described the *Irish Times* as "Arnott's organ of England's Faithful Garrison in Ireland", ibid. Arnott was the publisher and owner of the *Irish Times*.

48 *BMJ*, 4 February 1922, vol. 1, p. 206.

49 National Archives Kew, FD1/3562 MRC. Ireland and DD1/2754 Research in Ireland 1919–27.

50 Bigger (1891–1951) was also Dean of TCD's medical school until 1939 and Professor of Preventive Medicine and Bacteriology until 1950.

established at TCD as 'excellent', although they considered it unduly linked to the medical school. However, applications from elsewhere in Ireland were modest and small-scale, and it was not until 1939 that the Free State set up its own medical research body. By the 1960s the Rockefeller had awarded only around eleven grants to the arts and sciences in Ireland, of which several were minor awards for travel and equipment. There were only three scientific projects of importance. Two were awarded to the growing genetics programme at Trinity in the 1950s and 1960s. Queen's bio-chemistry in the 1950s received one and Arthur Conway, the physicist at UCD, another.[51] Although Conway was a physicist, he was using his equipment to look at cell structure, thus continuing a tradition by which the medical school played a crucial role in Irish scientific endeavour.[52] Conway was the only recipient in science from the RF within the National University of Ireland, apart from the occasional travel or training grant.

There were other fractures and diverging destinations in the medical profession. These are exemplified by Dr Leonard Kidd, a Protestant from Enniskillen educated at Foyle College and TCD. He was secretary of the Irish Medical Association (IMA) and played a leading role in the doctors' boycott of 1902.[53] In 1906 he decided to stand for the one seat on the GMC earmarked for an elected representative. He stood against Sir William Thompson, an important scion of the Dublin medical world. Kidd's platform was the needs of the provincial general practitioner. He won, though by the narrowest of margins: by 909 votes to the 901 cast for Thompson.[54] However, partition placed Enniskillen into Northern Ireland. Kidd continued to agitate on behalf of dispensary doctors, but now his attention refocused on Northern Ireland, inevitably given that the conditions of dispensary doctors in the North were determined by the Northern Ireland government at Stormont. Towards the end of his life, in the late 1930s, he discussed the greater involvement of the government in health, which he saw coming in Britain and to which he was on the whole favourable. The change in government involvement in health in Britain led to the foundation of the National Health Service, which caused further divergence

51 RF 403 A, 1.1 Projects. These records contain the folders on science research in Irish universities.

52 E.J. Conway FRS (1894–1965), appointed to UCD 1934–63.

53 Kidd died in 1941. As well as general practice, he was medical officer (MO) for Portora School, a keen fan of Irish rugby and the author of an article in the *Ulster Medical Journal*, vol. VII, no. 4, 1938, pp. 229–40, about the future development of the British Ministry of Health. His case illustrates the effect of the border in refocusing previously common interests on politically bounded ones.

54 *The Lancet*, 31 March 1906, vol. 1, p. 937. There were 2,800 eligible to vote.

between health systems in Northern Ireland and the Free State. Kidd had been a popular doctor and a leading representative of the provincial medical practitioner, but partition meant that his interests were directed to the state in which he now found himself.

Nonetheless, there were countervailing forces. Doctors continued to look to the Royal Colleges in Dublin for postgraduate qualifications and professional recognition. Some students from the North still went to Dublin for a medical education. A sense of the particularity of Irish medical history survived among the medical community. The public health systems in both states had common roots, even if they began to diverge. Migration also served as a unifying force. Many doctors in 1945 had experienced practice in Britain before the border and this tradition went on. Others from the South went on joining the British armed services and the colonial medical service. But undoubtedly the widening administrative and legislative divergences between Northern Ireland and the Free State had an effect on Irish medicine. So too did the cultural impact of partition on the practitioners of medicine.

6 The Notion of Being Irish and Emigration

Senia Paseta has discussed at length the impact of the rise of nationalism in Ireland in the late nineteenth century on the educated Catholic professional. It was assumed that they would be leaders in an independent Ireland, but, as *The Leader's* strictures on the medical profession show, a section of nationalism did not altogether trust them, believing them to be too British in their outlook and too integrated into the British institutions. This led *The Leader* to accuse Catholic professionals of "cringe and snobbery".[55]

On the outbreak of the First World War, the majority of Catholic doctors and some Protestants would describe themselves not only as Irish but also as Home Rulers. They may have believed that Home Rule would eventually lead to total separation, but, on the whole, they belonged to the moderate wing of nationalism. The war and the Sinn Féin rebellion of 1916 destroyed, politically at least, this wing of Irish nationalism. Just how significant this was can be seen from the involvement of many nationalist members of the medical profession in the First World War preceding 1916.

---

55 Senia Paseta, *Before the Revolution: Nationalism, Social Change and Ireland's Catholic Elite 1879–1922* (Cork: Cork University Press, 1999), p. 125, quoted in *The Leader*, 13 March 1901.

According to the UCD list of war service compiled at the conclusion of the Great War, 478 graduates and undergraduates of the college served in the war.[56] Of these 323 were medical.[57] They included ten on the college staff, of whom eight were medical. Sixteen of the forty-three killed in action are identifiable by a medical degree, and of the twenty DSMs (Distinguished Service Medals) awarded, sixteen went to doctors, who also took thirty-six of the forty-seven Military Crosses. Six OBEs all went to doctors, generally for administrative and organisational leadership. The Croix de Guerre was awarded to seven UCD graduates, often in addition to a British award. Six of these recipients were medics. The rallying to the flag happened on the expectation that, at the conclusion of the war, Home Rule for Ireland would ensue. But after the Rising of 1916 the mood of nationalist Ireland swung sharply towards more republican and extreme versions of independence. Already many medical students in Catholic colleges had signalled impatience with the aspiration of Home Rule and sought more radical solutions. However, after the new state was set up, Irish medicine remained still highly dependent on emigration and this affected even those who welcomed the nationalist revolution in Ireland. The impact of this can be revealed in brief biographies of those who went to Britain after 1922 to earn their living.

Richard Mulcahy came from a prominent nationalist family.[58] He graduated from UCD in 1939, and as he put it, "To follow a career in cardiology after leaving St Vincent's it was necessary for me to go to England."[59] There he "realised how inadequate my training had been".[60] Mulcahy was critical of his fellow Irish doctors in England. He considered that "Some of the Irish I met seemed to live in a fantasy world constantly aware of their origins and proclaiming nostalgia for Ireland."[61] The institution in which he first worked was "populated by NUI students all immigrants or birds of passage". Richard Mulcahy worked in cardiology at a private heart hospital run by a religious order. He believed that "many hospitals in England had the same experience as mine at St John's and Elizabeth's; once an Irish graduate had joined the resident staff he was

56 UCD Archives, *Graduates and Students in His Majesty's Forces 1914–1919. Roll of Honour.*

57 Sometimes the medics are classed as surgeon probationer, and these have been counted. If the roll of honour gives only a year of entry, their school cannot be identified and so they have been left out.

58 His father, also Richard Mulcahy, had taken part in the 1916 Rising and rose to a leading position in the army of the new Irish state.

59 Mulcahy, *Memoirs of a Medical Maverick*, Dublin, Liberties Press, 2015, p. 60.

60 Ibid., p. 67.

61 Ibid., p. 65.

followed by a succession of Irish graduates".[62] Mulcahy returned eventually to become a leading cardiologist in Dublin.

The Catholic Hospital was not, however, the only site of encounter. Michael P. Flynn, after graduating from UCD, left Ireland for a job in Birmingham in 1940. There he joined a practice which included a Dr Ryan from Cork, whom he described as "very English orientated".[63] Then moving on through the assistance of a medical agency, Philip Harris, he secured a job at Coleshill Hall Hospital, which in 1934 had become a certified hospital for mental defectives. At Coleshill was James Clark Rohan, who had graduated from Cork in 1920 and is part of the cohort examined in Chapter 4. Rohan had been appointed Deputy Medical Superintendent in 1935, the year he received a Diploma of Psychological Medicine (DPM) awarded by Cork.[64] In his time at Coleshill, Flynn acquired not just Irish friends and colleagues, but a sense of the liberal and progressive practices which characterised Rohan's contribution to the interpretation and management of mental deficiency.[65]

There is in fact a constant ambiguity among those Irish doctors with a background in nationalism who moved between Ireland and Britain or settled in Britain to pursue their professional career. An example of this is Gearóid P. Crookes, born in Cork in 1916 but brought up in Dublin. He came from a family strongly committed to the Irish cultural revival and to political nationalism. However, after graduating from UCD, he also contemplated emigration. This was the start of the Second World War and it occurred to Crookes that "one had to face the possibility of emigration to war-time Britain where the ultimate prospect of service with the RAMC was all too likely". Although this was "no ignoble ambition", not every young patriotic Irishman would regard it as his first choice.[66] On the fall of France, Crookes decided that Ireland might be in danger from a German invasion, and the best way to protect Ireland was to join the Irish army. He spent three rather boring and frustrating years in an army camp in Ireland, well away from the battlefields of the Second World War. Then he went to Birmingham, where he gained experience in ophthalmology. In 1946 he returned to Ireland and set up in private practice, acquiring several consultancies. His stay in England was short, but it did equip him with advanced education in his subject.

---

62 Ibid., p. 66.

63 Flynn, *Medical Doctor of Many Parts*, p. 5.

64 Rohan was also a consultant psychiatrist for Birmingham Regional Hospital and a member of the Medico-Psychological Association and well published in the area of mental deficiency.

65 Flynn, *Medical Doctor of Many Parts*, p. 11.

66 Gearóid P. Crookes, *Far Away and Long Ago: A Memoir* (Dublin: Tudor House Press, 2003), p. 145.

Identification with Ireland was important, even among those born in England who happily volunteered for military service in the British army. Charles Stewart Parnell Hamilton, born in 1891, was the grandson of an Irish emigrant doctor, Henry Hamilton, who had moved to England in 1854 at a late stage in his medical career.[67] Taking a fancy to Kent in southern England, Henry Hamilton took up a practice in Chilham. He retired there and eventually passed on the practice to his son, Henry Thomas. The family had political connections to the Irish nationalist movement. Charles's maternal grandfather was the founder of the *Waterford News*, a strong nationalist newspaper, and Henry Thomas named his son after the Irish nationalist politician Charles Stewart Parnell.[68]

Charles Stewart Parnell Hamilton received his education at Charing Cross Hospital. At the outbreak of the First World War he joined the RAMC. Hamilton joined the British army again in 1939, two exemplary contributions to the survival of the British Empire. At the same time Hamilton was sentimentally attached to the notion of his Irishness. He holidayed in Ireland and retired there in 1947, to a country in which he was neither born, educated, nor carried out his professional life but to which he felt a strong emotional attachment.

Hamilton himself pondered the significance of this. After touring the Dublin hospitals, he wrote a celebratory poem published in the *Journal of the Irish Medical Association* on the thoughts of an Irish medical graduate. In it he conjures up the famous medical schools of Ireland and the great figures in Irish medicine. But Hamilton was not a graduate of an Irish medical school. At the end of the poem he asks:

> Was I wrong to pen this theme? I, an exile from the scene?
> No, a father's memories never perish,
> His thoughts his sons must ever cherish.[69]

The political history of Irish nationalism formed a significant part of Hamilton's psyche, even whilst his career in England and abroad was typical of many of his English peers. But there was another dimension to Hamilton's Irishness: the importance to him of Catholicism. Where did this leave Protestant doctors? What implications were there for them if being Irish was to embrace a special position for the Catholic Church and the Irish language? The historiography of Irish identity and the views expressed above suggest that, even for

---

67 Henry Hamilton is recorded in the *Medical Register* of 1859 as a licentiate of the Apothecaries Hall London (1838) and member of the Royal College of Surgeons of England (1842).

68 Hamilton, *East, West: An Irish Doctor's Memories*, pp. 1–2.

69 From *JIMA*, vol. XXXIV, March 1951, p. 180.

Catholic doctors, understanding the meaning of all this, particularly if working in Britain, was not easy.[70] In 1943 the Protestant, nationalist doctor Robert Collis set out his views. In politics he was an Irish nationalist, by birth and upbringing Protestant. His sense of nationality was built on the specificity of Irishness in medicine. He commented that "Irish medical education emphasises 'the personal, the intimate' ... it reflects the soul of the people ... It is carried by migrants and ensures them a good reception throughout the world."[71] But just what was this sentiment, and how did it affect those Irish doctors who left Ireland to work in Britain?

7 Conclusion

Partition in 1922 represented a major cataclysm in the political history of Ireland. Its reverberations were political, economic and personal. The fact that since 1922 both new jurisdictions produced their own political and social histories reflects this. All-Ireland histories since 1922 are rare, though interesting and instructive.

In the case of health there are clear demarcations which arose after partition. The economic depression in the inter-war years hit Northern Ireland industries particularly hard - Ireland's heavy industries were concentrated in Ulster. Northern Ireland was less economically successful than it had been in the prosperous years before the First World War. The new state of Northern Ireland, as well paying for its own domestic upkeep, was expected to contribute annually to the Imperial Exchequer. In fact the political violence in its early years followed by economic depression made this impossible. The Government of Northern Ireland regularly approached the Westminster government for subventions and were, in many instances, successful. Additionally, the National Insurance system in Northern Ireland covered health but not in the Irish Free State. However, the Northern Ireland insurance fund in this period was insufficient to provide their insured population with benefits equivalent

70 The problem of conflicting identity is discussed in Oonagh Walsh, ed., *Ireland Abroad: Politics and the Professions in the Nineteenth Century* (Dublin: Four Courts Press, 2003); Louise Ryan and Wendy Webster, eds., *Gendering Migration: Masculinity, Femininity and Ethnicity in Post-War Britain* (Aldershot: Ashgate Press, 2008); and D.A.J. MacPherson and Mary J. Hickman, eds., *Women and Irish Diaspora Identities: Theories, Concepts and New Perspectives* (Manchester: Manchester University Press, 2014). The books cited include discussions on migrants to the British National Health Service.

71 Robert Collis, *The State of Medicine in Ireland* (The Carmichael Lecture) (Dublin: Parkside Press, 1943), p. 12.

to those in the rest of the United Kingdom and this shortfall was also made up from the central United Kingdom insurance fund. Though serious medical problems arose among Belfast's working-class communities often linked to poverty, the difference in living standards between the two jurisdictions was still important in the inter-war period and was to become even more marked with the arrival of the National Health Service.

In other respects Northern Ireland diverged from the state in the South who used the opportunity afforded by Partition to reform the health service. The workhouse system was abolished and County Health Boards were created to run public health. This attracted the attention of the RF who lent support to this experiment. Hospital development was on parallel lines in both states and, with the introduction in the South of the Irish Sweepstake in 1930, money found its way into hospitals in the Free State. The dispensary doctor remained a distinctive feature of both jurisdictions.

Both new states were a combination of inheritance from the old United Kingdom system before 1922 but with distinctive features reflective of their particular social and religious concatenations. By the 1940s, however, the coming of the National Health Service drew Northern Ireland's health system closer to that of the British Isles and away from that in the Republic of Ireland.

The impact of Partition on the profession of medicine was more complex. First medical emigration from Ireland to Britain continued to be a major factor which survived the Irish War of Independence, the Treaty which followed in 1922, the unilateral declaration of a Republic of Ireland in 1949 and subsequent decades. Professional and educational alignment was still important to facilitate emigration and – whilst it was questioned by some Irish nationalists in the 1920s and led to the creation of a separate *Medical Register* for Ireland – it had minimal impact. The Irish medical schools, North and South, continued to educate students for export to Britain and the British Empire, after graduation entrance onto the United Kingdom *Medical Register* was routine and all Irish medical schools received visits of inspection from the General Medical Council of the United Kingdom. The British Medical Association and the Irish Medical Association, though separate organisations, frequently worked together and offered joint membership, of particular value to those contemplating emigration. In Northern Ireland medical emigration also remained a significant feature. In that respect both jurisdictions shared models of medical education while its students had similar aspirations. This meant the fracturing of medicine was limited.

But it did occur. The degree of interaction between the North's medical school, Queen's University Belfast, and schools in the south remained roughly the same – all medical schools in Ireland were in competition with each other for students. But there is some evidence of increased self-segregation along denominational lines. The mitigating factors were the professional ties which survived and were important in maintaining links. But from time to time politics intruded in medicine. In Northern Ireland it led to measures to try and reduce access to public health jobs for Southern-born or educated citizens of the Irish Free State. In the Free State it took the form of attempts to tighten denominational control over medical education and medical practice.

CHAPTER 6

The Irish Doctor in Interwar Britain

Between 1860 and 1960 Britain was the chief destination for Irish medical migrants.[1] During 1900–5 52 per cent of Irish medical emigrants from our cohorts were in Britain, but in the interwar years the proportion rose. The total number of medical migrants from Ireland every five years between 1920 and 1940 was 528; and of these, 398 or 75 per cent went to Britain.[2] Some of this rise can be attributed to the gradual decline of medical opportunities in the colonial service and armed forces. They were still an important resource for the Irish medical graduate, and during the Second World War and shortly afterwards the numbers of Irishmen and women in the services rose. But as the British Empire entered its twilight years, so too did the chances of making a medical living there. Table 14 shows the extent of migration to Britain for three years 1920, 1925, 1930, and the schools from which they came. The three cohorts will become the main focus of this chapter. Emigrants in 1935 and 1940 were arriving in Britain very close to 1939 so their experience, whilst similar in many respects to the typical 1920s and 1930s emigrant, was interrupted by the outbreak of the Second World War.

For the years 1920, 1925, 1930, Irish medical schools exported around 38 per cent of their graduates in total to Britain.[3] In 1930, due to the uncertain economic situation, numbers of emigrants fell but recovered in 1935. The University of Dublin (Trinity College Dublin) remained a high exporter of graduates. For example, 76 graduates from the sample of 1920–40 were practising in England after ten years, but a further 61 were in colonial service, the IMS, army and navy or other destinations. This was by far the highest number of any of the schools examined for the interwar years. In contrast QUB and UCD had 34 medical graduates between them in colonial or military service or in destinations other than Britain for the same period.

1 Emigration to Scotland from Irish medical schools was very low, only 5 out of the total of 326 for the three years selected. Scotland was an exporter of graduates to Britain, easily overtaking Ireland in the numbers who set up practice there after graduation.
2 See the table in the Appendix.
3 In these calculations the total number including the untraceables are included.

 | DOI:10.1163/9789004324466_008

TABLE 14 Numbers of medical graduates from Irish schools migrating to England, Scotland and Wales for 1920, 1925, 1930

	1920	1920	1925	1925	1930	1930			
School	Grads	Migrants to Britain	Grads	Migrants to Britain	Grads	Migrants to Britain	Total grads	Total migrants to Britain	Percentage
Galway	9	4	16	7	7	1	32	12	37%
Cork	29	11	61	26	21	8	111	45	40%
RCS	46	22	49	25	17	3	112	50	45%
TCD	52	16	100	37	34	9	186	62	33%
UCD	77	27	71	26	69	25	217	78	36 %
QUB	63	36	82	27	53	16	198	79	40%
Total	276	116	379	148	201	50	856	326	38%

SOURCES: GRADUATE LISTS OF IRISH MEDICAL SCHOOLS AND THE *MEDICAL REGISTER* AND *MEDICAL DIRECTORY*

1 The National Insurance Act and Migration

Emigration was affected by significant changes to medical provision in England and Wales arising out of the implementation of the British National Insurance Act of 1911. Among its provisions the Act set up a compulsory insurance scheme, including medical benefit, for "all workmen over sixteen and earning less than £160 per annum".[4] At first it applied to certain designated trades but by 1920 it had been extended to cover over 11 million workers in the United Kingdom, and over the years more occupations were gradually drawn into the scheme. By 1938 it covered over 16 million people.[5]

Out of this fund certain benefits were available to the insured person. They included unemployment benefit, the main purpose for which the scheme had been devised but also certain medical benefits,[6] including the provision of a doctor and medical treatment. Under the scheme doctors could register to work under the National Insurance Act and claim back fees for the work they performed. Work was delegated and supervised by a local Insurance Committee, popularly known as 'the panel', appointed under the act. The fee scale was set by central government. Populous towns and poor rural areas had previously been regarded as less remunerative for a doctor than a wealthy suburb or a seaside town. However, the act made working-class industrial towns and cities more desirable for the doctor by creating an insured population there.

The coming of National Insurance had its opponents among doctors, particularly in Ireland where it was considered, like the dispensary system, a means to squeeze the doctor's income from private practice. Together with the opposition of the Catholic Church to any intervention by the state in matters of health, this meant that Ireland never developed the medical benefits available in the British Insurance scheme. There was also opposition in Britain from private insurance companies and from doctors wary of becoming, in the view of some of them, employees of the state. In contrast Joseph Daniel McFeely, an Irish doctor who had worked in Britain for many years, described himself as very much in favour of the National Insurance Act, believing that 'Medical Clubs and Tontines' were not enough to secure satisfactory medical services for the poor. He described Liverpool where he had worked, as hotbed of opposition to the act,

4 Bentley B. Gilbert, *The Evolution of National Insurance in Great Britain: Origins of the Welfare State* (London: Michael Joseph, 1966; second impression 1973), p. 355.

5 Hermann Levy, *National Health Insurance: A Critical Study* (Cambridge: Cambridge University Press, 1944), p. 123.

6 The provisions for medical benefit under the National Insurance Act of 1911 did not apply in Ireland.

but noted that "two days afterwards [after its introduction] there was a regular stampede to join the panel".[7] Nonetheless, McFeely expressed concern about the amount of red tape in the life of a panel doctor and the frequently disagreeable tone of his negotiations with the Insurance Committee on the subject.[8]

Mr Brock from the Ministry of Health gave evidence to the Royal Commission on the Workings of National Health Insurance in 1925, estimating that around 18,000 doctors were engaged in Insurance work. Most doctors had some panel practice: 35 per cent had lists of patients of 600 or less; another 35 per cent had between 1,200 and 2,000; while the remaining 30 per cent fell somewhere between the two.[9] A panel list of 1,000 patients, at a capitation fee of 11 shillings per person, could net a salary of over £500 per annum; a list of 2,000 could net over £1000,[10] which provided a reasonable income. Those whose panel lists were much lower still benefited from the additional income that the Insurance system brought. The panel list could be increased to well over 2,000 by employing an assistant, or setting up a joint or group practice. This became more common in the interwar years.

Brock went on to describe the distribution of panel work:

> In the mainly industrial areas where you do not get any considerable well-to-do population, it may be taken that probably 100% of the active general practitioners are on the panel. I find, in fact, that in Walsall, West Bromwich, Dudley, Burnley, Rochdale and Wigan, practically all the general practitioners are on the panel but when it comes to bigger cities such as Birmingham and Sheffield which both have medical schools, there is of course a larger proportion of consultants and border line men who are partly general practitioners and partly consultants.

He went on to calculate that the proportion of panel doctors in Birmingham was 64 per cent and 66 per cent in Sheffield. The more rural or well-to-do an

---

7 Joseph Daniel McFeely, *Reflections of an Old and Observant General Practitioner* (London: Edward O. Beck, *c.*1930), p. 84.

8 Medical benefit under the Act was distributed by the Insurance Committees from a panel of doctors registered with them for that purpose. Hence, they were called panel practices or panel doctors.

9 Brock, Minutes of Evidence taken before the Royal Commission on National Health Insurance, vol. 1, (London: HMSO, 1925), p. 52, paras. 1038–42 and 1047–8.

10 The rate was 11 shilling in 1925, but the BMA was pushing for this to be raised to 13s.6d. Another issue at this time was the transfer of panel practices. They could not be bought, but 'goodwill' and recommendation by the retiring doctor might play a part in helping a candidate accede to a practice; see "The Insurance Practice Settlement", *The Lancet*, 24 June 1920, vol. 1, p. 205; and ibid., 7 February 1920, p. 331.

area, the fewer panel doctors there were, and "in Devonshire (a rural area) there are only 54 percent, in Cambridge, it drops to 41 percent and in Kent 61 percent." In Bournemouth and Torquay (seaside towns) it fell well below 40 per cent.[11]

The coming of health insurance did not resolve the large disparities between areas in the provision of doctors. Southport, a commuter and seaside town in Lancashire, had one doctor to every 598.6 inhabitants in 1930. Torquay and Bournemouth were similar seaside towns, and Brock singled them out for having low numbers of panel doctors but a high number of doctors per population, one to 555.36 and 424.8 respectively. The high proportion of retired elderly in these towns contributed to this, but they were also wealthier towns and the difference in number of doctors between the better off areas and most industrial and urban conurbations is still striking. The ratio of doctors to the population in middle class towns such as Chichester and Harrogate was respectively one to 653.3 and one to 381.2,

In the towns described by Brock as being largely served by panel doctors the ratio of doctor to the population was much lower. In Dudley it was one to 3287, in Walsall one to 3028.9 and West Bromwich one to 2727.66. Interestingly in 1926 the three towns of Wigan, Burnley and Rochdale were better supplied with doctors than the other towns singled out as having a high concentration of panel doctors. They were older industrial areas where mining (Wigan) and textiles (Burnley and Rochdale) were concentrated. In these places there was an insured population but additionally an established tradition of voluntary clubs and insurance societies catering to a working-class population. Burnley and Rochdale were textile towns, which meant that a high percentage of the female population was also insured; and miners, before the First World War, were among the higher paid industrial workers. There were more doctors to population in these towns than in the other areas of high concentration of panel doctors though not as favourable as the better off towns quoted above.[12]

How did the changes affect the new Irish medical graduate? In his evidence to the Commission on National Health Insurance in 1925, Dr Comber, the

11 Brock, Minutes of Evidence, p. 53.

12 Before 1911 medical provision was offered by friendly societies, trade union clubs and private insurance companies; doctors' fees were sometimes collected weekly by 'the doctor's man' door to door in an urban or industrial working-class community. That may be why Wigan in 1908, a town with a significant mining industry, which was then a prosperous and relatively well-paid part of the economy with a tradition of friendly societies, had a ratio of doctors to population more favourable in 1908 at one to 1,381 of the population than in 1926 at one to 2,292.8. The ratio fell in Walsall too. Rochdale, West Bromwich and Dudley showed an improvement, while Burnley was largely the same. Calculated from the *Medical Directory* 1926 and 1930.

representative of the National Medical Union, an organisation hostile to the principle of state insurance, complained that 'The competition at the commencement of this Act was of course very terrible indeed. You see at this time a lot of down-at-heel practitioners rushed into the panel before anybody else and they are now doing pretty well.'[13]

The attraction of panel work was also, he believed, 'because of the large numbers of newly qualified men who have been turned out by the medical schools'.[14] Certainly Irish medical schools could be included in this description, for they produced annually far more graduates than Ireland could herself absorb. There was an additional incentive in the insurance scheme. *The Medical Yearbook* of 1925 averred that 'The National Health Insurance Act in establishing the panel system modifies the need for a capital sum at the outset, as it provides a certain living from the start of private practice and from which an income of £600-£1,000 may be reasonably expected'.[15]

In spite of the feeling that panel practice brought opportunities for the newly graduated doctor, the situation was not straightforward. Brock pointed out in his evidence that of the 18,000 doctors that he calculated were engaged in Insurance practice, 12,000 were working as assistants to panel doctors. This way of acquiring a practice by assistantship would have been familiar to new graduates in the nineteenth century, and as then it often involved long, arduous hours and frequent moves between practices. Practices were still up for sale, even if they were based partly on Insurance work. Panel practices could not be sold outright, but this had also applied in pre-Insurance times to a doctor's part-time public health and Poor Law appointments. In the same way as the transfer of 'goodwill', a doctor could inform his panel patients about his successor with a recommendation in their favour. In a practice with a mixture of private and insured patients, there would be some recognition of this 'goodwill' in the price.[16] One doctor in 1923 advised that the purchase price of a practice with a high number of panel patients would be worth eighteen months' remuneration to the doctor's successors.[17]

Added to this was the fact that panel practice was not always a fresh field for the new graduate. Many established doctors such as Joseph Daniel McFeely

13 Dr Charles Thornton Comber of the National Medical Union, Minutes of Evidence taken before the Royal Commission on National Health Insurance, vol. III, (London: HMSO), p. 759.

14 Ibid., p. 759.

15 "The Profession of Medicine", in *The Medical Yearbook*, 1925, p. 53.

16 Leonard Shoeten Sack, "Starting a Panel Practice", *The Lancet*, 23 February 1924, vol. 1, pp. 396–7.

17 "The Situation in East Anglia", *The Lancet*, 10 November 1923, vol. 2, pp. 1048–9.

took on panel patients after 1911. He himself claimed to have 2,200 panel patients, although he was in dispute with the Insurance Committee about the numbers.[18] In the towns identified by Brock as almost wholly panel towns, nine of the sixteen Irish-educated doctors identified for 1926 who were in practice there had graduated before 1900, five before 1914 and only two after 1914, the latest date being 1918. Although undoubtedly the Insurance Act opened up possibilities for the new graduate, increasing the amount of work available, establishing oneself in general practice could still be hard work.

An examination of the impact of the insurance scheme in this research supports the conclusions of Digby and Bosanquet.[19] The lower distribution of doctors in poorer areas indicates a continued disparity of outcome between rich and poor in health care. Insurance by no means solved the problem of health and poverty. Private practice was still important, and most practices were a combination of the two. Whilst not all the problems of setting up a medical practice were solved by the insurance system, in the thirties the combination of price deflation and an expanding private market for health care as well as insurance, meant doctors' incomes were buoyant during the period. A panel doctor might find it necessary to employ assistants to expand his or her Insurance practice, and in rural areas the costs of maintaining contact with patients were larger, but nonetheless Insurance became an important resource for making a medical living in the interwar period.

2 The Distribution of Graduates from Irish Medical Schools

The dynamics of settlement of Irish graduates in England were often very particular. For example, in St John's Wood, an affluent part of London, there were four graduates from Irish medical schools among its eighty-one doctors in 1930. On closer examination, all of them were women who had been part of the late-nineteenth and early-twentieth-century feminist assault on medical privilege. Whilst women were allowed to study in English colleges, not all of these institutions permitted them to graduate. Irish medical schools did provide this facility, so that a number of medical women, after studying in Britain,

18 McFeely, *Reflections of an Old and Observant General Practitioner*, p. 84. The Insurance Committee considered he had only 1,800 panel patients.

19 Anne Digby and Nick Bosanquet, 'Doctors and Patients in an Era of National Health Insurance and Private Practice', *Economic History Review*, second series, vol. XL1, 1988, pp. 74–94.

crossed the Irish Sea and graduated from Irish medical schools.[20] The group were not therefore typical of Irish medical graduates.

By contrast, in the poor inner London areas of Camden, Bethnal Green and Bermondsey, there was a much higher number of graduates from Irish schools together with immigrant doctors from more distant places. In 1930 seven out of twenty-two doctors in Camden, a third in total, were Irish graduates; and in Bermondsey six out of seventeen together with two doctors from the Indian subcontinent, almost half of the medical establishment there. Bethnal Green had four identifiable Irish migrants out of thirty-seven doctors, combined with two other migrants, one Indian and one Russian. Poorer inner-city areas were generally less attractive to those setting up practice, but easier to access for that reason. However, neither St John's Wood nor the poor inner London areas cited above were representative of the experience of most Irish-educated doctors.

In studies of distribution it must be borne in mind that time, place, personality, opportunity, connections or luck all influenced where an Irish-educated doctor might set up practice. However, some conclusions about general patterns of migration emerge in comparative studies of settlement. In 1930, for a selected number of towns identified by certain common factors, an estimate was made of the percentage of Irish-educated doctors practising there. Table 15 shows towns with a high ratio of doctors to population, a smaller than average amount of panel work and relative affluence. Note the percentage of Irish-educated doctors.

In the towns singled out by Brock as predominantly panel towns, the percentage of Irish-educated doctors is shown in Table 16.[21]

However, higher numbers of Irish-educated doctors appear in urban and industrial areas where there was a significant Catholic population. Towns expanding in the interwar years would also be areas where opportunities for setting up panel practice were higher, and they were also places which attracted immigrants.

Around 200,000 men and women moved to Britain from Ireland between 1924 and 1937.[22] The Irish immigrant population in Britain was not exclusively Catholic, and immigration was by no means as high as it was to become in

20 One of the women graduated in 1901 and two in 1909. The exception was Julia Bell, who qualified in 1926. She worked at the Galton Laboratory in London, and her decision to take a medical degree was because of her research interest in medical genetics, to which she made a significant contribution. See Greta Jones, "Bell, Julia (1879–1979)", *Oxford Dictionary of National Biography* (Oxford: Oxford University Press, 2004).

21 For Walsall, James Francis O'Meara has been left out. He is a graduate of Edinburgh 1892, but also mentions Cork where he may have prepared for the Edinburgh exam.

22 Delaney, *Demography, State and Society: Irish Migration to Britain 1921–71*, Table 2.3, p. 45.

TABLE 15 Percentage of Irish-educated doctors in selected towns wealthier than the average

Town	No. of doctors	Population	Ratio of doctors to population	No. of Irish-educated doctors	Percentage of Irish-educated doctors
Torquay	71	39,431	555	5	7
Harrogate	102	38,885	381	6	6
Southport	128	76,621	599	5	4
Bournemouth	218	91,761	421	9	4
Chichester	19	12,413	653	3	15
Cheltenham	75	48,430	645	7	9
Richmond, Surrey	44	35,639	809	4	9
Total	657			39	6 %

SOURCE: *MEDICAL DIRECTORY* 1930

TABLE 16 Percentage of Irish-educated doctors in selected panel towns

Town	No. of doctors	Population	Ratio of doctors to population	No. of Irish-educated doctors	Percentage of Irish-educated doctors
Walsall	32	96,926	3028	4	12.5
Wigan	39	89,421	2292	3	7.6
Burnley	57	103,157	1809	3	5
Rochdale	48	90,816	1892	1	2
Dudley	17	55,894	3288	2	11.76
West Bromwich	27	73,647	2728	3	11
Total	224			16	7%

SOURCE: *MEDICAL DIRECTORY* 1926

the 1940s and 1950s.[23] Nonetheless, the *Catholic Directory* of 1926 gives a list of districts in which there is a high concentration of Catholic priests and churches.[24] They list sixteen, of which five were examined together with three

23 Ibid., Fig. 4.1, p. 164.

24 *The Catholic Directory of England and Wales 1926* (London: Burns, Oates and Washbourne Ltd), p. 622. Besides the five districts examined here is Westminster, for which, in com-

TABLE 17 Percentage of Irish-educated doctors in selected towns with a high concentration of Catholic churches and priests

Town	No. of doctors	Population	Ratio of doctors to population	No. of Irish-educated doctors	Percentage of Irish- educated doctors
Brentwood	17	6853	403	2	12
Cardiff	189	200,184	1059	22	12
Birmingham	680	919,444	1352	55	8
Preston	85	117,406	1381	7	8
Bootle	41	76,487	1866	5	12
Northampton	57	90, 895	1595	9	16
Chorley	17	30,581	1799	2	12
Middlesbrough	68	131,070	1927	15	22
Forest Gate*	41			10	24*
Total	1,195			127	11%

* There are no population figures in the *Medical Directory* for individual London boroughs.
SOURCE: 1930 *MEDICAL DIRECTORY*. TOWNS MENTIONED IN THE *CATHOLIC DIRECTORY 1926* ARE IN ITALICS

northern towns, Chorley, Bootle and Preston, all regarded as strongholds of Catholicism and which figure prominently in the campaigns carried out by the Catholic Church in the interwar years in support of Catholic education and against birth control. Several, such as Bootle and Chorley, were sites of older Irish immigrant population, and in Preston's case of an indigenous historic Catholic population as well. Forest Gate is an area of east London adjacent to Stratford and East Ham.[25]

Irish-educated doctors could therefore be found in practices in the general population in the proportion of from 4 to over 20 per cent.[26] The average

mon with other districts of London, the *Medical Directory* does not give population figures. Also identified are Portsmouth, Clifton, Plymouth, Shrewsbury, Menevia (Wales), Liverpool, Hexham and Newcastle, Lancaster, Leeds and Salford.

25 See coverage of these issues in the 1929 election at Preston reported in *The Catholic Herald*, 3 August 1929, p. 9. For Chorley, see the political ructions between Catholic-supported candidates and their opponents reported in ibid., 6 December 1930, p. 7.

26 The importance of Scottish-educated doctors in Britain is clear from any perusal of the *Medical Directory*, and they normally exceed the number of Irish-educated doctors. In Walsall 10 of its 32 doctors in 1926 were Scots-educated as compared to 4 Irish-educated. In Wigan 14 of its 41 doctors were Scots-educated in 1927 as opposed to 3 Irish.

distribution ranged between 6 to 11 per cent.[27] There was a high concentration of immigrant doctors of all kinds in poor inner-city areas and a lower percentage in the better-off areas with high doctor to patient ratio. The urban industrial areas had a slightly higher percentage of Irish doctors than the well-to-do, but not by much. The highest overall percentage of Irish-educated doctors tended to be in Catholic areas. Some of this must have been due to the perceptions of the graduates from Irish schools in Éire that there would be institutions in these places which would facilitate the settlement of their graduates. The Insurance Act would also open the door for them. In particular a group practice could lessen the difficulty in setting up a practice serving a predominantly working-class population.

3 Friendship and Collegiality

As the chapter on the British Empire shows, some schools had particular traditions in supplying doctors for the army (TCD) or the navy (RCSI). Many of the routes by which Irish graduates travelled to Britain were, however, formed by friendship and collegiality frequently through the experience of the medical school. For example, five of the seven Irish-educated doctors in Cheltenham in 1930 were graduates of Trinity College Dublin. All had graduated within eight years of each other, in 1896, 1901, 1902, 1907 and 1915. The two exceptions to the Trinity connection were post-war appointments, a graduate of the RCSI in 1918 and Queen's University Belfast in 1922.

Informal networks could determine the place of practice. This is illustrated by King's Lynn, a town in East Anglia. King's Lynn also illustrates another post-war feature: the greater number of joint or even multiple practices which made the networks created during medical school, or shortly after, even more important. In 1925 John Valentine Horgan graduated from the National University of Ireland (Cork). By 1935 he was in practice in King's Lynn and had been joined in the same practice by Edmond Fogarty from NUI (UCD), who had also graduated in 1925, and John Sexton, another 1925 graduate of UCD. In 1935 the practice now included Thomas Hutton, educated in Canada. In 1957 it still was home to Fogarty, Horgan and Hutton with the addition of Graham

27 For the 1950s, when Irish immigration to Britain increased, one study of the 1951 Census calculated that the proportion of Irish doctors in Britain was around 11 percent. 'Arrangements for the Integration of Irish Immigrants in England and Wales by A.E.C.W Spencer', ed. Mary Daly (Dublin: Irish Manuscripts Commission, 2012), Table 12, p. 40. Report commissioned by the Catholic Archbishop of Dublin, John Charles McQuaid, for the International Catholic Migration Commission and presented 1960.

Leakey, a London graduate. In 1944 they were joined by a graduate from NUI, Thomas William Slattery. Fogarty and Horgan had an additional connection: in the interwar years they were members of the Guild of St Luke, SS Cosmos and Damian, an organisation of Catholic doctors in Britain. In the 1950s Fogarty had become Master and Horgan the honorary secretary of the East Anglia branch of the Catholic Medical Guild.[28]

4 The "Powerful Army" of Catholic Doctors and Practice in Britain

By the beginning of the twentieth century, a congruence was being suggested, though still disputed by some nationalists, between Irish national identity and Catholicism. The belief that this was important in medicine was clear from the following memorandum which Michael Tierney, President of UCD, wrote for the Irish government in 1948. He was alarmed at a proposal to locate a postgraduate medical school at St Kevin's Hospital. This he felt would divert resources from University College Dublin's medical school. In Tierney's opinion UCD was the largest and most significant of the Irish medical schools in the twenty-six counties. But he has an interesting insight into its role and value:

> The full history of the Medical school and of its contribution to the development of the Catholic medical profession in Ireland has never been written. When this is done, it will be found to constitute one of the finest chapters of Ireland's modern resurgence. In alliance with the great Catholic voluntary hospitals, especially the Mater Misericordiae and St Vincent's, the school may be fairly said to have given to Ireland the Catholic medical profession – and to Great Britain and its overseas dependencies – the powerful army of Catholic doctors who now constitute a large proportion of British practitioners.

UCD was, Tierney claimed, the heir to the Catholic Medical School founded by Newman in 1854. The struggles of that school paralleled the struggle of the Irish nation to free itself. But most pertinent to this study was Tierney's assertion that emigrating Catholic doctors had a missionary role abroad.[29] Certainly

28 See Digby, 'Shaping New Identities: General Practitioners in Britain and South Africa', in which there is a discussion about how personal connection and sometimes shared national identity shaped practice in the Cape Colony.

29 National Archives Dublin S14402A, Under Graduate and Post Graduate Medical Training 1945–51, Memorandum from Michael Tierney, 1948, p. 2.

the Catholic Church established institutions, hospitals and medical missionaries in many parts of the world in the nineteenth and twentieth centuries. They followed the migration of the Irish to America, Australia and other destinations including Britain. In addition, growing Catholic influence in Irish medical schools in the early twentieth century, leading to the introduction of Catholic holidays and rituals and sodalities, has been noted by historians.[30] Alfred O'Rahilly, who was Registrar at Cork in the interwar years and then President (1943–54), stated in 1943: "Our students are over 97% Catholic and we do not intend to ignore this fact. Negative non-denominationalism does not appeal to us in Cork."[31]

Medicine was already the site of conflict in the nineteenth century over certain medical practices forbidden by the Catholic Church. The most widely discussed issue before the First World War was craniotomy, a procedure well established in Dublin obstetrics and described in standard textbooks.[32]. The practice was not formally forbidden by the Papacy until 1884, and a further clarification on the ban was issued in 1888. From the 1850s, however, the tide of Catholic opinion was swinging against craniotomy.[33] After the Papal pronouncements of 1884 and 1888, the Catholic Church in Ireland actively campaigned against the practice in Irish hospitals and medical schools, sometimes by direct intervention and whilst Irish medical students continued to be trained in craniotomy, greater sensitivity on this subject in medical textbooks can be detected post 1880s.[34]

After 1922 doctors in the Éire had to operate within a legislative framework supportive of Catholic moral ideals exemplified by the ban on the advocacy of birth control in 1929 and, from 1935, the ban on the import and supply of contraceptives. The Offences Against the Person Act 1861 which made abortion illegal continued to be in force in both states on the island of Ireland; there appeared some relaxation of this rule among British doctors during the 1920s

30 John A. Murphy, *The College: A History of Queen's University College Cork 1845–1995* (Cork: Cork University Press, 1995), pp. 276–82.

31 Quoted in J. Anthony Gaughan, *Alfred O'Rahilly: Academic*, vol. 1 (Dublin: Kingdom Books, 1986), p. 126.

32 Henry Maunsell, *The Dublin Practice of Midwifery* (London: Longman, Rees, Orme, Brown, Green and Longman, 1834) Maunsell was Professor of Midwifery at the Dublin Wellesley Lying-in Institution.

33 U.E.U., "Craniotomy, The sacerdotal physician versus the medical", *Irish Ecclesiastical Record*, vol. IX, 1888, pp. 118–30. See Greta Jones, 'Craniometry in nineteenth century and twentieth century Ireland and Britain', unpublished paper.

34 For example, W.S. Playfair, *A Treatise on the Science and Practice of Midwifery*, 2 vols. (London: Smith, Elder and Co., 1893), vol. 2, p. 213.

and 1930s, even whilst the law of 1861 remained on the statute book, but this relaxation was not observable in either states in Ireland.[35]

Were Catholic medical ethics an issue for the medical student in Ireland and subsequently in Britain? The nationalist newspaper *The Leader* in 1910 welcomed a meeting of Catholic doctors at the conference of the British Medical Association held in Westminster Cathedral to propose the foundation of a Catholic Guild of St Luke. It claimed:

> Another field in which the teachings of the Church have triumphed over opposition is the question of craniotomy – a barbarous operation by which the bungling obstetricians of the English school (of medicine) killed the unborn child in cases of difficult labour – and at one time conscientious Catholic doctors were looked on with contempt because they were averse to the practice and thus were decried as practitioners who sought to save a babe at the expense of the mother's life. Now all has changed.[36]

Patrick Kane, the son of a farmer, was a Catholic medical student at Queen's University Belfast. He graduated in 1915 and subsequently left Ireland to become a general practitioner in Doncaster. This is his account of a class on obstetrics at Queen's from the memoir of his education deposited with his alma mater:

> The professor of gynaecology liked to propose impossible, difficult problems taking place at the "back of Binion", a North of Ireland expression for way out, that is the kind of place where you could not find a nearby lamppost to surreptitiously consult your "Medical aids to gynaecology". This particular problem could only be solved by removing the baby in pieces if the mother was to be saved. There were three or four other Catholics in the class. One was pale faced, fair haired and with glasses which pinched his nose giving him a nasal intonation. The professor turned to him and said "Mr Paul what would you do in this case? Your church does not allow you to kill the child to save the mother." Immediately the student replied, "I'd tell them to get the nearest Protestant doctor and let him do the killing."[37]

---

35 See John Keown, *Abortion, Doctors and the Law: Some Aspects of the Legal Regulation of Abortion in England from 1803 to 1982* (Cambridge: Cambridge University Press, 1988).

36 *The Leader*, 23 July 1910, vol. XX, no. 23, pp. 539–40.

37 Queen's University Belfast Archives. QUB/E/4/2/2/. Memoir of Patrick Kane.

5 The Guild of St Luke, SS Cosmos and Damian

The transition from education in Ireland to practising in Britain therefore presented to the practising Catholic doctor the possibility of conflict. One means to negotiate the problems was through the Guild of St Luke, SS Cosmos and Damian. The Guild was an organisation of Catholic doctors founded in Britain in 1910.[38] In a 1960 survey of Irish Catholic immigrants to Britain, the Guild was cited as one of the means by which Irish Catholic immigrant doctors found fellowship and assistance in Britain.[39] There was no Guild in Ireland itself until 1932, although before then the Guild had a branch in Dublin. In 1914 the Guild published a periodical, the *Catholic Medical Gazette*, but its production was hampered by the First World War. It returned again in 1922 as the *Catholic Medical Guardian*, which after 1951 became the *Catholic Medical Quarterly*.

A significant proportion of the Guild's members in Britain were graduates of Irish medical schools, a fact acknowledged in the 1952 Annual Report by the Master of the Guild, Dr W. B. J. Pemberton, in which he thanked Professor Alfred O'Rahilly, the President of University College Cork, for "bringing our Guild to the notice of Irish graduates coming to settle in this country. The Guild owes its present strength in no small measure to the support of its Irish graduate members."[40]

This was certainly true of the interwar years: between 1925 and 1937, 296 doctors from the membership lists can be identified as practising in Britain,[41] of which 145 were educated in Irish medical schools, or nearly half of the total. The Irish medical graduates in the Guild were generally from the National University of Ireland and its constituent colleges of Cork, Galway and UCD (a total of ninety); ten were from its predecessor, the old Royal University of Ireland (RUI) which was incorporated into the National University of Ireland in 1908; and

---

38 It was the inspiration of a graduate of the Catholic Medical School in Dublin, Thomas Maunsell (1839–1937). Maunsell entered the British army as surgeon in 1860, rising to become one of the last to hold the title of Surgeon General. He served with distinction in several colonial wars, was decorated with the Cross of Pro Ecclesia et Pontifice and received an honorary degree from the National University of Ireland. See his Obituary, *Catholic Medical Guardian*, vol. XVI, no. 1, 1938, pp. 33–4. The concept of the Guild owed a great deal to the revival of medievalism among English Catholics.

39 'Arrangements for the Integration of Irish Immigrants in England and Wales by A.E.C.W. Spencer', ed. Daly.

40 William Bernard Joseph Pemberton, 'Annual Report of the Master of the Guild of St Luke, SS. Cosmas and Damian' (London, 1952), pp. 1–42.

41 Compiled from membership lists in the *Catholic Medical Guardian* 1920–39. Student members, lay and religious, and those practising abroad or in the army and colonial service have been excluded. A number were untraceable.

twenty-six were graduates of the RCSI.[42] A further five were licentiates of the Apothecaries Hall and twelve were from Queen's College Belfast or its successor, the Queen's University Belfast. Only two were from Trinity College Dublin.

Seventeen members of the Guild were examined in this study from the cohorts of 1920, 1925 and 1930, and a further nine members from various five-year cohorts before 1920. The cohort of 1920 included W.J.B. Pemberton, the future Master of the Guild. He was unusual among the members for being a graduate of Trinity College Dublin. Pemberton began his medical career as a doctor in Bermondsey, the poor inner-city London borough mentioned before. He was still in practice in Bermondsey in the 1950s. Pemberton served as Master of the Guild c.1951–8 and as editor of the *Catholic Medical Quarterly* c.1962–7.[43] Four other individuals from the graduate cohorts of 1920, 1925 and 1930 became either Master or Honorary Secretary of their local branch.[44]

Besides propagating Catholic medical ethics, the Guild had other less overt functions. It provided help for those setting up practice, as exemplified by the experience of Fogarty and Horgan in East Anglia. This was largely through informal networking, for apart from posts offered in the Catholic missions abroad, there were only a few advertisements for practices in the *Catholic Medical Guardian*. However, in April 1932 there were three. They included an "Experienced Practitioner (convert) who would like to get in touch with Doctor contemplating selling partnership or retiring. Cash available good faith assured." A practice was advertised which could earn "£900 in a working class city area", and a request was made for an offer of "partnership or practice in a rural or semi-rural area".[45]

The Guild's broader purposes were described by Dr M.R. Walshe, an English Catholic and a member of the Council of the Guild, as a combination of "morals and miracles", referring in the latter instance to the Church's preoccupation with encouraging the Guild's members to verify instances of healing by divine intervention.[46] The Guild's chief remit, however, was in the realms of medical

42 It was common for students of the Catholic University, before it became the medical school of University College Dublin in 1908 and even for a while afterwards, to be prepared for the examinations of the RCSI.

43 William Bernard Joseph Pemberton (1896–1975). In addition to his practice, he acted as a surgeon to the Camberwell Metropolitan Police and was a member of the BMA; see "An Appreciation", *Catholic Medical Quarterly*, vol. XX, no. 1, 1967, p. 3.

44 Place and date of graduation are in brackets after the names. They were Terence Murphy (Cork 1920), Master at Plymouth; Edmond Fogarty (NUI 1925), Master East Anglia; J.V. Horgan (Cork 1925), Hon. Sec. E. Anglia; Charles O'Donovan (Cork 1925), Master at Leicester.

45 *Catholic Medical Guardian*, vol. X, no. 2, 1932, p. x.

46 M.R. Walshe, "The Role of the Catholic Professional Man in the Catholic Life of this Country", *Catholic Medical Guardian*, vol. XVII, no. 1, July 1939, p. 28. Martin Walshe OBE was a

ethics. The interwar years were a period of challenge to Catholic doctrine. The birth control movement had set up clinics in the 1920s, and the Local Government Act of 1929 allowed council-run Maternity and Child Welfare Clinics to give birth control advice in limited circumstances. The Catholic Church in Britain launched a campaign to stop local councils from implementing the birth control provisions of the Act. The interwar Eugenics Society also began to exert its influence over social legislation, especially in the recommendations of the Committee on Voluntary Sterilisation, set up by government and reporting in 1934 which proposed legalisation. Finally, the Bourne judgement in 1938, which permitted a doctor to induce abortion in certain defined situations, alarmed the Catholic Church.

The leaders of the campaigns in opposition to these developments were not Irish, but respectively an English and a Scottish convert, Dr Letitia Fairfield and Dr Halliday Sutherland, both prominent in the Guild and well known nationally.[47] Nonetheless, Irish Catholic migrant doctors were mobilised through the Guild to support them, and in this respect the Irish Catholic Church could claim to be conducting missionary work in Britain. But the Guild failed in its main aims. Even in the case of sterilisation, although the recommendations of the Committee on Voluntary Sterilisation were not enacted, the Guild conceded that their defeat owed as much to opposition by the Communist geneticist Professor J.B.S. Haldane as its own efforts.[48]

6 Professional Integration

The Guild illustrates the obstacles felt by many Irish Catholic doctors between the aims of the Catholic Church and their full integration into British medical practice. In general practice, particularly for those doctors working in Catholic areas, this may not have been an immediate problem. There was a catechism of

distinguished neurologist, educated at London, with a practice in Wimpole Street. He was knighted in 1953.

47 There are a considerable number of works on the birth control controversy. For a recent discussion, see Kate Fisher, *Birth Control, Sex and Marriage in Britain 1918–1960* (Oxford: Oxford University Press, 2006). On the sterilisation debate, there is an account in Jones, *Social Hygiene in Twentieth Century Britain*.

48 "Readers of his *Heredity and Politics* will have recognised that Professor Haldane has no prejudice in favour of the Church and yet his criticisms on sterilisation of the unfit are more in accord with her teaching … than the policy advocated by Dr Barnes." The reference is to Bishop Barnes, who revived the idea of sterilisation shortly after the end of the Second World War. *Catholic Medical Quarterly*, vol. XXII, no. 4, 1951, p. 105.

how to deal with a patient asking for a forbidden medical practice. They could be urged or advised against the practice, but they could not be forced one way or another. In the end, if obdurate, they would be advised to go to another doctor. This could all be conducted in the privacy of the doctor's surgery. Moreover, a Catholic, particularly one strongly rooted in Catholic medical ethics, would often practise in a Catholic area where there was less likelihood of conflict with the patient. There were other institutions in these areas, church and school, who were in a position to form expectations of what was allowed or not allowed by the doctor. Patients might, in these circumstances, never raise any questions of medical treatment with their doctor contradictory to the ethics of the Catholic Church.

The situation for Catholics working in hospitals was different. In the United Kingdom there was none of the legislative underpinning given in the new Irish State from 1922 to Catholic moral principles, nor as much religious segregation in schools or hospitals. Catholics worked alongside those who did not share their views, and this often put Catholic doctors under pressure. As the *Catholic Medical Guardian* said in 1925, "It cannot be denied that academic theology as applied to clinical medicine is viewed with some distrust by certain Catholic practitioners."[49]

A discussion in the Brentwood branch of the Guild at Forest Gate in 1933, following a paper on "Obstetrical Problems and the Catholic Conscience" by Dr P. Conlon (UCD 1921), illustrated the problems. Questions raised by the speaker were about:

> the lawfulness of sending patients to hospitals when it was known that evacuation of the uterus would be performed; the question of sterilisation of a woman who had already submitted to several Caesarean deliveries; the extraction of the foetus from a dead or dying mother.[50]

The advice from the Guild's chaplain, Father Alphonsus Bonnar, was to tell Catholic mothers that they should refuse abortion but "After giving such advice the Catholic doctor was not responsible for what hospital authorities might do."[51]

---

49 *Catholic Medical Guardian*, vol. III, no. 1, 1925, p. 10.

50 Fr Alphonsus Bonnar, Meeting of the Brentwood branch 1933, *Catholic Medical Guardian*, vol. XI, no. 3, 1933, p. 150. The audience included Henry Alphonsus Hannon (NUI Cork 1920), Michael McManus (LAH, UCD 1922), Joseph Patrick Robinson (UCD 1913), John Leo Bookey (NUI 1919). The secretary of the branch was Thomas Lawrence Dolan (RCSI 1918).

51 Ibid., p. 151. This contrasted with the position in Éire where ethics committees in hospitals were dominated by the Church and had the authority of legislation on abortion and birth control to back them up.

Questions arose as to the extent to which this would affect the standing of a Catholic doctor in a hospital and his or her career prospects. This was discussed at a meeting of the London branch in 1936, addressed by Dr Philip Hamill.[52] If a Catholic were asked to perform therapeutic abortion and refused, but was the only gynaecologist on the staff, would this mean that future employment of Catholics in the post would be put in jeopardy? How far was it morally right in the case where an abortion might potentially be carried out to transfer the patient to a less skilled colleague? Would therapeutic abortion in the case of TB or renal disease be justified? If a woman entered a clinic with this condition and was pregnant and this was reported, it 'will probably set in motion a train of machinery which may result in therapeutic abortion. It may be a standing order that such cases be reported.'[53] This might be considered to be complicity in the process, although on that question Father Bonnar assured the branch that both a Catholic anaesthetist who took part in a therapeutic abortion and a doctor who reported a problem pregnancy for which an abortion might be advised by others would not be excommunicated.[54] On the whole the Guild tried to reassure its members 'In England we are tolerant and respect the religious tenets of others. If a gynaecological resident medical officer were instructed by his chief to empty a uterus but demurred on religious grounds it is probable that his attitude would be respected and that his senior would himself operate.'[55]

The Church's teaching met a degree of resistance. Dr Reginald Miller believed that "it would make matters easier if the Church would condemn the taking of life in all circumstances including war and judicial execution". Dr Melmotte (UCD 1920) stated his opinion that "the question is purely a medical one, not theological". Whilst Dr King averred that "A medical superintendent must put his private ethical views aside and be influenced only the medical interests of the patient."[56] For some there was a feeling that the doctor was being pushed too far by the Church. Walshe returned to this theme in 1939. He considered that the clergy were often "wholly opportunist when they attempt to influence the moral verdict…"[57] Catholic doctors were sometimes the subject of

52 Dr Philip Hamill, Meeting of the London branch 1936, "The Position of Hospital Medical Officers in relation to Therapeutic Abortion", *Catholic Medical Guardian*, vol. XIV, no. 3, 1936, pp. 91–3. Hamill was educated at Cambridge and had a practice in Harley Street.

53 Hamill, ibid., pp. 91–2.

54 Bonnar, ibid., p. 93.

55 Hamill, ibid., p. 91.

56 Miller, ibid., p. 92; Melmotte and King, ibid. p. 23. James Henry Melmotte was a UCD graduate (1920). Reginald Henry Miller, educated at London (1905), was a paediatric specialist with a practice in Harley Street.

57 Walshe, "The Role of the Catholic Professional Man", p. 28. For Walshe see Footnote 46.

"intolerant abuse", the outcome of which was: 'I believe too often Catholic doctors have let themselves be persuaded to state conclusions before the Catholic body which they dare not try to substantiate before a medical tribunal.'[58]

Walshe raised the question of some of the wilder pronouncements made by members of the Church, including the deleterious effects of birth control on health and its contribution to maternal mortality. An article on birth control in the *Catholic Medical Guardian* by Dr Frederick J. McCann particularly aroused Walshe's ire. McCann believed that the use of contraception gave rise to a pathological condition he called the 'Malthusian uterus' which contributed towards maternal mortality.[59] Walshe considered Dr McCann's 'Malthusian uterus' to be "a figment of Dr McCann's imagination", and maternal mortality as in no way connected with it.[60]

In the end the Catholic Church in England was forced to concede that many of its aims were far from being achieved. Local councils continued to adopt the provisions of the 1929 Local Government Act, which allowed council-supported mother and child clinics to give birth control advice. The prominent Catholic prelate Monsignor O'Brien lamented in 1930 that in Bootle, "the most Catholic borough in England", the Maternity and Child Welfare Committee had voted for the provision of birth control information in what he described as "a public insult to the people of Bootle".[61] He advised the Catholic electorate at the next election to evict the 23 councillors who had voted in its favour. He then "read a letter from an eminent medical man, a friend, which related to the physical maladies that resulted from such practices".[62]

The Catholic Church continued to emphasise the missionary role of the Guild and the Irish Catholic doctor in England. Their successes in propagating Catholic ethics in medicine were nonetheless largely in Ireland itself.[63]

58 Ibid., p. 29.

59 Dr F.M.R. McCann, "The Effect of Contraceptive Practices on Female Sexual Organs", *Catholic Medical Guardian*, vol. V, no. 2, 1927, pp. 48–62. McCann was educated at Edinburgh (1888) and was consultant obstetrician at the Free Hospital for Women and West End Hospital. He had an address in Wimpole Street.

60 Dr Walshe replied in "Medical Views on Birth Control. Facts and Speculation", *Catholic Medical Guardian*, vol. V, no. 3, 1927, pp. 82–8. The controversy was renewed in the October issue, vol. V, no. 4, 1927, pp. 109 and 112.

61 "Bootle. Catholics want 'No Stopery'", *Catholic Herald*, 29 January 1930, p. 1.

62 O'Brien's opinion on the deleterious effects of contraception probably owed something to Dr McCann's views.

63 Dr A.P. Barry addressed the Sixth International Congress of Catholic Doctors in Dublin in 1954 on "Conservatism in Obstetrics", *Transactions of the Congress*, pp. 122–34. He suggested that ethical considerations indicated that symphysiotomy should replace the caesarean section, because the latter was associated with unethical post-partum practices,

Yet the Guild remained an important vehicle for the expression of Catholic moral views in medicine and it sustained individual faith. It also served to alert doctors to the realities of British medical life and the complexities of being a Catholic doctor in Britain. Overall, however, the experience of Irish Catholic doctors in Britain in this period was largely unproblematic. The respected and popular Catholic doctor serving a Catholic or Catholic Irish community or in a religiously mixed area in Britain was a well-known figure.[64] Patrick Kane, in spite of the questions which arose in his obstetrical training in Belfast, settled down to a respectable and integrated life in the area of Doncaster where he practised.

7 The Role of the State in Health Care

In the 1930s there was increased interest, including among medical professionals, about the relationship between poverty and ill health. This was accompanied by a debate about the reform of health care and the role the state should play in this. In Britain this led to the creation of the National Health Service in 1948, supported by general taxation and which provided medical treatment free at the point of delivery. The Act also nationalised the hospital system. In the 1930s neither jurisdiction in Ireland was either innovative in their medical provision or had sufficiently tackled the problem of ill health and poverty. However Northern Ireland and Éire were not immune from the debate about extending health care and the impact of class on health.[65] In Britain this debate often proved to be the beginning of political engagement for the migrant doctor.

---

meaning birth control or sterilisation. By 1956 an article by him in the BMJ claimed that no caesareans were performed in the National Maternity Hospital Dublin where he was Master, or in the Coombe Lying-in Hospital Dublin where his co-author of the article was Master. See Kevin Feeny and Arthur Barry, "Rupture and Perforation of Uterus in Association with Pregnancy, Labour and Puerperium", *BMJ*, 14 January 1956, vol. 1, p. 72. However, this practice is now the subject of considerable controversy among the women who underwent symphysiotomy in that decade; see "Symphysiotomy compensation is denied to 53 women", *Irish Times*, 14 April 2015, p. 1.

64 See the discussion of Dr Cornelius O'Doherty and his importance to the Manchester and Salford community in the earlier twentieth century in Neil Smith and Mervyn Busteed, 'The Emergence of an Irish Middle Class in Manchester', in *Irish Elites in the Nineteenth Century*, ed. Ciaran O'Neill (Dublin: Four Courts Press, 2013), pp. 206–7.

65 See John Privilege and Greta Jones, 'Crisis and Scandal: Government, Local Government and Health in Northern Ireland 1939–44', *Irish Economic and Social History*, vol. 42, 2015, pp. 33–52.

Eric St John Lyburn, a Protestant educated at Trinity College Dublin, was an enthusiastic nationalist and, as a schoolboy, had witnessed and taken part in events in Dublin during the Rising of 1916. During the decades he spent in England after graduating in 1930, first at a hospital in Birkenhead and then in general practice in the Midlands, his professional work drew him into the debate on preventative medicine and the state. Lyburn advocated the need for either the insurance system or, in default of that, the state itself to provide well-equipped diagnostic clinics for the population.[66]

Towards the end of the 1930s Lyburn's advocacy drew the attention of the Independent Labour Party (ILP), who invited him to join them. He spoke at public meetings on their behalf on the theme of health reform:

> I then went to Newport, where I had a most welcome meeting, and after this travelled to Norwich, where I spoke in the Keir Hardie Hall. I was rather impressed with the idealism of the ILP and their secretary at the time, Mr Fenner Brockway. He gave me plenty of support in the Independent Labour Party newspaper, *The New Leader*.[67]

But Lyburn was too mercurial to rise up in politics. He moved from the ILP to the Labour Party, and then in 1945 stood unsuccessfully as an Independent, polling 1,470 votes.[68] In the same election W.J. Pemberton, the future President of the Guild of St Luke and a critic of increased state intervention in health, stood as a National Liberal in West Bermondsey and saved his deposit with around 2,500 votes.[69]

Irish medical emigrants to Britain in this period espoused a variety of political and ethical causes. There were Irish members of the Socialist Medical Association as well as the Guild. Some like Robert McCarrison were drawn into the controversies over poverty and ill health; others stood for Parliament on both sides of the political divide. Nor was Ireland itself isolated from the broader controversies at the end of the 1930s about the role of the state in health.[70] During and following the war, changes in medical provision took place in both Irish states. Northern Ireland followed the British model and the changes there

---

66 E.F.St John Lyburn, *The Fighting Irish Doctor*, Dublin, Morris & Co., *c.*1950, pp. 28–33. Eventually, after various experiments, Lyburn opened up a private clinic in Tunbridge Wells, Kent.

67 Lyburn, *The Fighting Irish Doctor*, p. 172.

68 Ibid., p. 189.

69 See "An Appreciation", *Catholic Medical Quarterly*, vol. XX, no. 1, 1967, p. 3.

70 See Privilege, 'The Northern Ireland Government and the Welfare State 1942–8', for a discussion of the changes in Northern Ireland.

were radical. In Éire the Catholic Church's reluctance to contemplate increasing the power of the state in health was a brake upon change, as were the economic problems in Éire. Yet the Republic of Ireland (re-christened in 1949) also experienced substantial change.[71]

There was one issue arising out of the changes which affected the migrant Irish doctor. The British government, in contemplation of increasing expenditure on both education and health after the war, appointed the Goodenough Committee in 1944 to look at how a reformed health service would affect medical education. One conclusion of the committee was that more doctors were needed. In addition, improvements in clinical training to bring it much closer to the American model of medical education should be put in place.[72]

This brought about the first significant change to the position of the Irish medical emigrant in the Republic since the adoption of the 1858 *Medical Register*. Although negotiations went on through the late 1940s between the Irish and British governments to accommodate the changes, from 1950 Irish graduates seeking to work in Britain had to have 'P' for provisional beside their name in the *Medical Register*. Once they had completed a course of training in an approved hospital, it was removed.

8 The National Health Service and the Irish Migrant Doctor

The coming of the National Health Service (NHS) in 1948 and the enactment of its provisions on the 'appointed day', 5 July, brought about a substantial change to the health services in Great Britain. The legislation of 1946 applied only to England, Wales and Scotland but in 1948 its provisions were enacted in Northern Ireland. Éire did not adopt the British system largely because of the anticipated cost and Church opposition. Nonetheless the coming of the NHS accelerated change there. Under this influence the Republic of Ireland, as it became known in 1949, embarked upon a series of health reforms based on greater state involvement, a move which, given its tradition of Catholic voluntarism in health and education, was often controversial. It remained, however, in contrast to the system in Britain and Northern Ireland, where all medical care was now free at the point of delivery and the hospitals nationalised, a mixed private/public system combining a Voluntary Health Insurance scheme

71 For a discussion of the changes North and South, see Greta Jones, *"Captain of these Men of Death": The History of Tuberculosis in Nineteenth and Twentieth Century Ireland* (Amsterdam and London: Rodopi, 2001).

72 For a discussion of the Goodenough Report, see *BMJ*, 22 July 1944, vol. 2, pp. 121–3.

(VHI), private practice and some free treatment for the very poorest and for certain selected public health functions.

The first effect of the creation of the NHS in Britain was a rise of government investment in health. In his history of the NHS Charles Webster has pointed out that after 1948 spending by the government on health rose by fifty per cent between 1948 and 1956–7.[73] The most startling increase in expenditure was in dentistry where the British Government had grossly under-estimated demand. Investment in the dental services rose from £10 million in 1948 to £29.5 million in 1956.[74] According to one Irish commentator, 'Britain's social services (which) have created a mad rush for dental treatment are taking our dentists at £1000 a year and more, as fast as they can qualify.'[75] The number of medical practitioners also increased though more modestly, The Willink Committee on Medical Manpower 1954–7 talked of 'rapid recruitment to general practice' aiming to create an average patient list of 2,000–2,500. Between July 1948 and July 1955, the number of principals (practitioners) in general practice rose from 19,450 to 21,350.[76]

What effect did this have upon Irish medical migration to Britain? Certainly, it increased demand for doctors in Britain but was migration, as in the case of dentists, influenced by a significant rise in the remuneration offered? To return to the question posed in Chapter 2, was making a medical living during this period easier in Britain than in Ireland? Comparing rates of pay is relatively straightforward for those in public health, Poor Law and other government or local council supported roles. The salaries are often published. Remuneration for general practice is always more elusive, though for Britain, after the NHS was set up, the fact that it was the state that negotiated with and paid general practitioners makes it easier. The average salary of GP's in the early 1960s in Britain was £2,765. Even so GP's salaries varied, dependent on the size of a doctor's list and other emoluments.[77]

How did Ireland's doctors fare in the 1930s and 1940s? An editorial in the *Journal of the Medical Association of Eire* in 1947 stated "It has been said by

---

73 Charles Webster, *The Health Services Since the War, volume 1: Problems of Health Care. The National Health Service Before 1957* (London: HMSO, 1988), Table 1: Cost of the National Health Service, 1948–1957, p. 135.

74 Ibid., Table 1: Cost of the General Dental Service 1948–1956, p. 359.

75 RCSI Archives, Scrapbook. 'Cuttings of Interesting Information'. Quote from *Irish Times*, 27 September 1950.

76 Charles Webster, *The Health Services Since the War, volume 2: Government and Health Care. The National Health Service 1958–1979* (London: HMSO, 1996), p. 9.

77 The government attempted to control the size of doctor's lists but there was some variation. There was also work the doctor could contract to do for outside agencies for a fee. One example is medical examination for potential emigrants to Canada and other places.

many critics of the Association that the major purpose of its existence is only to talk about how badly paid doctors are."[78] In spite of this statement, the *Journal* was coy about doctor's remuneration in general practice but it did take up the cause of doctors in the public health service. In 1936 the salary of the Irish dispensary medical officer was £250 rising to £350 after two years of service though it must be remembered that this post was still often part time and many Irish doctors considered it as additional to their income from general practice.[79] The starting salary for medical officers in mental institutions in Ireland in 1938 was £250 rising to £300 after two years and then by increments to £500; a further £100 was granted for board. A superintendent in a mental hospital was paid initially £700 and this could rise to £800- £900 depending on the size of the hospital.[80] In Britain in 1935 the salary for junior medical assistants in mental hospitals was £350–£450 with an additional £50 for holders of the DPM. Senior assistant medical officers in mental hospitals in Britain received between £500–700 and superintendents £1,00-£1,500 depending upon the size of the hospital.[81]

However, it is clear that, particularly at the lower ends of the scale, salaries in the public health sector were lower in Ireland though not by much. The *Journal of the Medical Association of Eire* pointed out promises made by the Irish government in 1936 to raise starting salaries in the public health system to £300 had not been carried out and in 1947 they complained that 'There has been no important changes since so that we can imagine that a salary considered to be adequate in 1936 can nowadays be only described as grossly inadequate.'[82] A writer in *The Lancet* in 1941 argued that this was why, in spite of a drop in the numbers of Irish medical practitioners going to Britain at that time, so many posts in Ireland's public health and other medical services were still short of applicants. The county hospitals themselves were 'new and well-constructed but quite inadequately staffed' because of 'the reluctance of the central and local government ... to provide the required funds.'[83]

The lower salaries in Ireland at junior level were, in part, a reaction to the superabundant market there for newly graduated Irish medical men and women. But the coming of the NHS was to change this. The number of job advertisements in the *Journal of the Medical Association of Eire* was usually

78 'The Salaried Medical Man' (editorial), *Journal of the Medical Association of Eire*, vol. 20 no. 117, Jan.–June 1947, p. 227.
79 Ibid., p. 228.
80 'The Mental Hospital Service' *Journal of the Medical Association of Eire*, vol. 2 no. 8, February 1938, p. 19.
81 *The Medical Practitioners' Handbook* (1935), p. 56.
82 'The Salaried Medical Man', pp. 227–8.
83 'Surplus of Irish Doctors', *The Lancet*, vol. 238, no. 6173, 20 December 1941, pp. 772–3.

very sparse. Between the re-launch of the *Journal* in 1937 and 1948 there were scarcely any at all.[84] But two issues in 1950, September and November, carried between them around one hundred and fifty advertisements for posts in Britain.[85] In contrast there was only a meagre number of advertisements for jobs in Ireland and they were generally for more senior posts where the rates of remuneration were reasonably competitive. The impact of the surge in demand for doctors and dentists was commented on by the RCSI. A piece in the *Irish Times* of 1950 under the headline "Too few doctors, dentists, too many lawyers, chemists" proclaimed that the NHS had created a big demand for Irish medical graduates. Five hundred would leave Éire's medical schools for Britain that year and 'Everyone one of them will get a job.'[86]

Salary scales for the junior posts on offer in Britain and Ireland were not grossly divergent, partly as a result of planning in Éire for the new Health Act of 1947, one of the post-war reforming measures enacted by the government which the *Journal of the Irish Medical Association* believed would resolve the dispute over Poor Law pay promised by the government in 1936. But even in anticipation of this, the plethora of junior posts offered to the Irish graduate in Britain exercised a pull on the Irish medical migrant. By the late 1940s Great Yarmouth General Hospital was advertising for a house surgeon "within three months of qualification" on a salary of £350-£450 with £100 deducted for board, well within the range of junior posts advertised in Ireland.[87]

9 Conclusion

However, by the end of the 1960s, cutting across Irish medical emigration, was another migratory medical flow. This was from South East Asia. As Julian Simpson describes in his path-breaking book, migrants from this part of the world were becoming an increasingly indispensable part of the NHS.[88] Simpson points to the particularity of South East Asian settlement in Britain. The migrant doctors he described tended to be found in the less desirable practices

84 Unfortunately for historians, job advertisements have often been removed from medical journals lodged in archives. However, the National Library of Ireland has a relatively complete series of the *Journal of the Medical Association of Eire*.

85 *Journal of the Medical Association of Eire,* September 1950, vol. 27 no. 159, pp. 53–59 and November 1950, vol. 27, no. 161, pp. 93–100.

86 RCSI Archives, Scrapbook. 'Cuttings of Interesting Information'. Quote from *Irish Times*, 27 September 1950.

87 *Journal of the Medical Association of Eire,* vol. 27, no. 161, November 1950, between pp. 93–100 (un-numbered).

88 Simpson, *Migrant Architects of the NHS*.

in Britain, in working-class and industrial and ex-industrial areas, which had an historic legacy of low investment in surgeries and equipment compared with more affluent areas.

Simpson's work on the distribution of South East Asian doctors in Britain invites comparison with what we know of Irish doctor settlement in Britain. There were also fewer Irish doctors in affluent areas in inter-war Britain and slightly more in industrial and working-class ones; but not by much. The largest conglomeration of Irish doctors tended to be in Catholic areas. Irish educated doctors can also be found in poor inner cities but not more than other newly arrived immigrants who also found access to practice there easier to obtain. Many Irish medical graduates also followed the pattern of their South Asian colleagues taking first-step jobs in Britain in the public health service or hospitals and then graduating to general practice.

Irish doctors had several advantages over their South East Asian colleagues when it came to the transition to general practice. They were a long-standing medical migrant group and their medical institutions were relatively well integrated with those of British medicine. They were familiar in Britain and many of their compatriots, among past cohorts of Irish medical migrants, had achieved success there. The Irish were also advantaged to an extent, particular in the 1950s, by being able to access group practices already set up by medical graduates from Ireland in the inter-war years. Group practices were encouraged under the new NHS dispensation and in the 1950s some of those we have described earlier had been there since the 1920s providing a pre-existing network of opportunity and support for the Irish medical graduate.

Nonetheless there was some similarity in patterns of settlement with the migratory group identified by Simpson especially if we equate the religious distribution of Irish doctor settlement with distribution by ethnicity; the two, as Simpson shows, are also intertwined in the case of South East Asian doctor immigration. The tendency of Irish Catholic doctors to look to practices with Catholic and Catholic Irish populations point to the influence of cultural factors in doctor settlement. This was, of course, not true of Protestant doctors, but they replicated, with the Catholic medical graduates, other patterns familiar to the new South East Asian migrant. Friendships, the tradition of the medical school created pre-existing networks which could shape patterns of settlement though, in the case of the new migrants, these had been forged in very different circumstances.[89] But longstanding Irish medical migration within a community of nations that had some common shared history and in

89 See Chapter 8 for a discussion of the particular influences on medical migrants from outside Europe.

which the Irish and British medical elites were to a degree integrated, undoubtedly smoothed the paths of many Irish doctors in Britain.

Medical migration from Ireland to Britain was stimulated by the arrival of the NHS and the expansion of opportunities for the medical graduate. Irish doctors were invited to fill the shortfall in the British health service at a crucial juncture in its evolution. Nonetheless, although the flow of doctors to Britain from Ireland continued in the 1950s, overall the percentage of Irish medical migrants to Britain was beginning to fall. At the end of the 1960s Simpson calculates that 11.8 per cent of doctors in general practice in the UK were of South East Asian origin but the proportion of doctors born in Northern Ireland or the Republic of Ireland in general practice was falling.[90] Between 1920–40 Irish medical emigration was 39 per cent of the cohorts we examined for that period, the majority going to Britain. From 1945–60 it was 33 per cent.

Some of this was undoubtedly the attraction of the United States as an alternative destination. The pull exerted by America was not confined to Irish born and educated doctors. According to Abel-Smith's study of British doctors in the 1950s and early 1960s "a fifth of British born and trained doctors in their sample who registered in the 1950s were living overseas in 1963" and of these a high proportion were in North America.[91] Similarly Britain, whilst still an important destination, had been supplanted in the minds of many aspirant Irish medical graduates by the lure of America.

90 Simpson, *Migrant Architects of the NHS*, footnote 88, p. 168.

91 Ibid., p. 43 quoting Abel-Smith and Gates, *British Doctors at Home and Abroad.*

CHAPTER 7

The Lure of America

A guide written for the new medical graduate in 1935 had a section on practice outside the British Empire.[1] By this date, the issue of recognition of medical degrees in other countries was coming much more to the fore. It had always existed to some extent; for example, William Huggard had found it necessary to register with a Swiss board of accreditation on taking up practice in Switzerland in the late nineteenth century.[2] The writer of the guide warned the potential emigrant that "There are now local medical acts and registers for nearly all parts of the British Empire overseas." Entry in the *Medical Register* of the United Kingdom and the payment of a fee nearly always secured the doctor's future in these regions, but

> British Columbia, New Brunswick, Ontario Quebec, and Saskatchewan are exceptions. [Additionally] In respect of all other countries outside the British Empire persons registered or registrable [*sic*] in the United Kingdom require to pass the same, or nearly the same, examinations as those required of the natives of the country.[3]

Concerns of this kind were not new but were to arise in a particularly acute form when Irish medical emigration to the United States increased in the 1950s. Warning signs about the attitude of the American medical establishment towards Irish medical schools were demonstrated in the 1920s when the RF visited Ireland with the aim of assisting the newly founded state to modernise its medical education.

1 The Rockefeller Visit to Ireland

The RF was founded in 1913. A wealthy charitable organisation, one of its remits was to disburse funds for reform in public health, the eradication of

1 An earlier version of this chapter can be found in Greta Jones, '"A mysterious discrimination": Irish medical emigration to the United States in the 1950s', *Social History of Medicine*, vol. 25, no. 1, February 2012, pp. 139–56.
2 See Chapter 4.
3 *The Medical Practitioner's Handbook* (1935), pp. 62–3.

 | DOI:10.1163/9789004324466_009

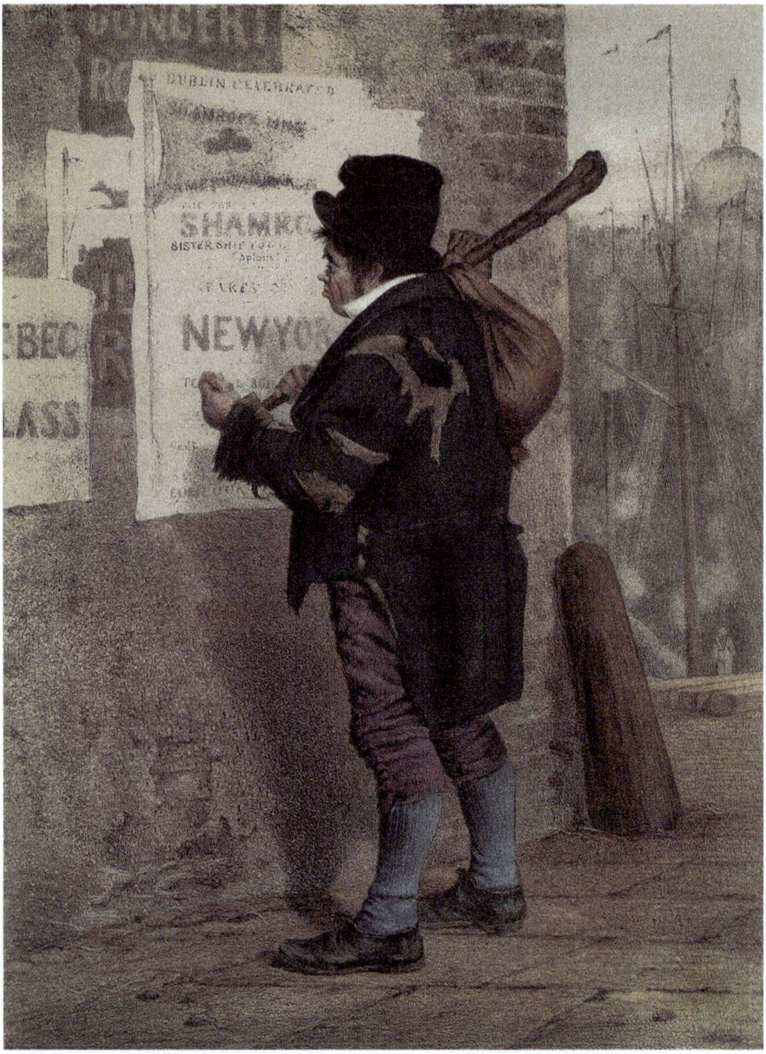

FIGURE 5 An Irishman looks at a poster advertising voyages to New York and resolves to emigrate. Coloured lithograph after E. Nicol, ca. 1840/1860
SOURCE: WELLCOME COLLECTION. ATTRIBUTION 4.0 INTERNATIONAL (CC BY 4.0)

disease, medical research and for the improvement of medical education. In 1919 Alan Gregg was appointed by the RF as head of its medical sciences division in Europe. Gregg was a Harvard-educated doctor, a member of the British Royal Army Medical Corps during the First World War and was based at Rockefeller's Paris office. The visit to Ireland was for two purposes. The first was to assist the reorganisation of public health by the government of the Free State and to train some of the newly appointed county medical officers.[4] The second aim was to reform Irish medical education. Although Gregg visited Northern Ireland, his chief concern was the new Irish state in the South. Thus began in Ireland, as in other parts of the world, chiefly through American philanthropic activity, an attempt to encourage the adoption of the American model of medical education based upon the Flexner reforms and the John Hopkins University Hospital.[5] In a relatively short time in the USA, Flexner had created a high prestige, scientifically based, intensive medical training based on the fusion of teaching and research. The reforms raised the status of American medicine worldwide and proved, partly because funding agencies such as Rockefeller took the gospel of Flexner with them in their excursions into other countries, extremely influential outside America itself.

Many of the problems in Irish medical education were financial, as previous visitors from the USA to Ireland had observed. In 1895 the *Journal of the American Medical Association* (*JAMA*) published an article titled "A Glimpse of Irish Surgery" by a Chicago doctor. His comment on Irish medical schools was respectful, but he noted that Trinity College Dublin (University of Dublin) "lacks many of the modern improvements which are so essential in the practice of ideal surgery". The old buildings and poor equipment were noted, and especially the problem of Dublin hospitals where:

> It is unfortunate that this old and otherwise enterprising city does not possess a general hospital where the clinical material could be centralised and made more available for clinical teaching. Not any of the hospitals contain more than 120 beds and those where the clinical teaching is done are often distant from the medical school to which they are attached.[6]

Gregg's conclusions about the state of Irish medical education in the 1920s were largely the same. On his visit to Ireland in 1925 he noted the proliferation of medical schools. There were four in Dublin alone (Trinity College, Dublin, the RCSI, University College Dublin and the Apothecaries Hall). This was not counting the number outside Dublin: two colleges of the National University of Ireland in Cork and Galway and the Queen's University medical school now

4 For a discussion of health reform in Eire post-1922, see Jones, *"Captain of all these Men of Death"*.

5 Ludmerer, *A Time to Heal*. Ludmerer suggests that, in spite of its great achievements, some patient care could be impersonal and over-technological, and the elites that were created in the leading medical schools were often exclusively male and white.

6 N. Senn, "A glimpse of Irish Surgery", *JAMA*, 17 August 1895, vol. 25, no. 7, pp. 281 and 282.

part of Northern Ireland. Gregg's recommendations were that two schools only should survive in Dublin (Trinity and University College Dublin) and that a large well-funded research hospital on the Johns Hopkins model should be set up, probably by the amalgamation of two existing hospitals. Although he was aware of the sectarian problems of uniting these two schools, nonetheless Gregg believed they could be encouraged to move towards closer cooperation and the sharing of resources. The negotiations towards this end took several years and were finally abandoned in the early 1930s. By then, however, Gregg had lost faith in the project. The problem was that a strictly rational distribution of resources in medical education seemed out of reach.

Gregg pointed out that in 1929 Ireland had one medical school to every 700,000 inhabitants (one to 500,000 if the Apothecaries Hall was included), compared to one to 2,600,000 in Norway, one to 2,100,000 in Austria and one to 1,700,000 in Holland. This was a wasteful multiplicity of schools in his view. The number of hospitals available to the Dublin population had been a source of pride in the nineteenth century and regarded as a particular advantage for the poor. But the very number, aggravated by the fact that many were either predominantly Protestant or Catholic institutions, meant that resources were stretched beyond what could support one state-of-the-art medical school and clinical teaching hospital in Dublin.

Gregg failed and one reason was that the medical schools operated to a different economic rationality. Basically the Irish medical schools sustained an export economy. Gregg's plan would have reduced the number of schools drastically, and consequently the fee income and the medical establishment in the hospitals. Moreover the plan demanded a level of good fellowship between the medical schools, which did not exist at that time. The sectarianism was disillusioning to Gregg. The RF kept press cuttings, and in their archive is one from the nationalist *Catholic Pictorial* on a story emanating from Sir William Thompson (1861–1926), the former Registrar General for Ireland, in the *Dublin Evening Standard*. The article, according to the *Pictorial,* stated "Dublin loses £1,250.00", which the *Catholic Pictorial* reckoned should have read:

> Dublin Protestant Hospital Fails to Pull Mr Rockefeller's Leg. Their hope of £1,250.00 subsidy disappointed. The catastrophe he (Thompson) sees coming is the loss of more of the loaves and fishes to those who have almost exclusively enjoyed them in the realm of medical science ... It is our turn for a spell of ascendancy.[7]

---

7 RF 1.1.403A, Boxes 7–8, Development Aid. Newspaper Cutting *c.*1931.

This example of mutual ill feeling together with the tendency for their confidential discussions to be subsequently openly debated in the press, was disillusioning to Rockefeller.

UCD and TCD felt some alarm when it was clear the RF was gradually distancing itself from assisting medical education in Ireland. Worried at the possibility of forgoing the generous assistance on offer, the heads of these two schools cobbled up a joint appeal to the RF in 1933. However, it still fell short of the objectives of Rockefeller, involving only appeals for funds for a joint trip to examine medical schools on the Continent. It was turned down.[8]

2 Medical Immigration to the United States

Immigration of foreign-educated doctors into the USA had risen in the late 1930s, peaking in 1938, 1939 and 1940. This was largely due to the political situation in Europe. After the USA entered the Second World War in 1941, doctor immigration tailed off but in 1945 the American Medical Association (AMA), the leading professional body for doctors in the USA, anticipated another rise in the immigration of both displaced persons and the 'displaced physician' into the USA. American medical schools had also been encouraged to recruit more heavily during the war, and these two factors led the AMA to anticipate a rise in doctor numbers.[9]

In fact, in the immediate post-war years, the numbers of medical professionals immigrating to the USA failed to rise to even the level of 1936–41. By 1951 the AMA's original estimate of an annual influx of 2,300 displaced physicians had been revised downwards to around 500–600.[10] In 1949, however, medical immigration started to rise again. Throughout the 1950s it climbed steadily each year, surpassing pre-war levels in 1957 and peaking in 1972, when it was estimated that 46 per cent of all new physicians that year were foreign-born and educated abroad.[11] The number of foreign-trained physicians actually in practice in the USA was 13.2 per cent in 1965 and 22.9 per cent in 1979.[12]

8 National Archives Dublin, Office of the Taoiseach, S6409, "Scheme for the Improvement of Irish Medical Education and Research".

9 Ludmerer, *Time to Heal*, Fig. 7, p. 272 and passim.

10 James Brunot, "Resettlement of Displaced Physicians: A New Approach", *JAMA*, 7 April 1951, vol. 145, no. 14, pp. 1059–62.

11 Bruce L.R. Smith, 'The Brain Drain Re-Emergent: Foreign Medical Graduates in American Medical Schools', *Minerva*, vol. 17, no. 4, 1979, p. 487.

12 Thomas D. Dublin, 'The Changing Role of the Foreign Medical Graduate in the Practice of Medicine in the US, Educational Commission for Foreign Medical Graduates), p. 5. Report presented 1980.

Some of this was due to a relaxation in immigration rules in 1965, which made it easier for foreign-trained physicians to obtain visas to enter the United States.[13] But the trend itself began before 1965, caused not just by ease of access but by the positive attractions of American medicine. Contrary to the AMA's expectations, demand for health care expanded in the United States after 1945, and the overcrowding anticipated by the AMA in the profession did not materialise. In fact there was a shortage of doctors in the less desirable parts of the American health care system, for example in state and county medical institutions, and it was in these posts that many overseas trained doctors could be found. The United States was not just comparatively wealthy compared with many other countries including those in Europe, but also its medical education was regarded as cutting edge. Hence many graduates of foreign medical schools made their way to America for postgraduate training. As was pointed out at the time, a substantial number of these remained after their courses ended and settled down to practise in the USA.

Among the flow of foreign-trained physicians into the USA were a small proportion of its own citizens. In most cases this was because they had failed to get a place in an American medical school so had tried abroad, mostly in Europe. In 1960–1 this was calculated as 2,520 students, mostly in European schools.[14] However, the majority of physician immigrants to America were foreign-born and trained.

TABLE 18 Number of graduates from foreign medical schools entering the USA 1930–60

Years	Number	Number passing licensing exam
1930–5	1,429	881
1936–41	8,168	4,220
1942–7	4,923	2,446
1948–53	5,852	2,957
1954–9	12,828	7,730

SOURCE: TAKEN FROM "MEDICAL LICENSURE STATISTICS FOR 1960", *JAMA*, 17 MAY 1961, VOL. 176, NO. 8, TABLE 30

13 Dr Robert M. Politzer, 'The Impact of Foreign-Trained Doctors on the Supply of Physicians', Undertaken for the US Department of Health and Human Services, 1983. The change was to allow high-priority visas to be issued to physicians.

14 David M. Greely, 'American Foreign Medical Graduates', *Journal of Medical Education*, vol. 41, no. 7, July 1966, pp. 641–50.

3 The AMA, Doctor Immigration and the Approved List

Faced by increasing migration of medical professionals into the country, the AMA took action. Publicly the AMA in 1950s expressed its worries in terms of equivalence of training and competence of foreign doctors, although alarm at the possible impact of immigration on the income of indigenous doctors undoubtedly played a part.[15] The Flexner Report had revolutionised the status of the physician in American society, and it was to Flexner that they turned. Abraham Flexner's report had created an alliance between himself, the Carnegie Institute, the Council on Medical Education, the AMA and the leading American medical schools. It led to the issuing of a list of approved and graded medical schools, which became a guide to their quality. Additionally the Flexner reforms encouraged charitable and state investment in the medical schools high on the 'approved' list and it influenced student choice. The approved list represented the benchmark of what was considered to be an acceptable medical education and it was this that the RF had brought to Ireland in 1925 in an attempt to reform Irish medical schools.

The approved list did not have the force of law. Individual state legislatures determined the licensing of physicians. But the approved list influenced state and federal legislatures, aspirants to a medical degree and public opinion. By these means many of the smaller private schools, tributes to entrepreneurial spirit but not necessarily to the highest academic standards, had closed down. Presence on an approved list became essential for a self-respecting American medical college and for ambitious medical students. In many cases states would only admit medical graduates to their licensing exam if they had graduated from a school on the approved list.

This passage in American medical education influenced the American attitude to foreign medical schools. European schools had traditionally been viewed respectfully by the American physician. When comparisons were made prior to 1912, it was generally to assert that whilst the best in the USA were comparable with anywhere in the world, foreign medical education illustrated the particular shortcomings of the US system: namely the survival of private proprietary schools, the divorce of school from university, the lack of a central controlling professional body and the poor level of preliminary

---

15 The economist Milton Friedman observed the activities of the AMA from the University of Chicago in the 1950s in this rather brutal fashion: "The American Medical Association is perhaps the strongest trade union in the United States." *Capitalism and Freedom*, Chicago, University of Chicago Press, 1962, p. 158.

education in basic science.[16] The reforms in medical education carried out through the Flexner Report in 1910 changed this view.[17] Whilst European schools retained a degree of respect, even though deficient in some respects in the opinion of American medical educators, by 1945, in the words of the AMA, twenty years of political turmoil, the devastation of war and the relative isolation of many Continental medical schools had put back medical education in Europe.[18]

Worried, therefore, by the rising immigration of foreign graduates into the USA, the AMA used the experience which had been so successful in transforming American medical education. They could exercise no direct control over the immigration of foreign doctors, but they could influence political and public opinion. This they attempted to do by producing an 'approved list' of foreign medical schools, which they hoped would influence the bodies responsible for licensure in the states of the USA and also public opinion about which foreign doctors could be safely permitted to practise. In the words of one commentator, "The policy of rating the school rather than the individual was an extension of a successful policy initiated by the Flexner Report of 1910." In that writer's view, however, "But what had succeeded for American medical schools failed when applied to foreign medical schools."[19]

If we look at events from a purely American perspective, the history of the approved list for foreign medical schools was brief: it was tried in the 1950s and abandoned as a failure by the end of that decade. But the impact upon those countries that were at the receiving end was significant. One of these countries was Ireland. Doctor emigration was a very significant part of the outcome of Irish medical education, and the refusal of the AMA to put five of the six Irish medical schools on the approved list had considerable internal repercussions in Irish medicine.

---

16 See J.N. McCormack, "Conclusions from a Comparative Study of the Status of the Medical Profession in Great Britain and the United States", *JAMA*, 29 September 1906, vol. 47, no. 13, pp. 1043–4; and "Medical Colleges in the United States and Abroad", *JAMA*, 14 August 1909, vol. 53, no. 7, pp 541–4.

17 Described in Ludmerer, *Time to Heal*; also in Thomas Neville Bonner, *Iconoclast Abraham Flexner and a Life in Learning* (Baltimore: Johns Hopkins University Press, 2002).

18 AMA Archives, Chicago, Minutes of Meeting of the Committee on Foreign Medical Credentials, 25 March 1949, in Minutes of the Business Meeting of the Council on Medical Education and Hospitals, 8–9 February 1949, Appendix H, p. 5.

19 AMA Archives, Chicago CHM5926/71, Melvin Lurie, 'Physician Licensing Policy', First National Congress on Health Manpower (sponsored by the Council on Health Manpower of the AMA), 22–4 October 1970, p. 92.

4 The Irish Medical Emigrant and the USA

The majority of emigrating Irish doctors went to Britain in the 1950s, but doctor emigration to the USA and Canada began to rise in the interwar years and even further after the Second World War. A survey of emigrating medical graduates from our cohorts 1860–1960 shows that three-quarters of the emigration to the USA and Canada was in the decade 1950–60.[20] Of those who were practising outside Ireland in that decade, 19 per cent were in North America. This was less than the 60 per cent emigrating to Great Britain in the same period, but more than for any other destination.[21] Doctor emigration was a feature of Irish medical schools throughout this period, but emigration to the USA was characteristic of the 1950s.[22]

The AMA set up the Committee on Foreign Medical Credentials in the autumn of 1947 to examine the issue of doctor immigration. The situation was complex. Foreign graduates could not sit the exams of the National Board of Medical Examiners (NBME), which was generally accepted throughout the USA. This left them dependent on acceptance by individual states. Some states excluded all foreign graduates from practising in their territory. In others the regulations which admitted foreign graduates to sit the licensing exam or be licensed differed according to their citizenship or immigration status, length of time in the USA or other considerations.

In 1949 thirty-two states of America stated that candidates for licensure had to be US citizens, with the exception of Canadians.[23] One state granted temporary licensure until full citizenship had been granted. Twenty-three states did

---

20 A total of 1,732 emigrant doctors were examined during 1860–1960, of which 56 went to the USA. These comprise 2 before 1920, 15 in 1920–40 and 39 in 1945–60. This is not of course the total figure of emigrants to the USA, but the figure from the selected cohorts. The migration to Canada was less than that to the USA, but still significant; see D. Wright, S. Mullally and M.C. Cordukes, '"Worse than being Married": The Exodus of British Doctors from the National Health Service to Canada c.1955–1975', *Journal of the History of Medicine and the Allied Sciences*, vol. 65, no. 4, 2010, pp. 567- 77; and D. Wright and S. Mullally, '"Not everyone can be a Gandhi": South Asian-trained physician immigration to Canada c.1961–1971', *Ethnicity and Health*, vol. 21, no. 4, 2018 (online 2015).

21 The next highest destination was Africa at 7.7 per cent. Some may have been African doctors returning home, having trained in Irish schools.

22 There were of course those who stayed only for a few years for postgraduate training and then returned, or who retired back to Ireland after completing a career in the USA.

23 Reciprocity existed between the medical schools of Canada and the USA. The AMA in fact inspected Canadian medical schools. This meant that emigrants to the USA from Ireland sometimes arrived there via Canada.

not accept any graduates of foreign schools except Canada. Eight states maintained this rule, but only after a fixed date had passed. Two had few restrictions.[24] A significant number of states, however, were prepared to take the advice of the AMA Council on Medical Education and Hospitals about which graduates of American and Canadian medical schools should be eligible to sit their licensing exams. It was with the purpose of extending this influence to foreign medical schools that the AMA set up the Committee on Foreign Medical Credentials.

The Committee functioned essentially as a subcommittee of the AMA's Council on Medical Education and Hospitals. At the first full-scale meeting on 25 March 1949, representatives from the Association of Medical Colleges, the AMA's old ally in the fight to improve medical education, the Advisory Board on Medical Specialities and bodies from the licensing world were present. They included the NBME, the Federation of State Medical Boards and the registration bodies of Connecticut, Illinois, Wisconsin, all states with more than average experience of immigration issues.[25] Representatives from the US Office of Education attended, as did various international and charitable organisations. Among them were the World Health Organization (WHO), the Pan-American Sanitary Bureau, the World Medical Association and the Institute of Inter-American Affairs. The Kellogg Foundation and the Rockefeller Foundation also took part. Three members of the Council on Medical Education and Hospitals were particularly important in the Committee on Foreign Credentials: Victor Johnson, H.G. Weiskotten and Donald G. Anderson. It was Donald Anderson who, as secretary to the committee, was to conduct the bulk of its business and receive most of the correspondence in connection with its deliberations.

In 1949 the main source of foreign doctors was seen to be displaced persons, and this was a delicate subject. There were political and humanitarian considerations involved, including the danger of alienating immigrant communities in the USA who gave hospitality to refugee physicians, encouraged them to set up practice and generally acted as their advocates. The committee was, however, resolute in its opinion of the importance of maintaining the standards of American medical education. It pointed out:

> The present high standards of medical practice in the United States has been the direct result of the recognition by the licensing boards, that evaluation of the school from which a physician graduates is equally important as evaluation of the physician himself. Before this principle

---

24 Creighton Barker and Grace Mooney, 'Licensing of Foreign Medical Graduates in the United States', *JAMA*, 7 May 1949, vol. 140, no. 1, pp. 10–12.

25 New York and Minnesota were invited but unable to attend.

> was generally recognised, the country was overrun with physicians who, armed with a degree from a low grade school or outright diploma mill, succeeded in one way or another, in passing the examinations for licensure. The needless suffering and injury perpetuated by the incompetent and, at times, fraudulent practices of many of these inadequately trained men constitute a dark chapter in the history of medicine.[26]

However, the committee was anxious not to appear too restrictive. Its aim, it claimed, was to facilitate the resettlement of the physician in America by removing prejudices against foreign graduates in the minds of some state licensing boards. A list was seen as encouraging state boards to adopt "an enlightened view towards the foreign-trained physician".[27]

The difficulties of producing reports on foreign medical schools soon became apparent. The first avenue explored was visitations, but it was quickly recognised that the cost would be prohibitive and the process time-consuming.[28] Questionnaires might be substituted for actual visitation, but the experience of these had not been encouraging. The Federation of State Medical Boards, the World Medical Association and the Committee on Displaced Persons had sent out 350 questionnaires to medical schools, but received back only 150. Of 300 sent out by the Department of State, only 132 were returned. Eventually it was decided to proceed by seeking detailed information about foreign medical schools in personal interviews "with qualified and disinterested persons who have knowledge of the school in question". It was particularly useful if this had been obtained by a visit. Written reports on graduate performance and other individual assessments and, where appropriate, "the status of the school with the General Medical Council of Great Britain" also formed part of the strategy.[29] However, visitations themselves could only be arranged on an informal and *ad hoc* basis when a trusted member of the AMA happened to be in the vicinity.

A small committee comprising Harold S. Diehl, chairman, Loren R. Chandler and Stanley Dorst visited Great Britain for a conference in October 1949,

---

26 AMA Archives, Minutes of the Meeting of the Committee on Foreign Medical Credentials, 25 March 1949, Appendix H to the Minutes of the Business Meeting of the Council on Medical Education and Hospitals, 8–9 February 1949, p. 4.

27 Ibid., p. 6.

28 AMA Archives, Minutes of the Council on Medical Education and Hospitals, 8–9 February 1949, p. 25. It was calculated at $60–90,000 p.a.

29 AMA Archives, Council on Medical Education and Hospitals, Appendix G of the Minutes of 20, 22, 23, October 1949. This would of course only be relevant to schools within the jurisdiction of the GMC, but in 1949 this included a number in former or remaining British colonies in Africa and Asia.

returning in February 1950. Harold S. Diehl broke off the visit to Great Britain to visit Ireland, and it was on the basis of his observations that Irish schools were assessed. A report was mailed back to the council and received in December 1949. During that period, Creighton Barker visited Copenhagen, Stockholm, Uppsala and Oslo. Knowledge of Switzerland was contributed by Freddy Homburger of Boston; and Vernon Lippard, who had visited Italy recently, provided information on their schools.[30]

The report on 'Classification of Foreign Medical Schools' presented to the committee was the basis of the list of 'approved' schools which was first issued in February 1950. The approved list comprised twenty-seven schools in, respectively, Denmark (one), Finland (two), Netherlands (four), Norway (one) and Sweden (three). The United Kingdom had sixteen approved schools: ten in England, four in Scotland, one in Wales and one in Northern Ireland, the medical school of Queen's University of Belfast.[31] In the first list drawn up for the Council on Medical Education on 7 February 1950, the names of the National University of Ireland and the University of Dublin (Trinity College Dublin) appeared. But, according to the deliberations of the Council on Medical Education and Hospitals, subsequently "the schools in Eire had been removed on the basis of later information".[32]

The actual reports on the medical schools presented before the council were brief and uninformative, but something of their direction can be gathered from the guidance given to the delegation before it departed on the British visit. Crucial to the view of the AMA on the suitability of a medical school was affiliation to a university and clinical facilities at all stages of medical training. Laboratory facilities, the qualifications of the faculty, size of class, entrance qualifications and the state of the library were also examined. The failure rate of the graduates of different foreign schools in American licensing exams was also raised. Less tangible measures, such as appraisal of students, reputation of the school and comparison with US schools were included. Finally, language is mentioned, presumably competence in English.[33]

30 AMA Archives, Business Meeting of the Council on Medical Education and Hospitals, Minutes of 4 and 5 December 1949. Freddy Homburger was a native of Switzerland and obtained his medical degree there. He headed the Cancer Research unit at Tufts. Vernon W. Lippard was President of the Association of American Medical Colleges and in 1952 became Dean of Yale Medical School.

31 AMA Archives, Meeting of the Council on Medical Education and Hospitals, 3–8 February 1950.

32 AMA Archives, Council on Medical Education and Hospitals, Minutes, 3–8 February 1950, Appendix B, p. 14.

33 AMA Archives, Minutes of the Council on Medical Education and Hospitals, 20, 22, 23 October 1949, Appendix G.

These reports raised serious issues for the Republic of Ireland's medical schools. Though alerted by the negotiations with the British government in 1949 about the new criteria for British medical education originating in the Goodenough Report, they had simply accepted the designation of 'provisional' (P) for their graduates on the UK *Medical Register* pending later clinical experience in a hospital approved for training.[34] Nothing substantial had been done to increase scientific facilities and unite university and hospital as one functioning medical school. Clinical teaching was still seriously impeded by organisational problems. In the schools in Cork and Galway, outside Dublin, the situation was less complicated because there were fewer hospitals and often ones with traditional links to the medical schools in those cities. However, there was frequently an insufficient variety of medical cases to allow the students a comprehensive education. In Dublin there were, and it was often to Dublin that students went to acquire their clinical experience.[35] However, the hospitals in Dublin were under the general advisement of the medical school, but not under their control.[36] Clinical teachers were appointed by the hospital, not the medical school, and this frequently militated against an ethos of research achievement.

5 The Approved List and the Foreign Medical Schools

In 1949 the US State Department became involved when a representative of the AMA asked Mr Paul Dompke, a State Department official, whether the issuing of a list of approved foreign medical schools would embarrass the State Department. The answer was:

> opinion was divided in the State Department. Some feared unwanted attention from the governments of the unlisted schools; others were in favour of taking a calculated risk. But it was not discussed at the highest level in the State Department.[37]

---

34 This was put into effect by the United Kingdom Parliament in the Medical Act of 1950.

35 See Kelly, *Irish Medical Education and Student Culture c.1850–1950*, pp. 123–4.

36 In a later comment in reply to a protest from Dr Bigger at TCD, this was made explicit by Dr Harold S. Diehl. He thought "it unwise to recognise the school since there is no supervision given in the clinical years". AMA Archives, Council on Medical Education and Hospitals, Minutes of the Business Meeting of the Council, 23–4 June 1950, p. 13.

37 AMA Archives, Minutes of Business Committee of the Council on Medical Education and Hospitals, 4–5 December 1949, Appendix G, p. 4. Interviews on 16 November 1949 and a subsequent telephone conversation on 28 November 1949 with officials.

In fact there was considerable 'unwanted attention' from certain governments, and Irish schools were not the only ones discomforted by their non-inclusion by the AMA in the list of approved foreign medical schools. In a meeting of the Committee on Foreign Credentials in 1952, the AMA was informed that:

> The Diplomatic services of France, Italy and the Irish Free State have protested the absence of schools in these countries from the lists. Other representations indicate that there are schools in Mexico and India which desire to be included in the list.[38]

By 1953 the AMA had received requests for visits from medical schools in West Germany, Italy, South America and China. The prospect opening up for the AMA was not only pressure to accede to requests for first-time visitation, but also for follow-up visits from disappointed medical schools. It was pointed out in one meeting that there were approximately 566 medical schools in the world, so this was a daunting task.[39]

6 Ireland and the Approved List

With regard to Ireland, the AMA Council on Medical Education and Hospitals was told in December 1950 that "The medical schools of Southern Ireland are disturbed that they have not been recognized by the Council. Considerable correspondence has been received from the Schools and other interested agencies."[40] From 1950 to 1953 a campaign of politico-medical lobbying took place on behalf of Irish medical schools. The Department of External Affairs (DEA) of the Republic of Ireland (later the Department of Foreign Affairs, DFA) was drawn into this and most of the extant correspondence between the AMA and interested parties in Ireland has survived, primarily in Irish government files.[41] Successive reports on the position of Irish medical school graduates in the USA were commissioned by the DEA from Ireland's Consul Generals in New York and Chicago and relayed to Ireland via the Irish Embassy in Washington, D.C.

---

38 AMA Archives, Minutes of the Meeting of the Committee on Foreign Medical Credentials, 25 April 1952, vol. 1, Appendix F, p. 11.

39 AMA Archives, Minutes of the Business Committee of the Council on Medical Education and Hospitals, 29–30 November 1953. Dr Turner pointed this out.

40 AMA Archives, Minutes of the Meeting of the Council on Medical Education and Hospitals, 2–4 December 1950, pp. 24–5.

41 National Archives Dublin, Office of the Taoiseach, File S14402B, 'Undergraduate and Postgraduate Medical Training'.

The DEA, together with the Department of Health, attempted to negotiate their way through this issue, and the Irish Medical Association and the Medical Registration Council of Ireland entered into correspondence with the AMA. So did luminaries from the Roman Catholic Church in the USA and Irish immigrant doctors in New York and Chicago, organised into a loose grouping called the Irish Universities Medical Club of America. The Council on Medical Education felt the impact of this pressure. In December 1950 it was stated that, as far as the Irish were concerned, "the situation is under control but if it becomes acute it may be necessary to consider personal inspection of the schools".[42]

For a time the Irish sought a backdoor means of evading the consequences of non-listing by the AMA. This emanated principally from Irish representatives in New York, and consisted of an attempt to secure recognition by the New York State Licensing Board. Mr Christianson of the United States Embassy believed, according to Irish officials, "that, as the other States of the Union practically always took their medical standards from New York, recognition by the New York Board of Regents must automatically mean recognition throughout the U.S.A.".[43] In May 1951 a report was sent from the Consul General in New York to the DEA via the Republic of Ireland's office in Washington. A friend of the Consul General, Dr Leo Kelly, a Brooklyn doctor, had visited him to tell him about Dr Maurillo, a member of the Board of Regents of New York, who reputedly got Swiss and Italian doctors recognised by New York.[44] They believed that a visit by Dr Maurillo to Europe was imminent in June 1951 and that he could be put to the same use on behalf of the Irish medical schools. A proposal to defray his expenses was sent to the AMA by the Irish Medical Association, but Dr Manlove turned down the offer on the grounds that "since Dr Maurillo was not known to the Council on Medical Education and Hospitals of the AMA, a report furnished by him would not be accepted as a basis for the Council's decisions".[45]

The proposal to use the New York Board of Regents to secure recognition in New York was pursued throughout 1952. In January 1952 a representative of Cardinal Spellman, the Most Reverend William A. Scully, chairman of the National Catholic Welfare Committee of New York, suggested to Ambassador

---

42 AMA Archives, Minutes of the Meeting of the Council on Medical Education and Hospitals, 2–4 December 1950, pp. 24–5.

43 National Archives Dublin, Office of the Taoiseach, File S14402B, 'Undergraduate and Postgraduate Medical Training', p. 11.

44 He is referred to in the documents produced by the Irish government as Dr Vincent Maurillo, but in the *New York Times*, 14 September 1951, p. 23 col. 8 as Dr Dominick Maurillo. His name is also occasionally spelt as Mauriello in Irish government documents.

45 National Archives Dublin, Office of the Taoiseach, File S14402B, 'Memorandum on the History of AMA and Irish Medical Schools', May 1953, pp. 7–8.

Matthews, the US ambassador to Ireland, that "an unofficial visit to the Irish medical schools by a Catholic member of the Board of Regents of Education in New York" could be arranged as a preliminary to securing a second official visit by the Board of Regents. In November 1952 the Irish Universities Club of New York was still urging the claims of Dr Maurillo, who had "approved the graduates of the medical schools of twenty Italian universities and of the University of Paris as acceptable for licensure in New York".[46] New York was the recipient of the largest number of medical immigrants applying for licensure, so the strategy made some sense. In 1955 New York State, along with Ohio, Illinois and California, had the largest number of graduates of foreign medical schools applying for licensure.

7 The Irish Medical Schools and the Irish Doctor

The omission of the medical schools of the Republic of Ireland from the approved list in USA caused considerable resentment among leading medical and academic luminaries in Ireland. Michael Tierney, President of University College Dublin, the largest of the three colleges making up the National University of Ireland, described the decision as "an undeserved and unexpected slur" and "invidious treatment" in a letter to the AMA. A letter protesting the decision was also received from Professor J.W. Bigger of the Medical Faculty of the University of Dublin (Trinity College Dublin).[47] Tierney's initial letters to the AMA in 1950 were inclined to hide behind recognition by the GMC of Irish medical schools. Ireland, he averred, "as you know, is a federal land North or South", a statement which might have caused some surprise in Northern Ireland; and UCD's medical degrees were:

> accepted for immediate admission to the British *Medical Register*. Its Extern Examiners are among the most distinguished teachers in British University Medical Schools, and its examinations and curricula are in entire conformity with the Regulations of the British General Medical Council.[48]

---

46 Ibid., File S14402B, Annex C, 'Present Condition of Medical Education in the Republic of Ireland', p. 1. Report attached to a letter from the Irish Universities Medical Club of Chicago to the Consul of the Republic of Ireland in Chicago, November 1952.

47 Minutes of the Council on Medical Education and Hospitals of 22–4 June 1950. J.W. Bigger represented Ireland on the General Medical Council 1936–41. He was Professor of Bacteriology at Trinity College Dublin.

48 National Archives Dublin, Taoiseach's Office, File S14402, Annex B. Copy of a letter from Tierney to Dr Donald Anderson of the AMA, 13 September 1950. The existence of a fed-

This was not, however, seen by the AMA as circumventing the difficulty. According to the AMA report of its discussions in 1952:

> Dr Manlove pointed out that should graduates be accepted whose qualifications are recognized by the General Medical Council of Great Britain, this would include graduates of schools in Eire, Australia, South Africa and India. From the information on file, he stated, there was doubt as to the quality of training offered in some of the schools in these countries.[49]

Not all Irish medical educators and doctors took the same view, however. One effect of the AMA intervention was to open up divisions about the recent history and conduct of Irish medical education. A strain of opinion existed in Ireland best expressed in a letter to the AMA from James O'Donovan, Dean of University College Cork's medical school. He believed that the failed inspections:

> will have an exceedingly good result in shaking the Governing authorities out of their Rip van Winkle sleep … it gives some of us who are willing to do the right thing a weapon with which to castigate those who were obstructing us and whom our personal and local weapons were not powerful enough to hurt.

The writer included with his letter his own memorandum drafted in 1941 to illustrate his point:

> we are not all unaware of the discrepancies between our standards and those required by modern medical teaching. No notice whatever has been taken of this report but I have now published it to my students and, armed with the results of your recent inspection, I think that we shall succeed in effecting the necessary reforms.[50]

---

eral Ireland might have come as a shock to the Republic of Ireland's citizens, given that legislation enacted there in 1949 finally severed any remaining and largely symbolic connections with the United Kingdom and therefore also with Northern Ireland, which still remained part of the UK.

49 AMA Archives, Minutes of the Meeting of the Committee on Foreign Medical Credentials, 25 April 1952, vol. 1, p. 8.

50 AMA Archives, Minutes of the Meeting of the Council on Medical Education and Hospitals, 28–30 November 1953, Appendix H, 'Reports on Medical Education in Ireland'. Letter to the AMA, 3 October 1953, from James M. O'Donovan, Dean of the Medical Faculty of Cork.

Since 1950 a number of Irish immigrant doctors in the USA had been active in trying to get a resolution to the problem. Disappointed at the omission of the Irish medical schools from the 2 November edition of the approved list, a number of them loosely organised themselves into a body called the Irish Universities Medical Club of America, predominantly doctors from Chicago and New York. In November 1952 they drafted a letter supporting the criticisms of the AMA and included with it their own memorandum on the state of Irish medical education. This was circulated to interested parties with copies to the Irish consulates in Chicago and New York. In their covering letter the authors of the Chicago memorandum claimed to be addressing the concerns of the majority of Irish emigrant doctors in general, not just the signatories. They felt that what they called "a petty jurisdictional dispute between the Irish medical schools and the Irish Medical Association" was putting in jeopardy a proposed revisit by the AMA. They urged:

> The Irish government and the Irish Medical Association to hold public inquiries at an early date to expose and correct the abuses which have brought our universities and the Irish medical profession into worldwide disrepute. [In particular] the Irish medical schools [should] assume control and supervision of the clinical teaching of their students in the same fashion as European, British and American medical schools.[51]

The letter elicited angry responses in speeches at the winter graduations of the National University of Ireland in December 1952 from both Dr Tierney, President of University College Dublin, and Alfred O'Rahilly, President of Cork. Tierney described the letter and the allegations in the memorandum as "so erroneous as to be in some cases positively grotesque. Certain of them are of such a character that they could constitute grounds for an action for slander."[52]

Pressure was applied, including a threat to expunge the names of the signatories from the list of NUI graduates. In January 1953 a small victory was secured for the official stance when Tierney announced to the *Irish Independent* newspaper that four of the signatories to the Irish Universities Medical Club claimed never to have seen the report or letter, much less signed it, and

51 National Archives Dublin, Office of the Taoiseach, File S 14402B, Annex C, 'Present Condition of Medical Education in the Republic of Ireland', p. 1. Report attached to a letter from the Irish Universities Medical Club of Chicago to the Consul of the Republic of Ireland, November 1952.

52 'Alleged Abuses in Medical Schools. U.C.D. President's Denial', *Irish Times*, 20 December 1952. See also O'Rahilly, 'Attack on Irish Medical Schools "Unjustified"', ibid., 22 December 1952.

two others were told of it but claimed that they had had insufficient time to study it.[53] This was something of a pyrrhic victory. Four months later the Irish Universities Medical Club of America issued a second letter. The letter was published on 23 May 1953 in the *Western People*, a newspaper widely read in the west of Ireland, and it referred directly to their intention "not to let the conferring address go unchallenged".[54] By going public, the letter writers aroused a great deal of interest in Ireland.[55] The possibility of this becoming a serious political issue led the government of the Republic to commission its first full-length account of the preceding two years of negotiation:

> The Minister spoke to me on Saturday, 23 May, regarding an editorial and a letter from the Irish Universities Medical Club of America which appeared in the issue of the *Western People* of that date and instructed me to prepare, for the information of the Taoiseach, a memorandum setting out the developments in the recent controversy between the Irish doctors in America and the Universities and Medical Profession here on the subject of the non-inclusion of the medical schools of the Irish Universities in the approved list of schools issued by the American Medical Association.[56]

The article in the *Western People* ensured that the AMA's second visitation to Irish medical schools which was to follow in September 1953 would be headline news in Irish newspapers.

The doctors in the Irish Universities Medical Clubs of Chicago and New York who drafted the letter and memorandum could be criticised on a number of counts. Tierney's attack on them was not, as they claimed, "still reverberating around Ireland and the civilised world".[57] They were guilty of inaccuracies and carelessness in the presentation of their case. Also, the government's account of the proceedings referred correctly to the fluid and amorphous nature of the Irish Universities Medical Club, its *ad hoc* character and the lack of a real organisational centre which could validate memoranda issued in its name.

The signatories were, however, representative of the generation of Irish emigrant doctors who experienced the problems of emigration to the USA in

53 'Doctors Repudiate Document', *Irish Independent*, 3 January 1953.
54 'Irish Doctors in America', *Western People*, 23 May 1953.
55 'U.S. Medical Club Replies to Dr Tierney', *Irish Times*, 25 June 1953.
56 National Archives Dublin, Office of the Taoiseach, File S14402B, Letter to Mr Fay from 'TVC' accompanying the 'Memorandum on the History of AMA and Irish Medical Schools', 30 May 1953.
57 'Irish Doctors in America', *Western People*, 23 May 1953.

the 1950s. They were thirty-seven in total. Each letter had twenty-three original signatories, but nine doctors signed both letters and these nine doctors are traceable. They were slightly older, in their thirties, and with two exceptions licensed to practice in America. The two exceptions, who belonged to the 1950 cohort of NUI graduates, received their licenses in 1956 and 1957. One of the double signatories was in his fifties: this was Thomas E. Hardy, the only one who had not gained his medical degree at NUI. He had got a BA there in 1915 but emigrated to Chicago where he obtained an MA at Loyola and then an MD from the University of Chicago in 1925.

Of the remaining doctors, the fourteen who signed the Chicago letter and another different fourteen who signed the New York letter some months later cannot be found for sure. But of those traceable, most were in their twenties and the rest in their early thirties; the oldest was thirty-six at the time of the letter. They were recent graduates. All bar three had graduated post-war. At the time of the Chicago letter, four had been licensed to practise in America, but thirteen were still unlicensed and in some cases were not subsequently licensed until the late 1950s or early 1960s.[58] These doctors were, given the profile of most of them, likely to have been at the rough end of the process of getting established in the USA but we cannot necessarily extrapolate from their experience to other Irish medical emigrants whose stories may have been different.[59]

The peculiar organisational vagueness of the group did not detract from the substantive issues they raised. The protesting emigrant doctors were in a position to evaluate both their education and their recent experience in the United States. It was not, as outlined in the memorandum on the state of Irish medical education, just the control and nature of clinical teaching that was at fault. They referred also to the teaching of basic science, the poor facilities of UCD dissection rooms and the overcrowding and understaffing. They complained that "at least 300 students were graduated yearly from the Irish medical schools, a number three times as large as that graduated yearly in any corresponding population area in England or the United States".[60] The refusal

58 Therefore, a total of 15 of the 26 signatories whose licensing details can be found were as yet unlicensed.

59 A full picture of the experience of Irish doctors in the USA would be extremely valuable but to do full justice to the history of Irish medical emigrants would require a separate study. This is because it involves a very substantial range of archives including individual state's licensure histories and the responses of state legislatures; an examination of the public hospitals and health resources in individual states and also access to the archives of the American Catholic Church and to some important medical/postgraduate medical schools.

60 National Archives Dublin, Office of the Taoiseach, File S14402B, Annex C, 'Present Condition of Medical Education in the Republic of Ireland', p. 1. Report attached to a letter from

of the Deans of medical schools to listen to their complaints and answer letters was indicative of "cynical and callous indifference". There was in Irish medical education, they claimed, "a small group of permanent officials who have a vested interest in medical education and are chiefly concerned with keeping the student body at a numerical level to insure their continued employment".[61] This was in effect a criticism of the established practice of packing the medical schools to produce doctors for export, which in the case of the United States in the late 1940s and early 1950s had gone badly awry.

The criticisms of the AMA applied also to Trinity College medical school and the Royal College of Surgeons in Ireland, but notably there were no signatories of students from these institutions. The protesting doctors were overwhelmingly from the predominantly Catholic National University of Ireland and most from University College Dublin, the largest medical school of the three in the National University of Ireland. This reflected a shared experience of undergraduate medical education, but also reflected the religious separation in Irish medical education which, at that time, militated against cooperation. This was so even though many of the misgivings about the treatment of Irish medical education by the AMA were shared by Trinity College's medical school.

The second visit of the AMA to Irish medical schools took place in September 1953. The report itself was not received by the medical schools until the end of November 1953, but to avoid speculation and the likely leaking of the contents, the university authorities made the reports available to the newspapers in the first week of December. The headline in the *Irish Times* of 30 November was "Irish Medical Schools not condemned in Report of U.S. Doctors. Different methods stressed", and the language of the AMA report was indeed conciliatory, referring to Irish medical education as in a "state of transition". However, the *Irish Times* was disappointed in the report:

> [a generation ago] rightly or wrongly Dublin was supposed to rank with Edinburgh and Vienna ... Is it conceivable that our schools have been resting on their laurels complacently disregardful of modern advances in the science and practice and medicine, while the schools of Great Britain and Northern Ireland studied and toiled to keep abreast of the times? We do not believe it for one moment.[62]

---

the Irish Universities Medical Club of Chicago to the Consul of the Republic of Ireland, November 1952.

61 Ibid., p. 2.

62 'Irish Medicine' (editorial), *Irish Times*, 30 November 1953.

But the criticisms of the first visitation were upheld in greater detail in this second report and approval was not given.

Though a great deal of bluster accompanied the reception of the second report, it gave rise to a reconsideration, albeit only briefly, of what the medical schools of Éire should be about. Tierney of UCD repeated that:

> There seems to me to be here a mysterious discrimination against Ireland which the Report does nothing to explain ... One of the conclusions to be drawn, in my opinion, from the Report is the un-wisdom of any attempt on our part to train for practice under American conditions.[63]

O'Rahilly of Cork maintained that "Whilst we are anxious to help Irish medical graduates in the USA, it is not the primary job of our medical schools to equip doctors for America."[64] Underlying the comments was apprehension, because the AMA report served as a warning in the light of a forthcoming inspection by the GMC scheduled for 1954. Failure to pass this would have had serious consequences for the ability of Irish doctors to move to Britain. On 1 December 1953 the *Irish Times* reported that "Whilst the heads of Irish medical schools are considering the report of the American doctors, they are preparing for what one doctor suggested yesterday is a much more important visit."[65]

The visit of the General Medical Council of the United Kingdom to the Irish schools came on 26 April-23 May 1954.[66] They found a number of unsatisfactory aspects to Irish medical education, most of which concurred with those criticisms of the AMA, but in some respects went further. They found too loose an arrangement between hospital and medical school, exacerbated in the case of Dublin by the multiplicity of medical schools. This prevented satisfactory arrangements in clinical teaching being set up. Cork and Galway could negotiate with one hospital, but even there the hospitals were often too small to accommodate sufficient variety of cases to reach the best standards of clinical training. No professor at a medical school had a clinical department or laboratory in any hospital. Clinical pathology was particularly neglected, and there was a serious shortage of autopsy material. Likewise, library and museums were lacking.

The university calendars were often unreliable guides to the teaching programmes. In both Cork and Galway they needed "Drastic revision in order to tally with and confirm the information with which we were supplied".[67] There

63 'Medical training in a State of Transition', *Irish Independent*, 30 November 1953, p. 7.
64 *Irish Times*, 3 December 1953.
65 'Medical Schools await visit No. 2', *Irish Times*, 1 December 1953, p. 7.
66 General Medical Council (GMC), Visitation Reports, V/M/1 and V/S/1.
67 Ibid., p. 9.

was a need for appointments in a number of areas where Irish medical schools were falling behind modern medical education.[68] In addition, shortages in medicine and surgery were sometimes covered by re-designation of a teacher's function at six-monthly intervals, a practice that the GMC thought pedagogically unsound. A lot of effort would be needed to remedy the situation. However, ties between Irish and British medicine in terms of personnel and also the dependence of Britain on Irish medical graduates meant that, strong as the criticisms were, the GMC extended their recognition of Ireland's medical schools.

The outcome by the late 1950s was that a more hands-on approach to medical education emerged. The AMA list and its effects on Irish medical attention had reached the highest political level. In 1955–6 Eamon de Valera, then leader of the chief opposition party in the Republic of Ireland but soon to become Taoiseach (Prime Minister) and then President of Ireland, asked his office to contact the current Taoiseach (John Costello) to inform him:

> that the situation regarding the deficiencies of the medical schools of the constituent colleges of the National University of Ireland had become extremely serious and that there was a danger of grave developments in the early future. Mr de Valera stated that further inspections of the medical schools from abroad are expected and that the time available in which to prepare for such inspections is only about a year.[69] [De Valera believed that] A bad name given to us now by such bodies as the American Medical Association and the General Medical Council would be hard to outlive. It would not only have a disastrous effect on our reputation abroad but would tend to lower our proper self esteem and our domestic standards … I trust therefore that you will give your personal attention to the claims of the Colleges of the University for financial aid, particularly for their medical schools and see that any short-comings here as regards medical teaching cannot be attributed to state indifference or neglect.[70]

8 The End of the Approved List

Throughout the early years of the approved list's operation, optimistic reports on its adoption appeared in *JAMA*. But by 1956 it was pointed out that only 25 per cent or thereabouts of state licensing boards accepted the list: "Thus

68 Radiology, dental disease, anaesthesiology and general practice were all cited.

69 National Archives Dublin, Office of the Taoiseach, File S132588B, 'University College Cork', Letter of 10 September 1956.

70 National Archives Dublin, Office of the Taoiseach, S14402B, Letter of 7 November 1955.

for more than half of all state medical licensing boards the listing has either been of no use or has lent itself to an unintended use." Moreover 75 per cent of all licensed foreign graduates were from unlisted schools (although the pass rate for graduates from listed schools in licensure exams was 68 per cent, as opposed to 46 per cent for those from unlisted schools.)[71]

The assessment procedures upon which the approved list was based had faults from the start. It relied too much on whether individual members of the AMA arrived, by chance, in a country with medical schools and were able to spare the time to examine them. This meant a degree of rather unjustified selectivity. But to conduct a thorough inspection by the mid-1950s of all foreign medical schools that exported graduates to the USA would have been impossible in terms of money and resources. The process relied on a degree of subjective opinion. The officers of the AMA felt that British schools were 'good' before they even examined them. Although non-appearance on a list did not, as the AMA guidance notes insist, mean disapproval of a school but only a judgement as to equivalence to US standards of medical education, this was not how it appeared to the recipients of an unfavourable judgement. Good individuals were therefore penalised because of poor schools, an issue raised early on. By 1956 this had become a widely expressed reason for abandoning the list.

By 1954 the AMA was already looking at alternatives to the approved list. A subcommittee of the Council on Medical Education and Hospitals, called the Cooperating Committee on Graduates of Foreign Medical Schools, was charged with coming up with an alternative. In 1956 the AMA announced that it was to offer an Examination for Foreign Medical Graduates (EFMG). Success in the exam amounted to accreditation by the AMA. The scheme opened on 1 October 1957 with the first exam scheduled for March 1958 and the second for August 1958.[72]

The AMA had stumbled into the situation not fully cognisant of the changes taking place in physician emigration. The Irish experience of the 1950s was an example of a general pattern. Physicians were on the move. The number of Irish medical migrants to the USA was already much smaller than non-European graduates moving to the United States in the 1950s and the numbers of these increased even more in the decades which followed. Additionally, students from outside Europe now seeking a medical training in schools in the

71 'Medical Education in the U.S. and Canada', *JAMA*, 25 August 1956, vol. 161, no. 17, pp. 1637–78 and 1661–2.

72 *JAMA* said that the number taking the exam was around 1,000 in 1958, and over 2,000 applications were received to enter the exam by February 1959; see T. Stewart, 'Foreign Medical Graduates', *JAMA*, 28 March 1959, vol. 169, no. 13, p. 1513.

developed world was also on the rise. The outcome of this in the 1960s and 1970s is discussed in the next chapter as is a second development; the increasing role of the state in investing public money in education.

9 Conclusion

The map of Irish emigration began to change in the 1950s. The prestige of American medicine had risen in the preceding decades and, in the post-war years, the demand for health care in the United States was buoyant. These two factors made it a desirable destination for medical emigrants. Consequently, the pattern of emigration into the United States post Second World War was rising numbers increasingly drawn, not just from Europe and South America, but from Asia and what was known then as the Third World. Compared to the total number of medical emigrants seeking to practice in the United States, the number of Irish doctors emigrating to the USA was small. Still, it represented – for the first time in the history of the Irish medical emigration – a substantial cohort of its yearly emigration.

A small number returned to Ireland but most settled. Usually, unless channelled through prestigious postgraduate schools, medical immigrants to the United States tended to start their careers in state institutions and, in the case of the Catholic Irish, in hospitals or districts attached to their own Irish American community. There was a sense in which the experience of many generations of medical emigrants into the USA, was refracted through the lenses of their own national communities already settled there. But one factor affecting Irish emigration was the problem of professional accreditation.

Accreditation provides particular insights into the nature of medical migration. The American Medical Association, the chief professional body for American doctors, was somewhat ambivalent about the pattern of rising emigration after the Second World War. This led to its failed experiment in adopting a system of grading of the medical schools of foreign-born and educated medical emigrants to control the flow and, they claimed, to ensure high standards in medicine were upheld. This experiment engaged the attention of the foreign ministries and diplomatic services of those countries whose rating was low. This process is instructive for the study of medical emigration. The movement of doctors across borders is often a highly political process determined by the views of the medical communities in the host country, demand and supply in the medical marketplace, the colonial history of the receiving or exporting country and often simply geographical proximity. It also crucially involves a certificate of educational achievement acceptable to the host country.

American medicine had from the end of the First World War acquired global prestige and, through the influence of its funding bodies such as Rockefeller, was influencing the organisation of medical education throughout the world. It was a model rather hostile to the over-production of doctors but its advice to cut numbers of medical graduates was not followed in Ireland. However, from the 1940s it influenced reform in British medical education to bring its training more into line with that of the best in the USA. The medical schools under the jurisdiction of the Irish Republic were slow to respond, leaving the first generations of Irish emigrants to the USA in the kind of difficulties described in this chapter. The somewhat muted but significant expressions of discontent from the Irish doctor in the USA reflect this. This resulted in demands for reform in Irish medical education and it illustrated that an undercurrent of medical reformers existed, bolstered by undergraduate medical student discontent at overcrowding and stretched facilities in medical schools. The movement of reform in Irish medical schools was of long gestation but was, by the 1960s, one of the factors leading to change in Ireland. If a medical school exported – and Irish medical schools did – it needed to pay attention to accreditation and reform required investment. Thus, at the end of the 1950s, a glacially slow but significant debate about what needed to be done in Irish medicine emerged. None of this, however, challenged the central part played in Irish medicine by emigration.

CHAPTER 8

Inward Migration

From 1945 a number of significant changes impacted upon medicine. In Britain and in many other parts of Europe, government investment in the health of their populations increased and this was reflected in the expansion of their health services. Ireland was not immune from the trend.[1] In the Republic there were health reforms in the late 1940s and early 1950s which involved the greater participation of the state in combating TB and providing for the welfare of mothers and children.[2] The Stormont government in Belfast legislated in 1948 to follow Britain and bring the provisions of the National Health Service (NHS) to Northern Ireland. The NHS increased demand for doctors and this kept migration of medical graduates from the Republic to Britain buoyant in the 1950s.

Greater state investment in health had the concomitant effect of increasing government involvement in medical education. This was signalled by the Goodenough Report of 1944, published in wartime Britain, one of whose briefs was to plan for the need for more doctors in the light of the anticipated health reforms after the war. A second was to improve the quality of medical education largely by bringing medical school education and hospital training closer. This was followed by the Robbins Report of 1963, which recommended the expansion of the university system as a whole in Britain. The involvement of the state in planning and allocating resources in medical education was the consequence, and whilst this did not lead to the complete demise of the old system of fee-supported education in the Republic of Ireland, it did lead to its attenuation.

This happened at a time when medical migration was on the rise and much of it taking place from the developing to the developed world, particularly to

1 For a discussion of the changes in Northern Ireland, see Privilege, "The Northern Ireland Government and the Welfare State 1942–8"; and Privilege and Jones, 'Crisis and Scandal: Government, Local Government and Health Reform in Northern Ireland 1939–1942'. For the Republic, see Jones, *"Captain of these Men of Death": The History of Tuberculosis in Nineteenth and Twentieth Century Ireland*, chs. 7 and 8.

2 The reforms were enacted by Noel Browne (1915–97), Minister of Health 1948–51. His first aim was the eradication of TB, followed by proposals for a state-supported scheme for maternity and child welfare. He was forced from office because of opposition, largely from the Church. A more modest proposal in reform of maternity services was eventually adopted after his resignation; see John Horgan, *Noel Browne: Passionate Outsider* (Dublin: Gill and Macmillan, 2000).

 | DOI:10.1163/9789004324466_010

the United States. The *Journal of the American Medical Association* reported in 1976 that the 57th session of the World Health Organization had stated that 6 per cent of the world's physicians were migrants.[3] All these trends impacted upon Ireland. There was increasing state investment and planning in higher education; Irish migration to North America increased and foreign-born medical students began to come to Ireland in significant numbers.

1 The State and Medical Education

Financial assistance to universities in Ireland was not new. The Queen's Colleges of Cork, Galway and Belfast were set up by government grant in 1845 and received recurrent assistance throughout the nineteenth century, although they were expected to help support themselves through student fees. Universities of ancient lineage, who had their own investment and endowment income, were less dependent on government assistance. The chief example of this in Ireland was Trinity College Dublin, but TCD was hit by inflation in the First World War and lobbied for government help. After 1922 the Free State started giving annual grants to University College Dublin and University College Cork in 1926, and to University College Galway in 1929. TCD also received grants in the 1920s. Money for the universities was divided into one-off capital grants for building and infrastructure, and 'grants in aid' to assist in the running of the universities, these being recurrent.[4] There was also financial support in Éire from local authorities for some students on designated courses.

After 1945 the university systems in most developed countries expanded both in numbers and in the variety of courses they offered. In 1938–9 the total number of students in universities in the Irish Free State was 5,141. After the war it rose to 6,934. It declined to 6,736 in 1953, but then increased, almost doubling in the 1960s. The total number of students in all faculties in 1962–3 was 11,836, in 1964–5 12,984, and in 1974–5 13,362, excluding students in the Royal College of Surgeons which was a private medical school.[5] Ireland remained a country which educated more of its population to tertiary level than many other nations. The percentage of full-time students to the population as a whole for 1965–6 in the Republic of Ireland was 1 to 201; the ratio for Northern

3 'International Comments', *JAMA*, 15 March 1976, vol. 235, no. 7, p. 1167; and 'International Comments', *JAMA*, 16 January 1978, vol. 239, no. 3, p. 244.

4 For a full discussion of University Finances, see 'Report of the Commission on Higher Education 1960–7', vol. 2, ch. 32, 'Public Aid for Higher Education'.

5 National Archives Dublin, DFA/2005/10/107. Estimates of student numbers, 1974/5.

Ireland was 1 to 326, closer to that of Britain at 1 to 407. Only Switzerland, Sweden and Finland had a higher ratio of students to population than Ireland.[6] Ireland therefore remained, as Professor Lyons of the Catholic University medical school had predicted in 1873, very dependent upon the universities for its intellectual resources.[7]

Ireland increased its investment in universities following the rise in student numbers. In the Republic 'Grant in aid' was under £2 million 1964–5, rising to £19.6 million 1966–75, and £28.9 million by 1978.[8] In Northern Ireland, the extent of government support was even greater after 1945 when university fees were abolished and the cost of a student's education now devolved upon the government. Means-tested subsistence grants were also available to poorer students. To sum up, in post-war Ireland the financial situation of the universities in the Republic was that government grants, both capital and recurrent, accounted for 55 per cent of their income. The remainder was investment income at 8.1 percent and student fees at 32.5 per cent (with 3.7 per cent from miscellaneous income). In Northern Ireland, government provided 57 per cent of Queen's University Belfast's income in 1947, rising to 76 per cent from 1955 and only dropping to around 50 per cent in 1990.[9]

The result was a keener scrutiny of higher education by governments. In 1960 the Irish Republic appointed a Commission of Inquiry into Higher Education which reported in 1966–7. The Commission recognised that it was necessary to break away from the old model: "The financing of institutions of higher education should be related not only to the numbers of their students but also to the range of their activities."[10] In Northern Ireland a Committee on Higher Education in 1965 also planned rationalisation and expansion of higher education.[11] The outcome of the practice of government planning and forecasting was not always successful. In 1957 the British Willink Committee, set up to discuss the numbers of students to be admitted to medical schools, recommended a cut back in intake.[12] It believed the demand for doctors would fall and foreign-

---

6 'Report of the Commission on Higher Education 1960–7', vol. 1, Table 57, p. 7. The figures for other nations are for 1963/4.

7 See Chapter 4.

8 National Archives Dublin, TAOIS/2008/148/224, 'University Finance', Appendix on State Expenditure on Third Level Education 1965/6–1978.

9 Leslie Clarkson, *A University in Troubled Times: Queen's University Belfast 1945–2000* (Dublin: Four Courts Press, 2004), p. 211.

10 'Report of the Commission on Higher Education 1960–7', vol. 2, p. 851.

11 Government of Northern Ireland, 'Report of the Committee on Higher Education in Northern Ireland' (The Lockwood Report), Cmd 475 (Belfast: HMSO, 1965).

12 'Report of the Committee to Consider the Future Numbers of Medical Practitioners and the Appropriate Intake of Medical Students' (The Willink Report) (London: HMSO, 1957).

born medical students then being educated in British medical schools would return to practise in their own countries. However, the demand for health care in the UK proved buoyant and some of the subsequent gaps in the NHS were to be filled by foreign-born doctors, among them a considerable proportion who had graduated from UK medical schools. Similarly, the Commission on Higher Education in the Republic of Ireland struggled to implement the blueprint they had developed for the reform of Irish medical education, though for different reasons.

2 Medical Education in the New Era

The effect of the expansion of the universities was that medicine ceased to be the faculty which sustained Irish universities. The number applying to medical school was still robust. In 1964–5 medical students were 10.5 per cent of all students studying at the four universities in the Republic of Ireland; and if we add the medical school of the RCSI at over 500 students, the figure rises to 14 per cent. But this was still a significant diminution from the days when, just before the Second World War, it was over 30 per cent.[13] From a peak in 1938–9, the number of medical students declined in all schools except UCD, which in 1938–9 was educating 587 and in 1964 664 medical students. There was a dip in the number of medical students in Ireland in the late 1950s, largely in response to the Willink Report in the UK which wrongly predicted a fall in the demand for doctors in Britain. However, by 1964 the University Colleges at Cork and Galway had recovered from their low point in 1959–60. The recovery also happened in TCD, although no medical school apart from Galway and UCD exceeded the number of medical students they had educated in 1938–9.[14]

Among the problems which faced the Commission of Inquiry into Higher Education in the Republic of Ireland was that of numbers, an issue which had previously been left to market forces, chiefly exercised through families and the deans of medical schools. Like Rockefeller, the Commission accepted that Ireland over-produced doctors. They calculated that Ireland could supply its own needs with 80–100 medical graduates a year, but in fact had produced 179 in 1964–5, excluding the 75 graduates from the RCSI.[15] Added to this was the fact that "Medical qualifications from the Apothecaries Hall would increase

---

13 'Report of the Commission on Higher Education 1960–7', vol. 1, Table 29, p. 52 and Table 23, p. 47.

14 Ibid., vol. 1, Table 29, p. 52.

15 Ibid., vol. 1, Table 74, p. 243.

the number probably to 255 at least."[16] Even if many students at the RCSI and Apothecaries Hall were now foreign-born and likely to leave Ireland to practise, this still left a surplus. In Northern Ireland it was also accepted that some diminution of medical graduates was advisable.[17]

However, in the Republic the Commission remained open to the idea that Ireland should continue to produce a surplus of medical graduates. It was put to them by the medical schools:

> that even permanent emigration of Irish doctors should not be viewed simply in terms of a "loss"; there was a shortage of doctors in many countries, both developed and developing, and Irish doctors not required for health services at home could ease that shortage. In particular emigration of Irish doctors to developing countries could be regarded as having a special character, humanitarian or even missionary; doctors who had emigrated to these countries had won respect and had carried abroad the reputation of Irish medicine and the benefits of a high standard of medical ethics and practice.

Their view was that "Ireland and Great Britain should be considered ... as an economic and cultural unit", with the apparent corollary that such education "should be provided for all who could be absorbed into this larger community".[18] Therefore the Commission accepted that:

> Recognising that emigration of Irish doctors has been a characteristic feature of modern Irish society and impressed by the evidence, we received on the subject, we think that in any calculation of the number of Irish doctors who should be trained, allowance must be made for emigration.[19]

In the spirit of political economy, the Commission puzzled as to the numbers this would imply. As it pointed out, it had no definitive set of calculations as to the number of medical emigrants from Ireland, even given its long-standing character. However, taking into consideration natural wastage and the extent to which emigration was built into the system, the Report recommended that 160–170 should graduate each year from medical school.[20] This was certainly

16 Ibid., vol. 1, p. 243.
17 See Government of Northern Ireland, 'Report of the Higher Education in Northern Ireland' (The Lockwood Report), p. 69.
18 'Report of the Commission on Higher Education 1960–7', vol. 1, p. 246.
19 Ibid., p. 246.
20 Ibid., p. 247.

still over-production. However, balanced against this was the fact that although the costs of a medical education were higher than that of all other faculties except for dentistry, it cost significantly less to produce a medical graduate in Ireland (£300) than in Britain (£1,061).[21]

The Commission also clearly hoped to allay the criticisms of medical education in Ireland made by Rockefeller and the AMA. It proposed that one large clinical school for medical postgraduates be created. This would be located in a well-equipped hospital selected for the purpose and staffed permanently with research-minded staff appointed by the clinical school itself. Unfortunately, the proposal immediately ran into difficulties, and whilst some rationalisation was achieved, the project found itself like Rockefeller and for much of the same reasons quickly mired in controversy. It proved impossible to merge the two largest university schools of medicine in Dublin, TCD and UCD, largely because of long-standing rivalries between them; and even the selection of the site for the proposed clinical hospital ran into difficulties. The government gradually backed off from the more radical suggestions and admitted that the initial favourable response from the institutions concerned had been "more apparent than real" as both had eventually rejected the proposals.[22]

Therefore, the new era of rationalisation and planning came up against some deeply rooted cultural expectations. Not all of the recommendations for the new era were successful, and the powerful social forces creating a migratory medical profession in Ireland survived the Republic's Commission of Inquiry.

3 Foreign Students

Foreign-born medical students existed in Ireland long before 1945. Many were sent by mission schools abroad. However, the numbers climbed in the 1950s. In 1964 the government of the Irish Republic was asked by UNESCO to estimate the numbers of foreign-born students in Irish universities.[23] The government calculated that they comprised 21 per cent of the total in 1962–3, which was unprecedented in the history of the Irish university. However, of the 2,537 foreign-born, over half were from the UK, from Europe or overseas territories largely settled from Europe in South and North America and Australia.[24] The

21 Ibid., p. 249. They took their figures from the Robbins Report, 1963, which was the engine for the expansion of university places in Britain.

22 See National Archives Dublin, DFA2005/7/352, Appendix A, 1974, p. 10.

23 Ibid., DFA2011/39/183.

24 A total of 59 per cent.

remaining 41 per cent of foreign students were from what the Irish government called the developing countries: Africa, the Far East, the Middle East and the Indian subcontinent. The largest contingent was from Africa (499) followed by the Caribbean (126). The Indian subcontinent and the Far East followed, with a smaller number from the Middle East and other places. This trend was also occurring in Northern Ireland. In 1949 only three 'colonial' students were admitted to the medical and dental faculties of QUB.[25] But in 1963–4 students from the Commonwealth and 'other countries' formed 8 per cent of the total student body and 14.5 per cent of medical students.[26]

In the 1940s and 1950s some at least of the migratory patterns were still dominated by European countries. This is true in the United States as well as Ireland. A good deal was migration generated by dislocation in Europe, both before and after the Second World War. Certainly political emigration on that scale receded in the latter half of the 1950s, but it would be a mistake to think that it disappeared. In the period 1946–55, for example, the National University at Galway hosted a number of Polish students. They were there because the Polish School of Medicine, which had opened during the Second World War in Edinburgh to serve Polish exiles from the Nazis, had now closed.[27] But many Polish exiles did not want to return to a Communist Poland and some among them sought a medical education. After the Cuban Revolution of 1959 there was an influx of doctors from Cuba into the USA, and the motivations of a significant number of them were political.

A second point to emphasise is that the place where medical emigrants start their journey does not always give an indication of the ethnic origin of the migrants. Some places like Mauritius, which sent a number of students to Ireland through the 1960s and 1970s, have something of an indeterminate status. It is both part of Africa, an island off its east coast, but its population is Indian, African and European. How this affected the cohorts of foreign-born students entering Irish medical schools will be explained below.

Of foreign students in Ireland during the 1960s and 1970s, a substantial number came for a medical education. There were 753 foreign-born students in Irish medical schools in 1963–4 and 859 the following year. This was around a third of all students from abroad in 1964–5, and 55 per cent of all medical

---

25 QUB Archives, Minutes of Academic Council, vol. XIV, 3 June 1949, 'Overseas Students'.

26 Government of Northern Ireland, 'Report of the Higher Education in Northern Ireland' (The Lockwood Report), Table 12: Geographical Distribution of full-time students, undergraduate and postgraduate by discipline 1963/4, p. 220.

27 Tadhg Foley, ed., *From Queen's College to National University: Essays on the Academic History of QCG/UCG/NUI Galway*, (Dublin: Four Courts Press, 1999), p. 151.

students in Ireland, whether foreign-born or Irish.[28] The Commission on Higher Education reported that "Our information from the medical schools was that the number of applications from foreign students for places in our medical schools would fill the schools many times over."[29] Indeed a steady increase in numbers occurred year by year until it began to decline in the 1980s.

They were not distributed equally among the universities. UCD produced the largest number of medical graduates of the three colleges of the National University, exceeded only by the RCSI in the Republic and Queen's University Belfast. However, in 1962–3 UCD introduced a policy which permitted only limited access to its arts, commerce, law and science faculties for foreign students, but excluded, except in exceptional circumstances, foreign students from certain other faculties including medicine. This ensured that the medical school in UCD retained its character as predominantly Irish and Catholic.[30]

TABLE 19 Distribution of foreign medical students in Irish medical schools[31]

1964–5	UCD	UCC	UCG	TCD	RCSI	Total
Medical students	–	32	53	146	522	753
Total foreign students all faculties	457	106	64	1,085	–	
% of foreign students who are medical	–	30%	83%	13%	100%	34%

SOURCE: *COMMISSION ON HIGHER EDUCATION 1960–7*[30]

The question for the Commission and the government of the Republic was that since the state now met some of the costs of medical education, why educate foreign students at all? According to the Commission on Higher Education, foreign students cost in total around £150,000 to the exchequer, and even if their contribution to taxation were taken into account, it was still around £75,000. To balance this, other benefits less available to the university itself but of value to the economy accrued to Ireland. They included the cost of subsistence paid by the students. Nonetheless, the Commission still calculated a shortfall, with around 48–50 per cent of the cost of the education of foreign students falling to the exchequer. It was also the case that "the universities are

28 Calculated from 'Report of the Commission on Higher Education 1960–7', vol. 2, Table 170, p. 793, and ibid., vol. 1, Table 73, p. 242.

29 Ibid., vol. 1, p. 242.

30 RCSI Archives Dublin, Minutes of the Education Committee, 1967, vol. 2, p. 803.

31 'Report of the Commission on Higher Education 1960–7', vol. 2, Table 170, p. 793. 30 Taken from 'Students from other countries' according to faculty 1964/5.

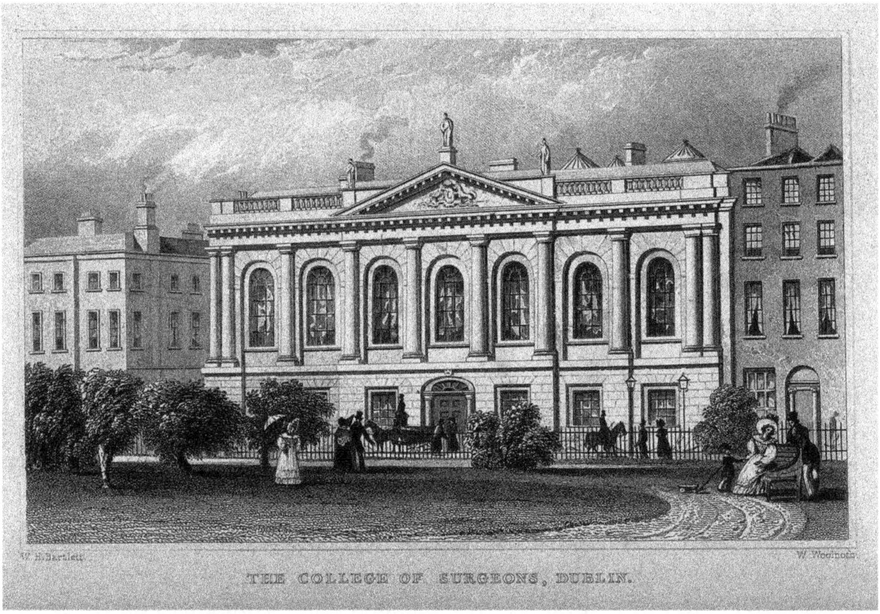

FIGURE 6 The College of Surgeons, Dublin, Ireland. Steel engraving by W. Woolnoth after W.H. Bartlett
SOURCE: WELLCOME COLLECTION. ATTRIBUTION 4.0 INTERNATIONAL (CC BY 4.0)

overcrowded; faculties are strained; the staff/student ratio is too high", and this meant that the possibility of controlling the entry of foreign students should be considered. In the end the Commission stated: "we strongly believe, however, that a place should be found in our system of higher education for students from abroad". This brought cultural benefits, and there was "an obligation to assist in training students from developing countries".[32]

4 A Private Medical School in the Age of Globalisation

In 1979 the World Directory of Medical Schools looked at the numbers of foreign students in the five Irish schools in the Republic during the period 1975–6. No school had more than a small fraction, except TCD which boasted 105 foreign-born students to 398 nationals;[33] while the Royal College of Surgeons in Ireland (RCSI) had 208 nationals and 417 foreign-born among its enrolled students.

32 Ibid., vol. 2, p. 807.
33 In TCD's case, this would cover students from Northern Ireland as well as from Britain. *World Directory of Medical Schools*, 5th edition (Geneva: WHO, 1979), pp. 156–9.

The reasons for this larger number at the RCSI, the second oldest medical school in Ireland, lay with the Commission on Higher Education.[34] It was the view of the Commission that the RCSI should abandon its undergraduate programmes and be reconstituted as a postgraduate licensing body similar to the Royal College of Physicians of Ireland. Under their recommendations, undergraduate teaching would disappear and the college's function change to that of examining students for a postgraduate licentiateship with candidates prepared for the examination by other medical schools. The Irish government accepted their recommendation, and suggested in the meantime that "the school of the Royal College of Surgeons continues to function mainly for expatriates until the College is able gradually to develop as a postgraduate institution".[35]

This was unacceptable to the RCSI, who considered that exclusion from its tradition of undergraduate teaching threatened its existence and was unjustifiable given the long and distinguished history of the RCSI's role in Ireland's system of medical education. After intensive lobbying of the government and employing legal advice, the government relented, if not completely at least partially. In a letter of November 1973 it signalled its willingness for the medical school of the college to be incorporated into government directives as a school providing medical education at university level.[36] This went some way to allaying the fears of the RCSI, but the college still bridled at what they felt was the government's failure to include it in the Education Act of 1971 which set up a Higher Education Authority comprising the other four Irish universities in the Republic.[37]

The RCSI rejected the recommendation of the Commission to transform itself into a postgraduate licensing body and, in spite of the fact that it was to receive only minimal government support, it survived. It did so because, although regarded by government as adhering to a superseded model of education – a private medical school almost wholly dependent on fees – the College sustained itself by recruiting overseas students. Lacking a place in a new modern world of medicine, according to the Commission and the government, it became arguably by today's standards the most modern of the Irish medical schools, implementing a global strategy for its survival and anticipating many of the trends in the universities of the developed world in the twenty-first century.

---

34 For a history of the RCSI, see J.D.H. Widdess, *The Royal College of Surgeons in Ireland and its Medical School 1784–1984*, 3rd edition (Dublin, Royal College of Surgeons, 1984).

35 RCSI Archives, Minutes of the Education Committee, 4 January 1968. Quoted in the minutes from an editorial in *JIMA*.

36 RCSI, Minutes of the Education Committee, 1 November 1973.

37 In 2010 the RCSI was finally given official university status.

Foreign students were vital for the survival of the RCSI. In whatever Irish university they studied, they paid higher fees than the native Irish, a 50 per cent surcharge on the fees normally charged to Irish undergraduates. In the case of the RCSI, the fees charged to foreign-born students more closely reflected the cost of sustaining their undergraduate education.[38] In 1962 the auditors told the college that "there is a loss of £138 on an Irish medical student, a loss of £67 on a dental student and a gain of £163 on an overseas student over the six year period of their training".[39] In 1977 the fees the RCSI charged were considerably higher for foreign-born students. Those from developed countries outside Ireland paid £800 per annum, those from developing countries £600 and Irish-born students £160. In 1974 the RCSI received only £18,000 per annum from government and no capital grants at all. This meant that the presence of foreign students was their guarantor of survival. Other forms of fundraising, for example capital grants for buildings, had to be met by the college itself, often with the assistance of their alumni in the developing world.[40]

The trajectory of the RCSI was set by these exigencies. During 1973–6 it admitted between 118 and 131 students each year to its medical school (excluding pre-meds) and graduated yearly between 100 and 119. The percentage of foreign student graduates in the college in that period was around 70–72 per cent.[41] Africa contributed the most, around half of the total, with the Caribbean, the Far East and the Indian subcontinent following. The peak of foreign admissions to the RCSI was in the early 1970s. When the RCSI examined admissions in 1987, it revealed an increase in applications from within Ireland, from 332 in 1977 to 675 in 1987; and a corresponding decrease in applications from developing areas, from 470 in 1977 to 352 in 1987.[42]

The RCSI rightly claimed that the education it provided contributed towards the development of poorer countries. Giving evidence to the Commission on Higher Education, they pointed out that "Nigeria has one doctor for forty thousand of the population; that would mean one doctor for the whole of Dublin."[43] The RCSI had strong links with West Africa, helping set up courses there for medical training and offering other forms of assistance. However, the picture was more complex than simply a medical school for the developing coun-

38 'Report of the Commission on Higher Education 1960–7', vol. 2, pp. 803–4.

39 RCSI, Minutes of the Education Committee, 11 December 1962.

40 For example, the South African Indian Commission supported the building fund. There were also donations from Mauritius, Zambia and Jamaica. Files from the Registrar's Office on the relationship between the RCSI and its overseas alumni are extensive.

41 RCSI Archives, RCSI/RO4/7, 2 January 1977.

42 RCSI Archives, Report of Admissions Board, 1987.

43 'Report of the Commission on Higher Education 1960–7', vol. 1, p. 251.

tries. Among foreign-born students there were still a small number of British, Europeans and the odd US or Canadian citizen.

A substantial number of Norwegians received an education at the college during the 1970s: around fifteen graduated in 1975. They attended the RCSI because of the inability of Norway's medical schools in the 1960s to produce enough doctors to meet the country's needs. According to the RCSI, the Norwegians "were extremely conscious of the fact that so many of their medical graduates have to be trained overseas".[44] However, given the shortage of doctors in Norway, the Education Committee of the RCSI was told that the "Norwegian Government are anxious that, if it is possible, they should be trained in this Island rather than some of the Continental Schools". Thus "no difficulties will be placed in the way of Norwegian students who wish to come to the College to study medicine".[45] The flow of foreign students to European schools did not therefore derive unequivocally from the developing world. Shortages of medical places within Europe could lead to peregrination of medical students. Switzerland's high number of foreign students, around 30 per cent in her universities, may very well have demonstrated continuing movements within Europe, not just from outside Europe.

However, the majority of foreign students conformed to the pattern of migrants from developing countries. Even here, however, the particularities of migrant experience should be noted. Both the Irish government and the RCSI recorded Africa as producing the largest number of students from developing countries, followed by the Caribbean and then the Far East. In the Irish government's survey in 1963–4, Africa sent 499 students to Ireland. Similarly high numbers of African students can be calculated for the RCSI. But a closer look at the students shows other factors at work. Many of the students from East Africa and South Africa were of Indian not African descent. This was also true of the Caribbean. Together with medical students from the Indian subcontinent and Indians from the Caribbean, this shifted the balance of RCSI students towards this ethnic group.[46]

---

44 RCSI/RO/375, Report of Professor Browne's visit to Norway, 4 October 1971.

45 RCSI, Minutes of the Education Committee, 7 April 1964. The Norwegian economy was in crisis in the 1960s, eventually improving after the discovery of offshore oil reserves. In 1960 only 5 per cent of men and 2 per cent of women had a university degree. This situation was transformed over thirty years. Until then Ireland helped meet some of their need for doctors.

46 The period of the 1950s and 1960s also saw a rise in doctor immigration into Britain from the Indian subcontinent. The particularity of this immigration is discussed in Julian M. Simpson, 'Diagnosing a Flight from Care: Medical migration and "dirty work" in the NHS', *History and Policy* (Cambridge: King's College and University of Cambridge, 8 December 2014).

A contributory factor was the political situation in the parts of Africa where there was substantial settlement from the Indian subcontinent, often going back to the nineteenth century. The coming of independence meant that the position of the Indian population in these places became increasingly politically precarious. We cannot look at migration of this group to the RCSI as entirely a response to the needs of the developing world or professional advancement. A medical degree acquired in a European country could act as an insurance policy against trouble ahead.[47] This became acute in 1972 when Idi Amin expelled the Uganda Asians from his country.[48] Political pressure existed on Asian settlers in other parts of East Africa and also the Caribbean. Finally, among the migrants from Malaysia were a number of ethnic Chinese who had also experienced political hostility during and after Malaysian independence.[49]

In their student profiles, graduates of the RCSI from the developing world generally described their ambition to return to their native land and practise there. Undoubtedly many saw themselves involved in patriotic nation building. But some at least of the graduates expressed their hope to go onto postgraduate work in the United States or Canada. Studying at the RCSI was often the first stage in a two-step or even three-step process of emigration.

In the late 1950s Brian Abel-Smith conducted an investigation into the migration of British doctors to the USA.[50] His study suggested that the attractions of the North American medical market place were not confined to the developing countries alone. Of his sample he found that the proportion of his British-born cohort living outside the UK was 12.5 per cent. For his Éire-born cohorts (including 314 persons educated in Britain) it was around 51.3 per cent. The remainder of Éire-born doctors, or 47.5 per cent, were resident within the UK and already emigrants to Britain.[51] But some of their compatriots had made an initial migration from the place they had graduated to Britain, and then a subsequent one usually from Britain to the United States. This was likely

47 A more thorough discussion of political refugees in academia can be found in Paul Weindling, Shula Marks and Laura Wintour, eds., *In Defence of Learning: The Plight, Persecution and Placement of Academic Refugees 1933–1980s* (Proceedings of the British Academy) (Oxford: Oxford University Press, 2011).

48 Michael Twaddle, ed., *Expulsion of a Minority: Essays on Ugandan Asians* (London: Athlone Press, 1975).

49 See Lee Kam Hing and Tan Chee Beng, eds., *The Chinese in Malaysia* (Oxford: Oxford University Press, 2000), pp. 201–9.

50 Brian Abel-Smith (1926–1996) was Professor of Social Administration at the London School of Economics.

51 Abel-Smith and Gates, *British Doctors at Home and Abroad*, Table 7, p. 30 (with the assistance of the World Health Organization).

to be the case for students from the developing world studying at the RCSI. In the 1960s and 1970s very few remained in Ireland, and the assumption must be that, for some, going to the RCSI was a step in a process which involved further migration in anticipation of greater professional advantage, escape from political danger or both.[52]

Because the RCSI was exporting graduates, they recognised that their licentiateship must be widely accepted across the medical world. It was recognised by the GMC, and its sister institution in Britain – the Royal College of Surgeons – made regular visits to the college; but the reach of the licence had to be much wider. As an alumnus in Australia advised them, the licence was not fully accepted in some states of Australia and in parts of South East Asia. This was a reflection of the general movement of medical qualifications into the university, a process beginning in the nineteenth century. The correspondent advised the college, "To its many junior graduates now living in Africa and Asia the door to academic advancement remains closed till a Bachelorship Doctorate replaces the present licence to practise."[53]

Some licentiates abroad accessed the qualification via schools in the developing world under the supervision of the RCSI. Thus the RCSI felt obliged to keep a strict supervision over the affiliated colleges, given some adverse comments on the misuse of the licence from licentiates from the developing world who left to practise elsewhere: "It was said that sixty percent of our fellows (in these countries) were emigrating within a short time of obtaining the Diploma." In some cases the licentiateship had been used ill-advisedly to claim consultant status in Canada.[54]

Because its licence was often the means to further migration, the RCSI followed closely the fate of its students. For example, it monitored the performance of its students in the United States' Examination for Foreign Medical Graduates (EFMG), which by the late 1950s had replaced the AMA list of approved medical schools. If performance fell below a satisfactory level, the RCSI conferred with, visited and invited a visit to the College from the officials of the American licensing board.[55] In turn it acted, particularly through the medium of those of its foreign students who returned to their original country, to assist in setting up equivalent licences and to examine and advise on them.[56]

---

52 A study of the subsequent destinations of the RCSI's foreign-born students would be very instructive in this respect.

53 RCSI, Minutes of the Education Committee, 4 January 1973.

54 RCSI, Minutes of the Education Committee, 8 May 1962.

55 RCSI, Minutes of the Education Committee, 12 May 1964 for a discussion of the issue and in subsequent meetings 1964–7.

56 RCSI Archives, RCSI /RO/377-380 for the files on Nigeria and West Africa. The RCSI established a close relationship with Nigeria, which involved mentoring and advising on the

This was essential for an institution that provided a qualification which had to be portable to all continents in a world which was increasingly sensitive to the reputation of medical degrees.

The number of foreign doctors who actually settled in Ireland was very small in the first decades after the Second World War. But it did sometimes happen that a foreign-born doctor stayed through marriage, or on obtaining a junior hospital position after graduation. We should also not assume that the appearance of a foreign-born doctor in Ireland was unknown till after the Second World War. In 1913 *The Leader* complained about the recent appointment of a house surgeon. Of the candidates:

> One was from fragrant Hollywood, County Down, and the other was an Indian! Colonel McCoghery, as an Imperialist, proposed the Indian… And so in this island suffering from a plethora of persons rushing to be medical gentlemen … a County Hospital has appointed an Indian as House Surgeon.[57]

Ireland produced more than enough native-born doctors to fill its vacancies, and the RCSI was careful to avoid the accusation of training foreign students to fill posts in Ireland. It discouraged the request that foreign-born graduates trained in Ireland should be eligible for postgraduate posts in hospitals, on the grounds that overseas postgraduates would compete with 'native' surgeons. Given over-production of doctors in Ireland, it was politically wise to do so.[58] The rationing of places for foreign medical students in the medical school of UCD was in part a response to the same worry. The fears faded somewhat as the numbers of foreign-born students seeking a medical education in Ireland dropped in the 1980s.[59]

5 The Future of Irish Medical Emigration

In 1960, at the moment when discussions were taking place on the establishment of a commission of inquiry for the purposes of modernising Ireland's universities, Seán MacEntee, a veteran republican and then Tánaiste (Deputy

---

suitability of hospitals for clinical training. But the Registrar's Office files contain many other examples of the college's contacts with their former students now overseas and their governments.

57 'Current Affairs', *The Leader*, 18 January 1913, vol. XXV, no. 23. p. 1.

58 RCSI, Minutes of Education Committee, 4 January 1968.

59 RCSI Archives, RCSI /RO/192, Report of the Admissions Board, October 1976–August 1988.

Prime Minister), wrote to P.J. Hillery, Minister of Education, on the subject of doctor emigration. Hillery's reply showed that he was clearly stung by MacEntee's claim:

> that our educational programmes still conform closely to the pattern set up in the middle of the last century, that is that they are still so framed as to produce surpluses of clerics, nuns (as teachers) and doctors: that we export large numbers in these categories; and that this old time pattern is not followed by the University of Dublin or by Queen's University Belfast.[60]

Hillery defended the Irish university system, first by emphasising its commitment to science teaching; and in support of this he pointed out that the three NUI colleges had only a third of their students doing arts subjects, whereas in Trinity College and Britain it was about 40 per cent. Moreover, it was not true that 30 per cent of TCD doctors got jobs in Ireland; in fact "the numbers of Trinity doctors in the hospitals and dispensaries in this country are a very small portion of the 60 or so doctors turned out annually by the Trinity medical school". But he went on to admit, "Nevertheless, though I say it myself, to my mind, all four University Colleges and the College of Surgeons as well are producing far too many doctors."[61]

Irish debate about medical migration at this time was shaped by the concerns raised by international organisations in the post-Second World War period around the impact of doctor migration. The assumption behind the discussion was that over-production of doctors was a waste of resources for the exporting country; it was an even worse case of 'loss' for poorer countries, since the flow of resources from the poor to the rich could not be defended on ethical grounds. The debate did not focus specifically upon Ireland, but Oscar Gish's 1971 overview of the economic impact of doctor migration included a chapter on Ireland North and South.[62] He pointed to the remarkable fact that in 1965–6 there were 3,650 Irish-born physicians working in Britain, compared

60 National Archives Dublin, TAOIS/S16803A, p. 2. Seán MacEntee, a participant in the 1916 Rebellion who narrowly escaped execution, had been trained as an engineer and obviously considered that he could bring a more modern scientific viewpoint to the education question.

61 Ibid., pp. 2–3.

62 Oscar Gish (1928–2004) was an American health economist who for much of his career worked abroad. From 1990 he was attached to School of Public Health and Community Medicine, University of Washington, Seattle. See online obituary, *Seattle Times*, 6–7 July 2004.

with 2,323 doctors in the Republic. Of the 3,650 in Britain, 950 were born in Northern Ireland, under 30 per cent of the total.[63] However, since the advent of the National Health Service, Northern Ireland was able to absorb a greater number of its medical graduates than the Republic. Gish considered it "ironic that the nationalists of the Republic of Ireland have been much more obliging about educating physicians for export to England and now to the United States than have the Orangemen of the North".[64]

In the spirit of bringing the supply of physicians into line with the demand for their services within Ireland (all on the assumption that the failure to do so was a waste of national resources), Gish considered that the Republic in particular faced three options. Two of them, to allow the free market to operate or to produce rigid controls on the emigration of doctors, were unattractive. Instead he proposed "an appropriate educational, manpower and employment strategy". This meant a combination of incentives for doctors to remain in Ireland, less training of physicians in favour of educating ancillary medical staff, and infrastructural development in the Irish health services.[65]

Gish was right about infrastructure, at least partially. The advent of the National Health Service did create more demand for doctors in Northern Ireland. Yet Queen's medical school still exported doctors, a fact confirmed by the study of our four cohorts during 1945–1960. They show that Queen's medical school produced more graduates for these four years than all the other medical schools in Ireland, 378, with University College Dublin's medical school a close second at 338.[66] Nonetheless 29 per cent of the Queen's Belfast medical school cohorts were working outside Ireland after ten years. QUB's medical school still exported an appreciable number of its medical graduates.

The view of emigration as an avoidable loss to a country seeped into official discussions at government level. In 1973 and 1974 two memoranda were drafted for the government by the Department of Health in the Republic on the issue of the present excess of the number of doctors trained. It was anticipated that the number would reach 532 in 1970–1 and 526 in 1972–3. Mitigating this, a rise in population from 3.6 million to 3.8 million was anticipated. This together with greater national prosperity and an increase in the proportion of the elderly in the population meant that the numbers of doctors who could be absorbed into Ireland, according to the Ministry of Health, had also risen to

63 Gish, *Doctor Migration and World Health*, pp. 669–70.

64 Ibid., p. 679.

65 Ibid., pp. 678–9.

66 Ibid. p. 670: "The Republic, with double the population of the North, can only support about 30 per cent more physicians".

around 200. Whilst it was certainly more than the numbers anticipated in the 1960s of around 80–100 doctors needed in Ireland, even so the numbers were still "far in excess of national requirements, even making liberal allowances for overseas students and a margin for the emigration of Irish graduates".[67] The memorandum went on to point out that the problem might become acute if it became more difficult for Irish medical graduates to find overseas work. Canada was increasing its output of doctors and the posts available in the UK were "less attractive than they were".[68]

The influence of the notion of national 'loss' is also illustrated by a letter received in 1978 by the Taoiseach's (Prime Minister's) office quoting the conference of the OECD in 1961 on the importance of investment in education to meet a country's scientific and economic needs. The letter approved recent rises in government funding for education, but it felt that "the benefits from education to society as a whole are reduced because many Irish graduates emigrate".[69]

On 1 January 1973 a significant change occurred in the terms by which migration was conducted for both Ireland and the United Kingdom. Simultaneously they joined the European Economic Community (EEC), then the Common Market. Following this a Medical Practitioner's Act was passed in 1978 in the Republic which altered the relationship between the Republic of Ireland and the General Medical Council. When the Act came into operation in 1979, over a hundred years of close relationships between the GMC and the Irish medical profession came to an end. Ireland's Medical Council was reconstituted as the sole authority in Ireland to supervise and register medical practitioners, under the general oversight of the EEC, whose laws ensuring mutual recognition between member states were now the guarantee for free movement for medical practitioners.[70] In Northern Ireland the GMC retained its authority to accredit and register doctors, although the European directive also applied there.

The European directive on doctors made practice across the borders of EEC countries possible, but not necessarily common at that stage. An article in the *Journal of the American Medical Association* in 1978 concluded that medical

---

67 National Archives Dublin, DFA2005/7/352, 'Reorganisation of Higher Education', Appendix C, Memo from the Department of Health, 31 August 1973, p. 2.

68 National Archives Dublin, DFA2005/7/352, Appendix A, Second Memo from the Department of Health to the Government, 11 September 1974, p. 1.

69 National Archives Dublin, TAOIS/2008/148/224, 1978, Letter on the Funding of Higher Education from V. Mulcahy, 9 November 1978, pp. 1–23.

70 Thanks to Ailbhe Enright of the Medical Registration Council of Ireland for help with this.

migration across Europe had not evoked much interest.[71] *JAMA* listed the issues which limited its appeal: language, the different cultural expectations of doctors, the relative unfamiliarity with different health systems and the adequate supply of doctors in many countries.[72] The European directive was created as a response to the idea of common citizenship rather than the actual issue of migration within Europe, and appeared to have made little immediate difference. In the long run, however, unequal development between European nations had the potential to create significant flows of medical personnel.[73]

More important was continuing migration into Ireland from outside the EEC. Gish had pointed out that in the mid-1960s there were already a number of foreign-born doctors in Ireland, but the number was small compared with the foreign-born student population: 100 compared to seven times that number of foreign-born students.[74] In the 1970s and 1980s the rise in non-EEC nationals, slow at first, began to accelerate. In the first decade of the twenty-first century the number of foreign-born students educated in Ireland's medical schools was now around 60 per cent of the total number, compared to 10 per cent in British medical schools.[75] Not many of them remained to practise in Ireland: usually a medical degree from an Irish school was a passport to further emigration. But foreign-born and foreign-educated doctors from outside the European Union (EU) now formed around 34–6 percent of new doctor registrations in the Republic of Ireland in the period from 2000.[76] Only one country in the OECD employed more foreign-born and foreign-educated doctors than Ireland.[77] This phase of Ireland's migration history deserves its own social historian.

71 'International Comments', *JAMA*, 16 January 1978, vol. 239, no. 3, p. 244.

72 'International Comments', *JAMA*, 1 December 1975, vol. 234, no. 9, p. 979.

73 In 2012, for example, 8.6 per cent of doctors trained overseas and practising in Ireland were from the European Union (Hungary, Poland and Romania); see 'Medical Workforce Intelligence Report' (Dublin: Medical Council of Ireland, 2012), Table 20, p. 60.

74 Gish, *Doctor Migration*, p. 669. He estimates that there were 100 overseas doctors practising in Ireland in the mid-1960s. However, in 1964/5 the number of medical students born overseas in Irish medical schools was 753.

75 'Medical Education in Ireland: A New Direction', Report of a Working Group on Undergraduate Medical Education and Training, Republic of Ireland, Department of Health (The Fottrell Report), 2006, p. 17.

76 The majority (35 per cent of the total of foreign-born and foreign-educated doctors) were from Pakistan or South Africa; see 'Medical Workforce Intelligence Report' (Dublin, 2012), Table 20, p. 60.

77 Ibid., p. 15. The figure in the UK was around a third of new registrants.

6 Conclusion

In the first decade of the twenty first century the numbers of Irish doctors educated in Ireland had increased, although it was pointed out that the percentage of doctors to population in Ireland had dropped slightly.[78] Even so, it was proving difficult to maintain the old system of an exclusively Irish-born and Irish-educated body of physicians serving the people of Ireland. The striking phenomenon to many observers was that Ireland, now an importer of doctors, still remained "the European country with the highest percentage of nationally trained doctors practising abroad". In other words, it still exported its own doctors.[79] This gave rise to discussion about how this might be, if not reversed, at least somewhat mitigated. Was it the quality of education, particularly postgraduate, or possibly the structure of the hospital system itself and lack of opportunities there? Whatever it was, it was not poverty or lack of opportunity, but rather comparative advantage which still influenced the decision of Irish-born and Irish-educated doctors to emigrate.

78 P. Bidwell, Niamh Humphries, Patrick Dicker, Steve Thomas, Charles Normand and Ruairi Brugha, 'The national and international implications of a decade of doctor migration in the Irish context', *Health Policy*, vol. 110, no. 1, April 2013, pp. 29–30.

79 Ibid., p. 31.

Epilogue

Where does Ireland stand in the overall history of medical migration? First, over the hundred years or so examined, forty per cent of its medical graduates left Ireland. This figure dropped over the hundred years or so of this study. In the latter half of the nineteenth century it was around 50 per cent. By 1960 it had fallen to 33 percent. Nonetheless the culture of emigration among Irish doctors continued into the twenty first century. The major destinations between 1860 and 1960 were Britain and the British Empire or ex-colonies, though not exclusively. After the Second World War, North America became an important destination and, as opportunities to work in the colonial service fell over the twentieth century, a higher percentage of medical migrants went to Britain. Of these medical migrants a few can be found clustered in Wales and some in Scotland, but Scotland – itself an exporter of graduates – was not as fertile a ground for the Irish migrant doctor as England. A few went back to Ireland on retirement but these returnees were rare. Most of those who went back were in fact Irish doctors who had served in the armed or colonial services and even here the rate of return was not high.

Medical migration was not just something that the Irish medical graduate fell into by happenstance. Over-production and consequently emigration was part of the strategy of Irish medical schools. Much of the preceding narrative has discussed the strong resistance evinced by the medical schools against reducing their intake. Neither the RF's strictures on the oversupply of medical schools in Ireland in the 1920s nor the Commission on Higher Education in the 1960s could shake the determination of the schools on the issue, even when the rationality of a supply-and-demand strategy was laid before them. The Irish medical school educated for export.

In this, Ireland was not unique but part of a conglomeration of medical schools crossing the world. There was never just one configuration for the export of doctors but many. There were schools which trained and exported their own citizens as Ireland did for most of the hundred years examined in this book. Others educated the citizens of foreign countries and then re-exported them as Irish medical schools began to do from the 1960s. Some specialised in a particular market and exported other forms of medical personnel apart from doctors. As Monnais and Wright point out, there are histories to be written about the migration of these health workers.[1] There were schools who

1 Introduction to Monnais and Wright, eds., *Doctors Beyond Borders*, p. 15.

 | DOI:10.1163/9789004324466_011

were, at one point in their history, 'predominately exporters of medical education as opposed to medical manpower'. These were "in proportional terms and descending order of magnitude: Spain (60 percent), Formosa (58 percent), Switzerland (52 per cent), Italy (49 per cent) France (47 per cent), Belgium (43 per cent) and Ireland (39 per cent)".[2] Some countries educated American citizens and exported them back to the USA, notably Italy, Austria and Belgium.[3] But what configuration of culture, ethnicity or opportunity determined this? Economics, culture, politics and even geography play a part in determining patterns of migration. During 1967–71 46 per cent of foreign-educated doctors granted a licence to practise in the United States were from the Philippines and Cuba.[4] Both countries had a geographical or a political relationship to the United States as Ireland had to Britain.

The former British or European colonies often developed their medical institutions through their links with the colonising powers. Medical schools in the colonising power, tended to have a residual reputation as centres of excellence among the colonised countries. Consequently, they attracted their postgraduate students. The situation also applies to Irish medical schools which, as we have noted in the case of the Royal College of Surgeons, developed links with institutions in overseas countries.[5] Sometimes Irish medical graduates also regarded a brief spell in English or Scottish medical school or hospital as useful aid to improving their experience and skill. But Ireland had its own medical culture, long standing institutions and overseas networks and felt no inferiority in this respect.

For much of the twentieth century the movement of postgraduates did not always lead to settlement. The example of New Zealand's medical postgraduate movement to Britain and then back to New Zealand is discussed in Monnais and Wright and some of the short-term medical migration discussed there also applies to other colonies and ex-colonies located outside Europe.[6] Only in the latter half of the twentieth century did certain schools in the developing world, often ex-colonies, start to export medical graduates on a large scale,

2 Mejia, Pizurki Royston, *Foreign Medical Graduates*, pp. 13–14.

3 Henry R. Mason, 'Foreign Medical Graduates: Profiles of those Qualifying for Practice in the United States', *JAMA*, 22 July 1974, vol. 229, no. 4, Table 1, pp. 428–30, p. 429.

4 Greeley, 'American Foreign Medical Graduates', Table 1: Countries in which American medical students studied 1963–4.

5 The process of creating the overseas networks deserves a history of its own.

6 See John Armstrong, 'A System of Exclusion: New Zealand Women Medical Specialists in International Medical Networks. 1945–1975', in *Doctors Beyond Borders*, eds. Monnais and Wright, pp. 118–41, footnote 1.

graduates who would eventually become part of the medical community in the European and North American societies in which they arrived.[7]

In that period, the latter half of the twentieth century, consciousness of the export of doctors from the poorer to the richer countries of the world influenced the way medical migration was seen. Economic market models were at the forefront of the debate about migration. It cost money to produce a doctor and for those who subsequently settled in another country, generally a richer one, this meant that there was no return on the capital expended on their education.[8] Irish governments pondered this dilemma, particularly at the time when government investment in higher education began to increase. But they did not attempt to limit medical migration.

Among the questions that has influenced this study are the reasons why. Did medical migration amount to an economic 'loss' for Ireland? Certainly Ireland's export of medical graduates has some classic features of conventional political economy. Ireland was next to a large market for doctors which experienced considerable economic development in the nineteenth and twentieth centuries. This led to an increase in the demand for health care both public and private in Britain, a demand met for a long time by Irish and Scottish medical schools. The Deans and Registrars of Irish medical schools were aware of the market and it influenced the numbers of graduates they produced, not precisely but generally. For long periods of her history Ireland lacked doctors and, certainly in the mid nineteenth century, was clearly under-supplied with doctors. However, estimates in the 1960s put Ireland's status, in four gradations of Gross Domestic Product (GDP), as in the second rank of developed countries. This was just below the UK, which was in the top category. But for most of the time we have examined, Ireland had the number of doctors that, given her economic position, she was considered to need.[9]

The determinant of her doctor production was the relationship between the medical school and the market. Over production may very well have produced a struggling tail of medical graduates for whom migration was an admission of defeat and who did not do well in the new circumstances in which they found themselves. For many others and for Ireland itself medical migration produced rewards. It buttressed medical institutions in Ireland, kept her university

7 Of the 17,000 foreign graduates making sponsored visits to the USA for postgraduate training in medical schools or hospitals in that period, 58 per cent stayed on in America after completing their courses. See Smith, 'The Brain Drain Re-Emergent', p. 487.

8 Ibid. and Hussain A. Ronaghy, Kathleen Cahill and Timothy D. Baker, 'Physician Migration to the United States: One Country's Transfusion is Another Country's Hemorrhage', *JAMA*, 4 February 1974, vol. 227, no. 5, pp. 538–542, p. 541.

9 Mejia, Pizurki and Royston, *Foreign Medical Graduates*, p. 117, footnote 1.

system reasonably healthy and offered a return on their investment in education for the middle-class family. It was also a ladder of social mobility into the professions and carried with it the chance of economic and sometimes social and political success for the medical migrant.[10]

Irish migration patterns changed over time becoming more global. After the Second World War medical migrants began to participate in wider migration movements particularly to North America. Easier travel, awareness of the rise of American prestige in medicine spread by research and philanthropic institutions and finally the economic boom of the 1950s offered prestigious postgraduate education and the chances of making a good medical living. Similarly the model of migratory pattern began to evolve in other directions. Ireland became a country which imported students from overseas and finally imported overseas born and educated doctors to supply their health service. However even this did not bring to an end Ireland's tradition of exporting doctors. It simply situated it in a more complex set of migratory relationships.

10 Rosemary Stevens and Joan Vermeulen have noted it was often the better off middle-class families who sponsored emigration to the USA from developing countries. See *Foreign Trained Physicians and American Medicine* (Bethesda: U.S. Department of Health, Education and Welfare, 1972).

Appendix

1 Methodology on Medical Emigration

The 'Report of the Commission on Higher Education' in the Republic of Ireland in 1967 commented that:

> Medical school authorities informed us that it was particularly difficult to place a figure on the rate of emigration of Irish doctors. A survey of the pattern of emigration over a long period involving the tracing of many individuals would be required to obtain accurate information and, in particular, to isolate the number of doctors who emigrate permanently. This we have not had the opportunity of doing.[1]

With the assistance of the Wellcome Trust, a study of emigration by graduates of Irish medical schools 1860–1960 was undertaken. At five-yearly intervals from 1860 cohorts of graduates were examined. The initial work was done over two years and involved the investigation of the destinations of these cohorts of Irish medical graduates ten years after graduation. The number of individuals traced was 4,246.

The *Medical Register* of the United Kingdom was used. The register was set up in 1858 by Act of Parliament and covered all the constituent parts of the United Kingdom including Ireland. Registration was the key to practice in Britain and in the British armed services and colonies. The register also included in this period a list of those in the armed or colonial services and those practising abroad. In the nineteenth century it listed doctors in the regions of the British Isles, those practising in Scotland, Wales, Ireland, and also a separate list of those in London and the English provinces.

The *Medical Register* is a good guide to the eventual destination of doctors, though not an infallible one. It can be supplemented by the *Medical Directory*, which is also published annually. The *Medical Directory* basically advertises the services of doctors. It generally includes more career information about individual doctors and often a list of their publications. The *Medical Register* by contrast contains only their name, year of graduation, school and licensing body and qualifications. Both publications include an address. Entry on the *Medical Register* is the most important act of a doctor after qualification, because it is the key to a recognised professional status and the authoritative guide when checking a doctor's credentials. Even after the partition of Ireland in 1922 and the creation of a separate Irish *Medical Register*, medical graduates from

---

1 'Report of the Commission on Higher Education 1960–7', vol. l, p. 246.

Ireland retained the right to be entered on the United Kingdom *Medical Register*. The majority did so and can still be traced there.

The research analysed the destinations of medical graduates from six Irish medical schools through 1860–1960: Trinity College Dublin also known as the University of Dublin, the Queen's Colleges of Cork, Galway and Belfast, the Royal College of Surgeons and the graduate lists of University College Dublin (UCD). Unfortunately, the graduate lists of the Apothecaries Hall were not available, although they have now been lodged in the archives of the Royal College of Physicians of Ireland.

University calendars and handbooks regularly list the year's graduates, and a few make it easy for researchers by producing, at intervals, cumulative lists of their graduates, the degrees they obtained and the year they obtained them. Trinity College Dublin (the University of Dublin) produced such a list in their annual University Calendar in 1901, 1906, 1913 and 1951. Even more helpfully, this was divided into faculties. Queen's University Belfast produced a similar list in 1919–20, in which many of the subsequent destinations of their graduates were inscribed in the footnotes. University College Galway produced a master list covering all previous graduates and their degrees in their calendar for 1954–5. University College Cork had a similar compendium of their graduates in their Sessional List for 1928–9. These lists supplemented examination of the annual lists of graduates. It was never necessary to examine newspaper reports of graduations in a systematic way, but for researchers without access to calendars or registers, Irish newspapers regularly report graduations and lists of graduates.

Graduations take place in summer and winter and this needs to be taken into account, as does the fact that those forced to retake exams or stopped from graduating because they have not paid their medical school fees have a later graduation date than would normally be the case. In a few other cases in the nineteenth century a name inscribed on a list of graduates may also be found in the list of another school in the same year. This does not happen frequently and scarcely at all after the First World War, but it does occasionally occur before then. This is because peregrination in search of a medical education at undergraduate level still occurred in the nineteenth century.

The remit of the study concentrated on the school and not the nationality of the student graduating; however, whilst there are students graduating from Irish medical schools who are from outside Ireland, this is rare until the 1950s. A survey done of Trinity school entrants to their medical school which examined the parent's address illustrates this. A very small number mention a parental address outside Ireland, and often in these cases it was an outpost of the British Empire. A similar investigation of Queen's University Belfast's medical students demonstrated that the vast majority of undergraduates were drawn from the surrounding counties.

Names are occasionally misspelled in the *Medical Register*, which complicates tracing but it rarely happens. Checking against place and year of graduation in the *Medical Register* for an individual means that this problem can easily be eliminated. The same is true for the fact that very rarely, but once or twice, the wrong year of graduation is given. The *Medical Register* was, however, good at recording women graduates who changed their name on marriage.

A number of points remain to be made in connection with the figures for destinations. First, a small number of doctors give a *poste restante*, usually a bank, rather than a place of residence in the register. The banks mentioned are usually Grindlays (associated with India) and Glyn and Mills. They were generally used by doctors on the move: places where letters, information and correspondence could be forwarded and into which salaries paid. This is confirmed by the increase in banks quoted as addresses during the First World War.[2]

The survey concentrated on cohorts of graduates from Irish medical schools through 1860–1960 examined every five years, and is confined to six of the seven medical schools in Ireland. The results given are therefore a sample of graduates between 1860 and 1960, not the total amount of students graduating from Irish medical schools between these years. This means that some short-term fluctuations in graduates would not be recorded. However, the number traced is sufficiently large to allow some general conclusions about the pattern of emigration over the period.

The place of practice of the graduate was examined after ten years. This takes into consideration the fact that new graduates may be unemployed or in a temporary job, or their professional direction may be as yet unclear. An assumption was made that the direction of their career was clearer after ten years. But of course there remain those who move or change their job after ten years. To test the extent of this, the destination of 566 graduates between five and ten years was examined, and a further cohort of 102 graduates between ten and twenty years. Five years after graduation, 36 per cent of the graduates examined, excluding those unregistered, were at addresses outside Ireland. By the tenth year this had risen to 40.79 per cent. Examination of the residence of a further 102 graduates between ten and then twenty years, as well as a small rise in the 'unregistered', reveals a further 10 per cent movement out of Ireland and a 3 per cent inward movement, mainly those returning from army or Indian medical service. This leaves further migration out of Ireland after the ten-year cut-off point as around 7 per cent.

Therefore, the number of individuals studied ensures a significant statistical insight into the movement of Irish graduates. The two World Wars are in themselves outside the scope of the study, but the key dates of 1915 in the First World War and 1940 and 1945 in the Second World War give some indication of their impact. Whilst important and interesting, the war years are exceptional years in the amount of doctor movement, much of it temporary. The study is more concerned with elucidating voluntary

2 Glyn and Mills' archives are in possession of the Royal Bank of Scotland, who kindly allowed me access.

migration in peacetime. The tables that follow are the outcome of the study. The significance of the tables is discussed in the main body of the text, which also contains other tables based on further analysis of the overall figures. The Appendix tables are computations based on the analysis of 4,246 graduates every five years during 1860–1960.

TABLE 20 Number of Irish medical graduates in Ireland or elsewhere ten years after graduation

	UCD 1910–60	RCS 1860–1960	QUB 1860–1960	TCD 1860–1960	Cork 1860–1960	Galway 1860–1960	Total
In Ireland	375	334	554	324	193	102	1,882
Unregistered	120	120	105	169	45	73	632
Outside Ireland	231	449	378	459	128	87	1,732
Total graduates traced	726	903	1,037	952	366	262	4,246
Percent outside Ireland	32	50	36	48	35	33	40.79

TABLE 21 Movement of Irish medical graduates 5 years after graduation compared with 10 years

	5 years	10 years	Difference
In Ireland	283	204	−79
Unregistered	77	93	+16
Outside Ireland	206	269	+63
Total	566	566	566

TABLE 22 Graduates not in the *Medical Register* ten years after graduation, 1860–1960

Period	Total no. of medical grads	Not in register	Percentage
1860–95	754	112	15
1900–15	618	85	14.5
1920–40	1,400	200	14
1945–60	1,474	235	16
Total	4,246	632	15

TABLE 23 Destination of medical graduates from Ireland by period
(The figures did not remain static, and the reasons for this are discussed in the text.)

1860–95

	UCD	RCSI	QUB	TCD	Cork	Galway	Total for all schools
Total no. of grads	–	260	174	239	15	66	754
In Ireland	–	99	54	68	9	14	244
No. outside Ireland	–	145	92	124	5	32	398
Unregistered	–	16	28	47	1	20	112
Percentage grads outside Ireland	–	56%	53%	52%	–	–	53%

1900–15

	UCD	RCSI	QUB	TCD	Cork	Galway	Total for all schools
Total no. of grads	77	191	126	171	36	17	618
In Ireland	40	79	41	42	17	9	228
No. outside Ireland	27	97	61	98	17	5	305
Unregistered	10	15	24	31	2	3	85
Percentage of grads outside Ireland	–	51%	48%	57%	–	–	49%

1920–40

	UCD	RCSI	QUB	TCD	Cork	Galway	Total for all schools
Total Number grads	311	208	359	305	161	56	1,400
In Ireland	142	85	213	110	84	26	660
No. outside Ireland	115	89	115	145	59	17	540
Unregistered	54	34	31	50	18	13	200
Percentage of grads outside Ireland	37%	43%	32%	48%	37%	–	39%

1945–60

	UCD	RCSI	QUB	TCD	Cork	Galway	Total for all schools
Total no. of grads	338	244	378	237	154	123	1474
In Ireland	193	71	246	104	83	52	750
No. outside Ireland	89	118	110	92	47	33	489
Unregistered	56	55	22	41	24	37	235
Percentage of grads outside Ireland	26%	41%	29%	39%	31%	27%	33%

Table 24 shows the percentage of women graduates in various decades from 1860 to 1960. Irish medical schools were generally open to admitting women students from the mid-nineteenth century. However, the first significant increase in women doctors was during and after the First World War, and the second surge was after the Second World War. Overall just over 10 per cent of doctors during the whole period were women, but the percentage rose over time.

Table 25 shows the number of medical graduates who disappeared off the *Medical Register* altogether after ten years. The percentage of unregistered throughout the period is remarkably stable at around 15 per cent. The interesting question is whether this is higher in Ireland than in England, Wales or Scotland. If so it might indicate particular pressure on the Irish graduate. There is, unfortunately, no estimate of unregistered medical graduates over a comparable length of time for England, Wales or Scotland. Crowther and Dupree, however, looked at 1,288 individuals graduating from Scottish medical schools in the late nineteenth century. Of these 29 were untraceable

TABLE 24 Women medical graduates 1860–1960

School	1860–95	1915–30	1935–45	1950–60	Total
UCD	1	43	29	63	136
TCD	2	32	24	52	110
Galway	-	5	10	26	41
RCSI	7	13	20	56	96
QUB	2	38	42	61	143
Cork	-	16	21	13	50
Total	12	147	146	271	576

TABLE 25 Percentage of cohort unregistered after ten years

Period	Total no. of medical grads	No. of unregistered	Percentage
1860–95	754	112	15
1900–15	618	85	14.5
1920–40	1,400	200	14
1945–60	1,474	235	16
Total	4,246	632	15

and a further 47 had dropped off the register after five years, about 6 per cent of the total.[3] If another 6 per cent of the Scottish graduates disappeared from the register after a further five years, this would mean a total for ten years of a dropout rate of 12 per cent, a figure within distance of the Irish one but lower.

Becoming unregistered is itself a complex phenomenon. There can be many reasons, and to produce a definitive social picture of the unregistered would require a detailed study of them, not an easy proposition. Error may account for some of the apparent dropouts, and that is the reason why the sample chosen is a large one. Of the causes, premature death, professional failure or emigration to places where registration is not an issue may all play a part.

One reason for being unregistered was premature death. John Herbert Sibthorpe graduated in 1905 from TCD but tragically died a year later in 1906 aged 26. Thomas Robert Lingard, born around 1859 and graduating from TCD in 1880 then died in 1890 aged 31, thus escaping by a hair's breadth the ten-year cut-off point. Another TCD graduate of 1885, Henry Moore Brabazon, was born in 1861 and died in Calcutta in 1891, four years before the cut-off date, whilst serving in the Indian Medical Service (IMS).

But one 1875 TCD graduate, Joseph Blood is in neither the 1885, 1883 nor 1887 *Medical Register* but appears in the 1911 England and Wales Census as a medical practitioner in Birkenhead. Whether the gap in his assuming a practice is due to ill health or to temporary emigration followed by his return is not clear. But emigration to the USA is the cause of absence for Peter Joseph Farrell, a graduate of TCD in 1875, who went to Rhode Island, USA. Born in 1848 he died there in 1906 at the relatively young age of 58.[4]

If the rate of the unregistered in Ireland is due to professional failure, then this would be significant; but it is as likely to be due to premature death. Ireland suffered a higher rate of tuberculosis than the rest of the United Kingdom during most of the late nineteenth and early twentieth century, and it is a disease which particularly affects

3 Crowther and Dupree, *Medical Lives in the Age of Surgical Revolution*, pp. 123–5.
4 Information assembled through the use of Ancestry.co.uk.

the young adult.[5] Also more women medical graduates were unregistered, around 25 per cent, but a proportion may have been in fact registered but at some point before the cut-off point have changed their name through marriage. However, there is also an observable pattern among women medical graduates of returning later to their medical careers after dropping out when getting married or when starting a family, a fact to which Laura Kelly draws attention; she also notes the professional difficulties that women medical graduates faced because of their gender.[6] Thus there may be an inflated drop-out rate for women in the first ten years after graduation which is, to some extent rectified in later years.

2 Cross-Referencing with Other Studies

How does the result of this study compare with existing surveys on medical migration? The Commission on Higher Education itself came up with a figure of medical graduate emigration of 25 per cent, but the value of this is reduced by the fact that they considered only 'voluntary migrants' as distinct from "graduates who might be obliged to do so owing to lack of employment opportunities at home".[7] The figure was extrapolated from a study by Cork medical school of 408 'responding doctors' for 1945–54. When the figures for voluntary and involuntary emigration are put together, 45 per cent of the sample were in the UK and 16 per cent elsewhere – figures much closer to those in this study, and in fact rather higher.

A survey was also done by Atkinson Stoney of the Medical Registration Council of Ireland on the destinations of medical students qualifying in 1948. He estimated that 90 medical graduates left annually, around 30 per cent of the total number of graduates. For 1945–60 my figure is 33 per cent.[8]

In 1965 a survey of higher education in Northern Ireland argued:

> traditionally it [QUB medical school] supplied not only local requirements but also sent graduates into the armed forces, to India, to the Colonial Medical Service to Great Britain particularly to the Industrial North of England.[9]

---

5 See Jones, *"Captain of all these men of death"*.

6 Kelly, *Irish Women in Medicine c.1880s–1920s*, p. 145.

7 'Report of the Commission on Higher Education 1960–7', vol. l, p. 247.

8 Quoted in the 'Report of the Committee to Consider the Future Numbers of Medical Practitioners and the Appropriate Intake of Medical Students' (The Willink Report) (London: HMSO, 1957), p. 29.

9 Government of Northern Ireland, 'Report of the Higher Education in Northern Ireland' (The Lockwood Report), p. 69.

The survey claimed that for the first twenty-five years of QUB's existence, presumably from 1908 when the medical school became part of the Queen's University, only 15 per cent of its graduates remained in Ireland, although in their view this had now increased to 40 per cent. These figures are in my view exaggerated and are contradicted by the earlier report on Northern Ireland medical manpower commissioned by the British Ministry of Health which gave a figure of 25–30 per cent of individuals emigrating, out of approximately 100 a year graduating, a figure which is in line with the results in this study.[10] A further table in the Report surveyed 2,177 Queen's medical graduates who took degrees up to 1953. Of these, 112 or 5 per cent were 'unregistered' or 'address unknown but probably abroad', and of the traceable ones 46 per cent were in Ireland, 42 per cent in Britain and 7 per cent abroad, mainly in Canada and the USA.[11]

Because no methodology accompanies the calculations in these reports, including no uniform date after graduation, strict comparisons are impossible. Except for the Queen's study which surveyed cumulative emigration of students up to 1953, they are also confined to the period after 1945 when, as after the First World War, there was a great deal more short-term movement of medical professionals, including some who would still be in the armed forces. Also, except in Atkinson Stoney's case, they survey single medical schools which sometimes have a higher emigration rate than others. In terms of sample size and consistency, the results of the present study are more reliable.

But a word of caution is needed. Emigration is dynamic, and the four years that separate each cohort over the hundred years of 1860–1960 might very well be affected by short-term events. Just as we cannot extrapolate from figures which are taken from one medical school, rely on 'opinion' or deal only with a particular short period of time, so the overall figures may disguise short-term rises or falls. Whilst reliable overall, there is still a need to measure the figures by the changes which war, economic dislocation, colonial politics and other factors bring about in particular periods. Thus whilst the figures show a decline in recruits for the Indian Medical Service in the 1930s, there is a sudden though temporary upswing in recruits in the Second World War and just after. The results in the research point to some conclusions overall, but they do not negate the importance of further more focused research for particular periods.

3 The Social History of the Irish Medical Emigrant

The study also aimed to produce a more in-depth social picture of the Irish emigrant doctor, including the profit and loss of emigration for the individual. There has been

10 'Report of the Committee to Consider the Future Numbers of Medical Practitioners and the Appropriate Intake of Medical Students' (The Willink Report), p. 28.

11 Government of Northern Ireland, 'Report of the Higher Education in Northern Ireland' (The Lockwood Report), Table 55, p. 271.

no systematic attempt to construct this for Irish doctors until Jones (2010) and none that focuses on the Irish emigrant doctor.

For those who entered the colonial medical or armed services, rates of pay and allowances are published. *Crawford's Roll* provides information on salaries and the length of service of Irish doctors and their final rank, all of which affected income. For those in other areas of medical practice, the information is less readily available; but rates of pay for various public posts are published in the nineteenth and twentieth century, including in advertisements in the medical press.

Income from private practice is less readily accessible, but there exist tax guides, guides to the purchase of practices, the records of firms which specialise in linking prospective buyers to medical livings, and medical journals which reflect the opinion of doctors about their remuneration and the difficulties of making a medical living. Occasionally, though rarely, medical publications contain job adverts for practices. Some of the information also found its way into reports by medical professional bodies and government reports. However, this study attempts to widen the scope of the investigation to establish two things: the overall situation of Irish doctors and their emigrant counterparts, and their general financial standing in middle-class society. The examination of their wills helped broaden the picture.

The *British Medical Journal* (BMJ) used to publish, before the First World War, a list of brief obituaries of doctors taken from the *Medical Directory*. They were published from 1876–7 until 1912–13, not always in a continuous series. They are useful because otherwise tracing the date of death of a doctor *ab initio* can be time-consuming. Although they give the date of death, they do not always give the date of qualification. Doctors chosen for the study of their wills had to be over fifty, as those who died before that age would not be reflective of a full working life. Where ages were not given, they were calculated from the date of the qualification (checked in the *Medical Register*). Two tables were produced using these lists, which identified 123 doctors who were graduates of Irish medical schools and whose address on death was in Ireland; and 123 counterparts, graduates of English or Scottish medical schools working in Britain. Consultation of the *Medical Register* established continuous practice in either Ireland or England over a substantial period of a career.

A subsequent table looked at the relative advantage for Irish-educated doctors who left Ireland to work in Britain or worked outside Britain primarily in the armed or colonial services though not always. A total of 114 doctors graduating from Irish medical schools were examined, including fifty abroad and sixty-four in general practice in England. The BMJ lists were used for 1911–12 and 1913, as these had not been previously mined. In addition, the wills of doctors from the cohorts of 1860, 1875, 1880, 1890, 1895 and 1900 were traced. For doctors working in the colonial or armed services including the navy, military records were used to track them down.

Information about legacies can be found in calendars of wills, which are published annually from the beginning of the nineteenth century. The modern form of probate dates from 1858, roughly coincident with the beginning of this study.[12] Probate registers publish the name, address and usually the profession of those leaving legacies. Probate records have been digitalised in both the Republic of Ireland, Northern Ireland and for England and Wales. But probate is not straightforward. The date of death is needed to trace the will. Even then, although a will is usually probated several months after death, a few take several years. In some cases the final figure may be raised or lowered. Moreover, an Irish doctor abroad could probate in either England and Wales, Scotland or Ireland, and sometimes an Irish doctor probated both in Ireland and England. Finally, because of the Troubles of 1919–22, wills probated for that period in the Republic of Ireland are patchy.

The research of probate was inspired by W.D. Rubenstein's examination of the wills of the wealthy in Britain in the nineteenth and early twentieth centuries.[13] Rubenstein identified the very rich as those leaving a legacy of over £500,000, around £40 million in today's figures. No medical men or women appeared in his list of the wealthiest in Britain.

As a method of estimating wealth, probate has further drawbacks. First, certain forms of property are excluded from probate. Second, a will does not tell the researcher whether money has been distributed among a family prior to death. It is an absolute figure which does not include certain exactions, such as income tax or death duties. As Rubenstein argues, a look at tax records would be an even better guide to estimating wealth, but these are closed to the researcher. Wills also reflect individuality, thrift, luck and often good fortune, because the will-maker themselves might be a beneficiary of legacies from other family members.

The second problem is those who left no record in the will calendars. Absence from a list may be an indication of penury and the failure of a medical practice. But in some cases the reasons for the absence from probate could be established. Premature death was a common cause. In a couple of cases, consultation of the *Medical Directory* and *Medical Register* established that a few were practising abroad and died there outside the jurisdiction of the United Kingdom or Irish probate office. Second, Irish probate records, although they have achieved a reasonable degree of maturity, are not always complete. It is also true that examining the probate calendars generally accesses the more successful doctor in settled practices. A few legacies were so small as to invite reflections upon the circumstances of the doctors and are discussed in the text. Wills therefore are only a rough estimate, and all that is claimed for the study is that in

12 A separate Probate Act was passed for Ireland. The provisions were the same as for Britain.

13 Rubenstein, *Men of Property: The Very Wealthy in Britain since the Industrial Revolution*.

addition to the examination in Chapter 2 of the financial situation of doctors in the area of Ballinasloe, it lays on the table a hypothesis about the financial situation of the medical profession in Ireland.

The conclusion is that both in Ireland, England and abroad a reasonable living was available to the Irish graduate. Some data exist to support this view. The income tax rate fixed by Pell in 1842 was based on an annual income of £150, and this excludes the majority of working-class wages and lower middle-class salaries. Olive Anderson calculates a clerk's wages in the mid-nineteenth century as around £99, a skilled manual worker £70–80, textile workers £50 and unskilled and agricultural workers £20–40.[14] Our calculation of a starting income for doctors places them around clerical level and above, but rising over a career to salaries which put them into the middle classes.

This work only briefly addresses broader economic changes affecting the doctor. Income tax was increased in 1894 by a tax on the capital value of land, but not much changed until Lloyd George's 1909 budget when a super tax was to be levied on incomes above £5,000 (£450,00). This would certainly have affected some doctors. Added to this was the impact of the First World War when income tax and inflation rose. First World War inflation means that whereas rule of thumb multiplies a pre-1914 income by a factor of eighty in order to compare with the present day, this is reduced to a factor of forty post-1914. This must be taken into account when looking at the value of legacies probated after the First World War. Death duties were introduced in 1909, although their implementation took longer, but they covered only the wealthier. However, attention is paid in Chapter 6 to the financial impact of the insurance system on Irish doctors in Britain. As in the case of other middle-class professions, the deflation of the 1930s raised the value of doctor incomes, and work has been done and referred to in that chapter which suggests a relatively prosperous period for most doctors.[15]

When it comes to the dynamics of family fortunes in the lives of medical practitioners, actual wills are a better guide. Some Irish doctor's wills have survived, and they are invaluable as a record of the professional middle-class medical family who earned a living or part of their living through medicine. They detail marriage settlements, provisions for children and also transfer of money between members of the family during the lifetime of those making the wills. They also detail property and other movable wealth and investments.

---

14 Olive Anderson, 'Wage Earners and Income Tax', *Public Administration*, vol. 41, Summer 1963, p. 189.

15 Digby and Bosanquet, 'Doctors and Patients in an Era of National Health Insurance and Private Practice'.

4 The Census

The social background of a selection of graduates was investigated using the Irish Census of 1901 and 1911. These two censuses are, however, the only ones to survive the Troubles of the early 1920s, and they cover only a small proportion of our cohort. They do, nonetheless, take in graduate cohorts during an important period in the development of the medical profession and show a progression of individuals into medicine drawn from the business, retail and clerical classes; in other words, they lend substance to the thesis of the central importance of medicine in creating a new professional class in Ireland which drew in Catholics who were previously under-represented in the professions.

Using the census is not straightforward, however. It was necessary to research not just graduates but fathers of medical graduates, and given the ubiquity of some Irish names, it was sometimes difficult to track down the household. This was compounded by the fact that many future medical graduates were in boarding school at the time of the census, or were new graduates who had taken up their first job often at some distance from their family home. Nonetheless, where they could be traced, the information in the household schedules gives a good idea of the social and financial status of the family, their occupation, religion and the place of residence in relation to the medical school. The sample was small but rich in illustrative examples of social mobility from business and retail into the medical profession taking place for many Catholic families and some Protestants in the period up to and after the First World War.

Bibliography

Primary Sources

Archives

Rockefeller Foundation Papers, Tarrytown, New York.
Papers of the American Medical Association (AMA), Chicago.
Royal College of Physicians of Ireland (RCPI), Dublin.
Royal College of Surgeons in Ireland, Dublin.
Public Record Office of Northern Ireland.
National Archives, Dublin.
National Library, Dublin.
Library and manuscripts of the Wellcome Trust Foundation, London.
The Central Catholic Library, Dublin.
New York Public Library.
New York Academy of Medicine.
Queen's University of Belfast Archives.
Glyn and Mills Archives, London, in possession of the Royal Bank of Scotland.
Trinity College, Dublin Archives.
University College Dublin Archives.

Parliamentary Papers: United Kingdom and Ireland

'Ninth Annual Report of the Colonial, Land and Emigration Commissioners,' Reports from the Commissioners, 1 Feb.–1 Aug. 1849, vol. XXII, Cmd 1082, pp. 1–97.

'Report of the Committee to inquire into the causes which tend to prevent sufficient eligible candidates from coming forward to the Army Medical Department', PP 1878–9, vol. XLIV. C. 2200 (44), pp. 304–5 (48–49).

'Final Report of the Queen's Colleges', PP 1908–9, vol. XX, Cd. 4825, p.13 (Cork) and Cd. 4883, p.10 (Galway), Cd. 4831, p. 24.

'The Royal Commission on National Health Insurance, Minutes of Evidence', vol. 1, London, Cmd 2595. HMSO, 1925.

'Report of the Committee on Higher Education in Northern Ireland'. Belfast: HMSO, Cmd 475, 1965 (known as the Lockwood Report).

Reports from Governmental Organisations

International

Organisation for Economic Co-operation and Development (OECD). 'Immigrant Health Workers in OECD Countries in the Broader Context of Highly Skilled Migration', Report. Organisation for Economic Co-operation and Development, 2007.

United Kingdom

'Report of the Interdepartmental Committee on Medical Schools'. London: HMSO, 1944 (known as the Goodenough Report).

'Report of the Committee to Consider the Future Numbers of Medical Practitioners and the Appropriate Intake of Medical Students' (The Willink Report). London: HMSO, 1957.

Webster, Charles. *The Health Services Since the War, volume 1: Problems of Health Care. The National Health Service Before 1957*. London: HMSO, 1988; *volume 2: Government and Health Care. The National Health Service 1958–1979*. London: HMSO, 1996.

United States

Dublin, Thomas D. *The Changing Role of the Foreign Medical Graduate in the Practice of Medicine in the U.S.* Philadelphia: Educational Commission for Foreign Medical Graduates, Report presented in 1980.

Politzer, Robert. 'The Impact of Foreign-Trained Doctors on the Supply of Physicians', Undertaken for the U.S. Department of Health and Human Services, 1983.

Stevens, Rosemary and Joan Vermeulen. *Foreign Trained Physicians and American Medicine*. Bethesda: U.S. Department of Health, Education and Welfare, 1973.

Ireland

Annual Reports of the Local Government Board (Ireland) 1872–1922. Dublin: Alexander Thom & Co. for His Majesty's Stationery Office (HMSO).

Census of Ireland. 1901, 1911 (online at <http://www.census.nationalarchives.ie/search>), 1936.

'Commission on Emigration and Other Population Problems 1948–54'. Dublin: Stationery Office, 1955.

'Medical Education in Ireland: A New Direction', Report of the Working Group on Undergraduate Medical Education and Training. Republic of Ireland, Department of Health, 2006 (known as the Fottrell Report).

'Report of the Commission on Higher Education 1960–7', 2 vols. Dublin: Stationery Office, 1967.

Reports from Non-Governmental Organisations

Annual Reports of the Board of Superintendence of Dublin Hospitals. Dublin: Alexander Thom & Co. for HMSO.

'Annual Report of the Master of the Guild of St Luke, SS. Cosmas and Damian'. London, 1952.

'Arrangements for the Integration of Irish Immigrants in England and Wales by A.E.C.W. Spencer', for the International Catholic Migration Commission, 1960. Published by the Irish Manuscripts Commission and edited by Mary Daly Dublin 2012.

The Catholic Directory of England and Wales, 1839–2014. Published by Gabriel Communications on behalf of the Bishops Conference of England and Wales. The current Directory is available online at <https://directory.cbcew.org.uk>, last accessed 22 April 2021.

'The Changing Role of the Foreign Medical Graduate in the Practice of Medicine in the US', Educational Commission for Foreign Medical Graduates, Report presented by Thomas D. Dublin in 1980.

Hart's Annual Army Lists, 1839–1915. Compiled by H.G. Hart. London: John Murray.

Irish Catholic Directory, 1836–1959. Dublin: J. Duffy & Co.

Irish Medical Directory. Medical Press and Circular, 1871–97.

The Medical Directory, 1870-onwards. London: John Churchill and Sons.

Medical and Dental Students' Register. General Medical Council, 1936.

The Medical Register of the United Kingdom and Ireland. General Medical Council.

'Medical Workforce Intelligence Report'. Dublin: Medical Council of Ireland, 2012.

The Medical Yearbook, General Medical Council, 1925.

Queen's College Belfast (QUB) Calendars and Sessional Lists.

Queen's College Cork (later University College Cork) Calendar and Sessional Lists.

Queen's College Galway (later University College Galway) Calendars and Sessional Lists.

'Report as to the Conditions under which Medical and Dental Practitioners registered or legally qualified in their own country may practice abroad'. London: General Medical Council (GMC), 1912, 1927 and 1933.

'Report by the Statistical Committee of the General Medical Council containing a Summary of Statistics regarding Medical Students in the year 1871'.

Royal College of Surgeons in Ireland (RCSI), Roll of Licentiates, Calendars and Sessional Lists.

Trinity College Dublin Calendars and Sessional Lists.

University College, Dublin, Calendars and Sessional Lists.

World Directory of Medical Schools, 5th Edition. Geneva: WHO, 1979.

Periodicals

British Medical Journal (BMJ)

Catholic Medical Guardian (later the *Catholic Medical Quarterly*)

Dublin Quarterly Journal of Medical Science

Dublin Review

Health Policy

Irish Ecclesiastical Record

Journal of the American Medical Association (JAMA)

Journal of the Irish Medical Association (JIMA)

Journal of the Medical Association of Eire

Journal of the Statistical and Social Inquiry Society of Ireland

The Lancet
Minerva
St Stephen's: A Record of University Life
Transactions of the International Congress of Catholic Doctors
Transactions of the Ulster Medical Society (Dublin: John Falconer)
Ulster Medical Journal

Newspapers

Belfast Newsletter
The Catholic Herald
Irish Echo
Irish Independent
The Irish Times (*online*)
The Leader
New York Times
Provincial Medical and Surgical Journal
The Western People

Secondary Sources

Online Resources

Ancestry.co.uk.
National Archives Ireland
Online Census Ireland and United Kingdom
Probate Calendars UK, Northern Ireland (PRONI)

Unpublished Theses

Kelly, Laura. 'Irish Medical Students at the University of Glasgow 1859–1900', M.Litt thesis, University of Glasgow, 2007.

Unpublished Articles

Jones, Greta. The Controversy about Craniotomy in Nineteenth-Century Ireland and Britain.

Jones, Greta. 'Thomas Henry Huxley, the Catholic Church and the founding of the University of London'.

Published Books and Articles

Abel-Smith, Brian, and Kathleen Gales. *British Doctors at Home and Abroad*. Welwyn: Codicote Press, 1964.

Akenson, Donald Harman. 'The Historiography of the Irish in the United States of America' in *The Irish Worldwide: History Heritage and Identity*, vol. 2, *The Irish in the New Communities*, ed. Patrick O'Sullivan. Leicester: Leicester University Press 1992, pp. 162–79.

Akenson, Donald Harman. *The Irish Diaspora: A Primer.* Toronto: P.D. Meany Co., 1996.

Anderson, Olive. 'Wage Earners and Income Tax', *Public Administration*, vol. 41, no. 2, Summer 1963, pp. 189–92. DOI: 10.1111/j.1467-9299.1963.tb01574.x.

Armstrong, John. 'A System of Exclusion: New Zealand Women Medical Specialists in International Medical Networks. 1945–1975', in *Doctors Beyond Borders: The Transnational Migration of Physicians in the Twentieth Century*, ed. Laurence Monnais and David Wright. Toronto: University of Toronto Press, pp. 118–41.

Arnold, David. *Science, Technology and Medicine in Colonial India.* Cambridge: Cambridge University Press, 2000.

Beck, Ann. *A History of the British Medical Administration of East Africa, 1900–1950.* Cambridge, Mass.: Harvard University Press, 1970.

Bidwell, P., Niamh Humphries, Patrick Dicker, Steve Thomas, Charles Normand and Ruairi Brugha. 'The national and international implications of a decade of doctor migration in the Irish context', *Health Policy,* vol. 110, no. 1, April 2013, pp. 29–38. DOI: 10.1016/j.healthpol.2012.10.002.

Bonner, Thomas Neville. *Iconoclast Abraham Flexner and a Life in Learning.* Baltimore: Johns Hopkins University Press, 2002.

Borjas, George J. and Barry R. Chiswick. *Foundations of Migration Economics,* ed. Benjamin Elsner. Oxford: Oxford University Press, 2019.

Bornat, Joanna, Parvati Raghuram and Leroi Henry, '"Without racism there would have been no geriatrics": South Asian Overseas-Trained Doctors and the Development of Geriatric Medicine in the United Kingdom, 1950–2000', in *Doctors beyond Borders: The Transnational Migration of Physicians in the Twentieth Century*, ed. Laurence Monnais and David Wright. Toronto: University of Toronto Press, 2016, pp. 185–207. DOI: 10.3138/9781442629622-011.

Bowley, A.L. *Wages and Income in the United Kingdom since 1860.* Cambridge: Cambridge University Press, 1937.

Bradley, James, Anne Crowther and Marguerite Dupree. 'Mobility and Selection in Scottish University Medical Education, 1858–1886', *Medical History,* vol. 40., no.1, 1996, pp. 1–24. DOI: 10.1017/S0025727300060646.

Brown, Spencer H. 'British Army Surgeons Commissioned 1840–1909 with West Indian/West African Service: A Prosopographical Evaluation', *Medical History*, vol. 37, no. 4, October 1993, pp. 411–31. DOI: 10.1017/S0025727300058750.

Browne, Janet. *Charles Darwin: Voyaging,* Volume 1 of a Biography. London: Jonathan Cape, 1995.

Bryder, Linda. '"A Health Resort for Consumptives": Tuberculosis and Immigration to New Zealand, 1880–1914', *Medical History*, vol. 40, no. 4, 1996, pp. 453–71. DOI: 10.1017/S002572730006169X.

Bunge, Wiep van (ed.). *The Early Enlightenment in the Dutch Republic 1650–1750: Selected Papers of a Conference held at the Herzog August Bibliothek Wolfenbüttel, 22–23 March 2001*. Leiden and Boston: Brill, 2003.

Burke, Helen. *The People and the Poor Law in 19th Century Ireland*. Dublin: Women's Educational Press Ireland, 1987.

Campbell, Fergus. *The Irish Establishment 1879–1914*. Oxford: Oxford University Press, 2009.

Cassell, Ronald D. *Medical Charities, Medical Politics: The Irish Dispensary and the Poor Law*, 1836–1872. London: Royal Historical Society, 1997.

Choa, Gerald H. *'Heal the Sick was their motto': The Protestant Medical Missionaries in China*. Hong Kong: Chinese University Press, 1990.

Churchill, Fleetwood. *Researches on Operative Midwifery, Etc.* Dublin: Martin Keene, 1841.

Churchill, Fleetwood. *A Handbook of Obstetric and Gynecological Nursing*, 5th edition of *Manual for Midwives*, edited by Thomas More Madden. London: Bailliere, Tindall and Cox, 1893.

Clarke, R.S.J. *A Directory of Ulster Doctors (who qualified before 1901)*, 2 vols. Belfast: Ulster Historical Foundation, 2013.

Clarkson, Leslie A. *A University in Troubled Times: Queen's University Belfast 1945–2000*. Dublin: Four Courts Press, 2004.

Coakley, Davis. *Medicine in Trinity College Dublin: An Illustrated History*. Dublin: Trinity College Dublin, 2014.

Collis, Robert. *The State of Medicine in Ireland* (The Carmichael Lecture). Dublin: Parkside Press, 1943.

Collis, Robert. *To Be A Pilgrim: The Autobiography of Robert Collis*. London: Secker and Warburg, 1975.

Cox, Catherine. 'Access and Engagement: The Medical Dispensary Service in Post-Famine Ireland', in *Cultures of Care in Irish Medical History 1750–1970*, eds. Catherine Cox and Maria Luddy (Basingstoke: Palgrave Macmillan, 2010), pp. 57–78.

Cox, Catherine and Hilary Marland (eds.). *Migration, Health and Ethnicity in the Modern World*. London: Palgrave Macmillan, 2013.

Cox, Catherine, Hilary Marland and Sarah York. 'Itineraries and Experiences of Insanity: Irish Migration and the Management of Mental Illness in Nineteenth Century Lancashire', in *Migration, Health and Ethnicity in the Modern World*, eds. Catherine Cox and Hilary Marland. London: Palgrave Macmillan, 2013.

Cox, Catherine and Maria Luddy (eds.). *Cultures of Care in Irish Medical History. 1750–1970*. Basingstoke: Palgrave Macmillan, 2010.

Crawford, D. G. *History of the Indian Medical Service 1600–1913*. London: Thacker and Co., 1914.

Crawford, D. G. (ed.). *Roll of the Indian Medical Service 1615–1930*. London: Thacker and Co., 1930.

Crowther, M. Anne and Marguerite W. Dupree. *Medical Lives in the Age of Surgical Revolution*. Cambridge: Cambridge University Press, 2007.

Crookes, Gearóid P. *Far Away and Long Ago: A Memoir*. Dublin: Tudor House Press, 2003.

Crossman, Virginia. *Poverty and the Poor Law in Ireland 1850–1914*. Liverpool: Liverpool University Press, 2013.

Crozier, Anna. *Practising Colonial Medicine: The Colonial Medical Service in British East Africa*. London: I.B. Taurus, 2007.

Cueto, Marcos (ed.). *Missionaries of Science: The Rockefeller Foundation and Latin America*. Bloomington: Indiana University Press, 1994.

Delaney, Enda. *Demography, State and Society: Irish Migration to Britain 1921–1971*. Liverpool: Liverpool University Press, 2000.

Delaney, Joyce. *No Starch in My Coat: An Irish Doctor's Progress*. London: Cox & Wyman, 1971.

Dictionary of Irish Biography, 11 vols. Cambridge: Cambridge University Press for the Royal Irish Academy, vols. I–X 2009, vols. X–XI 2018.

Digby, Anne. '"A Medical El Dorado?": Colonial Medical Incomes and Practice at the Cape', *Social History of Medicine*, vol. 8, no. 3, December 1995, pp. 463–79. DOI: 10.1093/shm/8.3.463.

Digby, Anne. *Making a Medical Living: Doctors and Patients in the English Market for Medicine 1720–1911*. Cambridge: Cambridge University Press, 1994.

Digby, Anne, 'Shaping New Identities: General Practitioners in Britain and South Africa', in *Medical Identities: Well Being and Personhood*, ed. Kent Maynard. New York–Oxford: Berghahn Books, 2007, pp. 14–35.

Digby, Anne and Nick Bosanquet. 'Doctors and Patients in an Era of National Health Insurance and Private Practice, 1913–1938', *The Economic History Review*, second series, vol. XL1, 1988, pp. 74–94. DOI: 10.1111/j.1468-0289.1988.tb00456.x.

Doherty, Richard and David Truesdale. *Irish Winners of the Victoria Cross*. Dublin: Four Courts Press, 2000.

Doolin, William. 'Medical Education in the Irish Free State', in *Irish State Hospital Year Book*. Dublin: O'Neill Publications, 1937, pp. 36–9.

Earner-Byrne, Lyndsey. *Mother and Child: Maternity and Child Welfare in Dublin 1922–1960*. Manchester: Manchester University Press, 2007.

Farmar, Tony. *Patients, Potions and Physicians: A Social History of Medicine in Ireland 1654–2004*. Dublin: A&A Farmar and the RCPI, 2004.

Feinstein, Charles. 'New Estimates of Average Earnings in the United Kingdom 1880–1913', *The Economic History Review*, vol. 43, no. 4, November 1990, pp. 595–632. DOI: 10.2307/2596737

Fisher, Kate. *Birth Control, Sex and Marriage in Britain 1918–1960*. Oxford: Oxford University Press, 2006.

Fleetwood, John F. *The History of Medicine in Ireland*. Dublin: The Skellig Press, 1983.

Flynn, Michael P. *Medical Doctor of Many Parts: Memoirs of a Public Health Practitioner and Health Manager, Spanning Sixty Years of Social Change*. Dublin: Colourbooks Ltd, 2002.

Foley, Tadhg (ed.). *From Queen's College to National University: Essays on the Academic History of QCG/UCG/NUI Galway*. Dublin: Four Courts Press, 1999.

Francis, Charles R. *On the Best Means of Preserving Health in India*. Bristol: J.W. Arrowsmith, 1889.

Francis, Charles R. *The Indian Medical Service*. London: Mitchell, 1898.

Friedman, Milton. *Capitalism and Freedom*. Chicago: University of Chicago Press, 1962. (Fifth Impression, Phoenix Books, 2002)

Froggatt, P. 'The Irish Connection' in *The Influence of Scottish Medical Education:* An Historical Assessment of Its International Impact, ed. Derek A. Dow. Carnforth: Parthenon, 1988, pp. 63–76.

Garry, Gerald T. *An African Doctor*. London: John Gifford, 1939.

Gaughan, J. Anthony. *Alfred O'Rahilly: Academic*, vol. 1. Dublin: Kingdom Books, 1986.

Geary, Laurence M. 'Australia Felix: Irish Doctors in Nineteenth-Century Victoria', in *The Irish in the New Communities* (*The Irish World Wide: History, Heritage, Identity*, vol. 2), ed. Patrick O'Sullivan. Leicester: Leicester University Press, 1992, pp. 162–79.

Geary, Laurence M. 'Australian Medical Students in Nineteenth-century Scotland: The Social Perspective', *Journal of the Royal College of Physicians of Edinburgh*, vol. 26, 1996, pp. 472–86.

Geary, Laurence M. *Medicine and Charity in Ireland 1718–1851*. Dublin: University College Dublin Press, 2004.

Gilbert, Bentley B. *The Evolution of National Insurance in Great Britain: Origins of the Welfare State*. London: Michael Joseph, second edition, 1973 (first published in 1966).

Gish, Oscar. *Doctor Migration and World Health: The Impact of the International Demand for Doctors in Health Services in Developing Countries*. London: Bell, 1971.

Gramaglia, Letizia. 'Migration and Mental Illness in the British West Indies 1838–1900: The Cases of Trinidad and British Guiana', in *Migration, Health and Ethnicity in the Modern World*, eds. Catherine Cox and Hilary Marland. London: Palgrave Macmillan, 2013.

Greely, David M. 'American Foreign Medical Graduates', *Journal of Medical Education*, vol. 41, no. 7, July 1966, pp. 641–50.

Grubel, Herbert G. 'Reflections on the Present State of the Brain Drain and a Suggested Remedy', *Minerva*, vol.14, no. 2, 1976, pp. 209–224. DOI: 10.1007/BF01107886

Hamilton, Charles Stewart Parnell. *East, West: An Irish Doctor's Memories*. London: Christopher Johnson, 1955.

Hamilton, Reginald. *Colony: Strange Origins of One of the Earliest Modern Democracies.* Kent Town (South Australia): Wakefield Press, 2010.

Harrison, Mark. *Public Health in British India: Anglo-Indian Preventative Medicine 1859–1914*. Cambridge: Cambridge University Press, 1994.

Haynes, Douglas M. *Fit to Practice: Empire, Race, Gender and the Making of British Medicine, 1850–1980*. Rochester, N.Y.: Rochester University Press, 2017.

Hing, Lee Kam and Tan Chee Beng (eds.). *The Chinese in Malaysia.* Oxford: Oxford University Press, 2000.

Hingston, R.W.G. *A Naturalist in Hindustan*. London: H.F. & G. Witherby, 1923.

Hingston, R.W.G. *A Naturalist in the Guiana Forest.* London: E. Arnold & Co., 1932.

Hingston, R.W.G. *A Naturalist in the Himalayas, Observations done on active service 1914–16*. London: H.F. & G. Witherby, 1920.

Hingston, R.W.G. *Nature at the Desert's Edge: Studies and Observations in the Baghdad Oasis*. London: H.F. & G. Witherby, 1925.

Horgan, John. *Noel Browne: Passionate Outsider.* Dublin: Gill & Macmillan, 2000.

Huggard, William Richard. *A Handbook on Climatic Treatment: Including Balneology.* London: MacMillan and Co Limited; New York: MacMillan Company, 1906.

Hutchinson, John. *The Dynamics of Cultural Nationalism: The Gaelic Revival and the Creation of the Irish Nation State*. London: Allen & Unwin, 1987.

'International Comments' *Journal of the American Medical Association*, vol. 235, no. 7, 15 March 1976, p. 1167.

Johnson, William. *The Modern Epidemic: A History of Tuberculosis in Japan*, Council on East Asian Studies. Cambridge, Mass: Harvard University, 1995.

Jones, Greta. '"A mysterious discrimination:" Irish medical emigration to the United States in the 1950s', *Social History of Medicine,* vol. 25, no. 1, February 2012, pp. 139–56. DOI: 10.1093/shm/hkr049.

Jones, Greta. *"Captain of all these Men of Death": The History of Tuberculosis in Nineteenth and Twentieth Century Ireland.* Amsterdam–New York: Rodopi, 2001.

Jones, Greta. 'Contested Territories: Alfred Cort Haddon, Progressive Evolutionism and Ireland', *History of European Ideas,* vol. 24, no. 3, 1998, pp. 195–211. DOI: 10.1016/S0191-6599(98)00018-7.

Jones, Greta. 'Eugenics in Ireland: The Belfast Eugenics Society, 1911–15', *Irish Historical Studies,* vol. 28, no. 109, May 1992, pp. 81–95. DOI: 10.1017/S0021121400018599.

Jones, Greta. 'Marie Stopes in Ireland: The Mother's Clinic in Belfast 1936–47', *Social History of Medicine,* vol. 5, no. 2, August 1992, pp. 255–77. DOI: 10.1093/shm/5.2.255.

Jones, Greta. *Social Hygiene in Twentieth Century Britain.* London: Croom Helm, 1986.

Jones, Greta. '"Strike out Boldly for the Prizes that are Available to You": Medical Emigration from Ireland 1860–1905', *Medical History,* vol. 54, no. 1, January 2010, pp. 55–75. DOI: 10.1017/s0025727300004312.

Jones, Greta. 'The Rockefeller Foundation and Medical Education in Ireland in the 1920s', *Irish Historical Studies,* vol. 30, no. 120, November 1997, pp. 564–80. DOI: 10.1017/S0021121400013456.

Jones, Greta. 'Women and Eugenics in Britain: The Case of Mary Scharlieb, Elizabeth Sloan Chesser, and Stella Browne', *Annals of Science,* vol. 52, no. 5, 1995, pp. 481–502. DOI: 10.1080/00033799500200361.

Keetley, Charles Robert Bell. *The Student's Guide to the Medical Profession.* London: Baillière Tindall and Cox, 1878.

Kelly, James and Fiona Clark (eds.). *Ireland and Medicine in the Seventeenth and Eighteenth Centuries.* London: Routledge, 2016 (first published 2010 by Ashgate).

Kelly, Laura. *Irish Medical Education and Student Culture c.1850–1950*. Liverpool: Liverpool University Press, 2017.

Kelly, Laura. 'Irish Medical Student Culture and the Performance of Masculinity c.1880–1930', History of Education, vol. 46, no. 1, 2017, pp. 39–57, published online 16 May 2016. DOI: 10.1080/0046760X.2016.1181794.

Kelly, Laura. *Irish Women in Medicine c.1880s–1920s: Origins, Education and Careers.* Manchester: Manchester University Press, 2015.

Kelly, Laura. 'Migration and Medical Education: Irish Medical Students at the University of Glasgow, 1859–1900', *Irish Economic and Social History*, vol. 39, no. 1, 2012, pp. 39–55

Keown, John. *Abortion, Doctors and the Law: Some Aspects of the Legal Regulation of Abortion in England from 1803 to 1982*. Cambridge: Cambridge University Press, 1988.

Kiely, Elizabeth, and Maire Leane. *Irish Women at Work 1930–1960: An Oral History.* Dublin: Irish Academic Press, 2012.

Krop, Henri. 'Medicine and Philosophy in Leiden around 1700: Continuity or Rupture?' in *The Early Enlightenment in the Dutch Republic 1650–1750: Selected Papers of a Conference held at the Herzog August Bibliothek Wolfenbüttel, 22–23 March 2001*, ed. Wiep van Bunge. Leiden and Boston: Brill, 2003, pp. 173–96.

Langley, John Baxter. *Via Medica: A Treatise on the Laws and Customs of the Medical Profession in Relation Especially to Principals and Assistants with Suggestions to Students on Preliminary Education.* London: R. Hardwicke, 1867.

Lankford, Nelson D. 'The Victorian Medical Profession and Military Practice: Army Doctors and National Origin', *Bulletin of the History of Medicine*, vol. 54, no. 4 (Winter), 1980, pp. 511–28.

Levy, Hermann. *National Health Insurance: A Critical Study.* Cambridge: Cambridge University Press, 1944.

Lloyd, Christopher and Jack S. Coulter. *Medicine and the Navy 1815–1900*, vol. 4 of J.J. Keevil's *Medicine and the Navy 1200–1900*. Edinburgh and London: E.S. Livingston, 1963.

Love, Alan C. and William Wimsatt. *Beyond the Meme: Development and Structure in Cultural Evolution.* Minneapolis: University of Minnesota Press, 2019.

Lucassen, Leo. 'Beyond the Apocalypse: Reframing Migration History', in *History, Historians and the Immigration Debate: Going Back to Where We Came From*, eds. Eureka Henrich and Julian M. Simpson. London: Palgrave Macmillan, 2019.

Lucey, Donnacha Seán and Virginia Crossman (eds.). *Healthcare in Ireland and Britain from 1850: Voluntary, Regional and Comparative Perspective.* London: Institute of Historical Research, 2014.

Ludmerer, Kenneth M. *A Time to Heal: American Medical Education at the Turn of the Century to the Era of Managed Care.* New York: Oxford University Press, 1999.

Lyburn, E.F. St John. *The Fighting Irish Doctor: An Autobiography.* Dublin: Morris & Co., 1950.

Lyons, Robert Spencer Dyer. *Intellectual Resources of Ireland: Supply and Demand for an Enlarged System of Irish University Education.* London: Smith, Elder & Co., 1873.

MacCarthy, Aidan. *A Doctor's War.* Cork: Collins Press, 1979.

MacPherson, D.A.J. and Mary J. Hickman (eds.). *Women and Irish Diaspora Identities: Theories, Concepts and New Perspectives.* Manchester: Manchester University Press, 2014.

Mapother, E.D. 'The Dublin Hospitals – their Grants and Governing bodies', *Journal of the Statistical and Social Inquiry Society of Ireland*, vol. V, Part XXXVII, 1869/1870, pp. 130–42 (Read before the Society on 22 June 1969).

Mapother, E.D. *The Medical Profession and its Educational and Licensing Bodies.* Dublin: Fannin & Co, 1868.

Margulies, Harold. 'The Foreign Medical Graduate and the United States', *Journal of Medical Education*, vol. 41, no. 9, September 1966, pp. 246–51.

Marland, Hilary. *Medicine and Society in Wakefield and Huddersfield.* Cambridge: Cambridge University Press, 1987.

Maunsell, Henry. *The Dublin Practice of Midwifery.* London: Longman, Rees, Orme, Brown, Green and Longman, 1834.

May, J. Henry. *Medical Practitioner's Accounts.* London: Gee and Co., 1903.

Marks, Shula, Paul Weindling and Laura Wintour (eds.). *In Defence of Learning: The Plight, Persecution and Placement of Academic Refugees 1933–1980s*, Proceedings of the British Academy. Oxford: Oxford University Press, 2011.

McCarrison, Robert. 'Foreword' to *National Fitness:* A Brief Essay on Contemporary Britain, ed. F. Le Gros Clark. London: Macmillan and Co., 1938, pp. vii–x.

McCarrison, Robert. *Nutrition and National Health: The Cantor Lectures.* London: Royal Society of Arts, 1936.

McCarrison, Robert. *The Nation's Larder and the Housewife's Part Therein: A Set of Lectures at the Royal Institution of Great Britain in April, May and June 1940.* London: G. Bell & Sons, 1940.

McCormick, Leanne. '"The Scarlet Woman in Person", The Establishment of a Family Planning Service in Northern Ireland 1950–1974', *Social History of Medicine*, vol. 21, no. 2, 2008, pp. 345–60. DOI: 10.1093/shm/hkn028.

McDowell, R.B. and D.A. Webb. *Trinity College Dublin 1592–1952: An Academic History*. Dublin: Trinity College Press, 2004 (First published 1982 by Cambridge University Press).

McFeely, Joseph Daniel. *Reflections of an Old and Observant General Practitioner*. London: Edward O. Beck, c.1930.

McLean, David. *Surgeons of the Fleet: The Royal Navy and its Medics from Trafalgar to Jutland*. London: I.B. Taurus, 2010.

Meenan, F.O.C. Cecilia Street: *The Catholic University School of Medicine,* 1855–1931. Dublin: Gill and Macmillan, 1987.

Megaw, J.W.D. 'Note on the Future of the IMS' (pamphlet), 28 July, 1933.

Mejia, Alfonso, Helena Pizuki and Erica Royston. *Foreign Medical Graduate: The Case of the United States*, WHO Division of Manpower. Lexington: Lexington Books, 1980.

Miller, Kerby A. *Emigrants and Exiles: Ireland and the Irish Exodus to North America*. Oxford: Oxford University Press, 1985.

Monnais, Laurence, and David Wright (eds.). *Doctors Beyond Borders: The Transnational Migration of Physicians in the Twentieth Century*. Toronto: University of Toronto Press, 2016.

Mulcahy, Risteárd. *Memoirs of a Medical Maverick*. Dublin: Liberties Press, 2015.

Mullally, Sasha and David Wright. 'Connecting to Canada: Experiences of the South Asian Medical Diaspora during the 1960s and 1970s' in *Doctors beyond Borders: The Transnational Migration of Physicians in the Twentieth Century*, eds. Laurence Monnais and David Wright. Toronto: University of Toronto Press, 2016, pp. 230–56. DOI: 10.3138/9781442629622-013.

Murphy, John A. *The College: A History of Queen's University College Cork 1845–1995*. Cork: Cork University Press, 1995.

Nevin, Monica. 'A Study of the Social Background of Students in the Irish Universities', *Journal of the Statistical and Social Inquiry Society of Ireland*, vol. XXI, Part V, 1966/1967, pp. 62–95 (Read before the Society on 27 January 1967).

O'Brien, Eoin. *Conscience and Conflict: A Biography of Sir Dominic Corrigan 1802–1880*. Dublin: Glendale Press, 1983.

O'Connor, Steven. *Irish Officers in the British Forces 1922–45*. Basingstoke: Palgrave Macmillan, 2014.

Ó Gráda, Cormac. *Ireland: A New Economic History 1780–1939*. Oxford: Clarendon Press, 1995.

Ó Gráda, Cormac. 'New Evidence on the Fertility Transition in Ireland 1880–1911', *Demography*, vol. 28, no. 4, 1991, pp. 535–48. DOI: 10.2307/2061421.

O'Neill, Ciaran. *Catholics of Consequence: Transnational Education, Social Mobility and the Irish Catholic Elite 1850–1900*. Oxford: Oxford University Press, 2014.

O'Neill, Ciaran (ed.). *Irish Elites in the Nineteenth Century*. Dublin: Four Courts Press, 2013.

Ortega, Francesco and Giovanni Peri. *The Effect of Income and Immigration Policies on International Migration*, NBER Working Papers 18322. Cambridge, Mass.: National Bureau of Economic Research, 2012.

Oxford Dictionary of National Biography. Oxford: Oxford University Press, 2004.

Packard, Randall M. *White Plague, Black Labor: Tuberculosis and the Political Economy of Health and Disease in South Africa*. Berkeley: University of California Press, 1989.

Paseta, Senia. *Before the Revolution: Nationalism, Social Change and Ireland's Catholic Elite 1879–1922*. Cork: Cork University Press, 1999.

Perkin, Harold J. 'Middle Class Education and Employment in the Nineteenth Century: A Critical Note', *Economic History Review*, vol. 14, no. 1, 1961, pp. 122–130. DOI: 10.2307/2591359.

Peterson, M. Jeanne. 'Gentlemen and Medical Men: The Problem of Professional Recruitment', *Bulletin of the History of Medicine*, vol. 58, no. 4, 1984, pp. 457–73.

Peterson, M. Jeanne. *The Medical Profession in Mid-Victorian London*. Berkeley: University of California Press, 1978.

Playfair, W.S. *A Treatise on the Science and Practice of Midwifery*, 2 vols. London: Smith, Elder and Co., 1893,

Privilege, John. 'The Northern Ireland Government and the Welfare State 1942–8: The Case of Health Provision', *Irish Historical Studies*, vol. 39, no. 155, 2015, pp. 439–59. DOI: 10.1017/ihs.2014.2.

Privilege, John and Greta Jones. 'Crisis and Scandal: Government, Local Government and Health Reform in Northern Ireland 1939–44', *Irish Economic and Social History*, vol. 42, 2015, pp. 33–52. DOI: 10.7227/IESH.42.1.2.

Rivington, Walter. *The Medical Profession: Being the Essay to which was Awarded the First Carmichael Prize of £200 by the Council of the Royal College of Surgeons, Ireland*. Dublin: Fannin & Co., 1879.

Rubenstein, W.D. *Men of Property: The Very Wealthy in Britain since the Industrial Revolution*. London: Croom Helm, 1981.

Ryan, Louise and Wendy Webster (eds.). *Gendering Migration: Masculinity, Femininity and Ethnicity in Post-War Britain*. Aldershot: Ashgate Press, 2008.

Shanley, John P. 'The History of the Irish Medical Association', The Doolin Memorial Lecture, *Journal of the Irish Medical Association*, vol. 62, no. 385, July 1969.

Simpson, Julian M. 'Diagnosing a Flight from Care: Medical migration and "dirty work" in the NHS', *History and Policy*. Cambridge: King's College and University of Cambridge, 8 December 2014.

Simpson, Julian M. *Migrant Architects of the NHS: South Asian doctors and the Reinvention of British General Practice (1940s–1980s)*. Manchester: Manchester University Press, 2018.

Sinclair, Edward B. and George Johnston. *Practical Midwifery: … an account of 13,748 deliveries … in the Dublin Lying-in Hospital during … seven years, commencing November 1847*. Dublin: M'Glashan & Gill, 1858.

Smith, Bruce L.R. 'The Brain Drain Re-Emergent: Foreign Medical Graduates in American Medical Schools', *Minerva*, vol. 17, no. 4, 1979, pp. 483–503.

Smith, Neil and Mervyn Busteed. 'The Emergence of an Irish Middle Class in Manchester', in *Irish Elites in the Nineteenth Century*, ed. Ciaran O'Neill. Dublin: Four Courts Press, 2013, pp. 206–7.

Spencer, A.E.C.W. *Arrangements for the Integration of Irish Immigrants in England and Wales*, ed. Mary E. Daly. Dublin: Irish Manuscripts Commission, 2012.

The Medical Practitioners' Handbook. London: British Medical Association, 1935.

Twaddle, Michael (ed.). *Expulsion of a Minority: Essays on Ugandan Asians*. London: Athlone Press, 1975.

Vaughan, Megan. *Curing their Ills: Colonial Power and African Illness*. London: Polity Press, 1991.

Vaughan, W.E. and A.J. Fitzpatrick. *Irish Historical Statistics: Population, 1821–1971*. Dublin: Royal Irish Academy, 1978.

Vbra, Elisabeth S., George H. Denton, Timothy C. Partridge and Lloyd H. Burckle (eds.). *Paleoclimate and Evolution with Emphasis on Human Origins*. New Haven: Yale University Press, 1995.

Walsh, Oonagh (ed.). *Ireland Abroad: Politics and Professions in the Nineteenth Century*. Dublin: Four Courts Press, 2003.

Whitelock, Derek. *Adelaide 1836–1976: A History of Difference*. St Lucia: University of Queensland Press, 1977.

Whyte, J. H. *Church and State in Modern Ireland, 1923–1970*. Dublin: Gill and Macmillan, 1971.

Widdess, D. H. *The Royal College of Surgeons in Ireland and its Medical School 1784–1984*. Third Edition. Dublin: Royal College of Surgeons, 1984.

Wilkinson, Susan (ed.). *Recollections of an Irish Born Doctor in Nineteenth-Century Argentina: Arthur Pageitt Greene (1848–1933)*. Washington, England: The Memoir Club, 2015.

Wilson, Edward O. *Sociobiology: The New Synthesis*. Cambridge, Mass.: Harvard University Press, 1975.

Wright, David and Sasha Mullally. '"Not everyone can be a Ghandi": South Asian-trained Doctors Immigrating to Canada, c.1961–1971.' *Ethnicity and Health*, vol. 21, no. 4, August 2016, pp. 340–54 (Epub 2015 Jul 20). DOI: 10.1080/13557858.2015.1054100.

Wright, David, Sasha Mullally and Mary Colleen Cordukes. '"Worse than being Married": The Exodus of British Doctors from the National Health Service to Canada c.1955–75', *Journal of the History of Medicine and the Allied Sciences*, vol. 65, no. 4, October 2010, pp. 546–75. DOI: 10.1093/jhmas/jrq013.

Index

www.ingramcontent.com/pod-product-compliance
Ingram Content Group UK Ltd.
Pitfield, Milton Keynes, MK11 3LW, UK
UKHW021627101026
15624UKWH00019B/76